DATE DUE

JUL 1 6 1993	
FEB - 6 1995	
FEB 2 2 1995	
MAR 1 3 1995	
MAR 2 7 1995	
APR 1 0 1995	
SEP 2 5 1995	
OCT 1 0 1995 19	
FEB - 8 1996	
NOV 1 7 1997	

BRODART   Cat. No. 23-221

Nursing Research with
Basic Statistical Applications

The Jones and Bartlett Series in Nursing

Adult Emergency Nursing Procedures, Proehl

Basic Steps in Planning Nursing Research, Third Edition, Brink/Wood

Bone Marrow Transplantation, Whedon

Cancer Chemotherapy: A Nursing Process Approach, Barton Burke et al.

Cancer Nursing: Principles and Practice, Second Edition, Groenwald et al.

Chemotherapy Care Plans, Barton Burke

A Clinical Manual for Nursing Assistants, McClelland/Kaspar

Children's Nutrition, Lifshitz/ Finch/Lifshitz

Chronic Illness: Impact and Intervention, Second Edition, Lubkin

Clinical Nursing Procedures, Belland/Wells

A Comprehensive Curriculum for Trauma Nursing, Bayley/ Turcke

Comprehensive Maternity Nursing, Second Edition, Auvenshine/Enriquez

Concepts in Oxygenation, Ahrens/Rutherford

Critical Care Review, Wright/Shelton

Emergency Care of Children, Thompson

Essential Medical Terminology, Stanfield

Family Life: Process and Practice, Janosik/Green

Fundamentals of Nursing with Clinical Procedures, Second Edition, Sundberg

1991-1992 Handbook of Intravenous Medications, Nentwich

Handbook of Oncology Nursing, Johnson/Gross

Health Assessment in Nursing Practice, Third Edition, Grimes/Burns

Health and Wellness, Fourth Edition, Edlin/Golanty

Healthy People 2000, U.S. Department of Health & Human Services

Human Development: A Life-Span Approach, Fourth Edition, Freiberg

Instruments for Clinical Nursing Research, Oncology Nursing Society

Intravenous Therapy, Nentwich

Introduction to the Health Professions, Stanfield

Introduction to Human Disease, Third Edition, Crowley

Journal of Perinatal Education, ASPO

Management and Leadership for Nurse Managers, Swansburg

Management of Spinal Cord Injury, Second Edition, Zejdlik

Math for Health Professionals, Third Edition, Whisler

Medical Terminology, Stanfield

Memory Bank for Chemotherapy, Preston

Memory Bank for IVs, Second Edition, Weinstein

Memory Bank for Medications, Second Edition, Kostin/ Evans

Mental Health and Psychiatric Nursing: A Caring Approach, Davies/Janosik

The Nation's Health, Third Edition, Lee/Estes

Nursing and the Disabled: Across the Lifespan, Fraley

Nursing Assessment: A Multidimensional Approach, Third Edition, Bellack/ Edlund

Nursing Diagnosis Care Plans for Diagnosis-Related Groups, Neal/Paquette/Mirch

Nursing Management of Children, Servonsky/Opas

Nursing Pharmacology, Second Edition, Wallace

Nursing Research: A Quantitative and Qualitative Approach, Roberts/Burke

Nutrition and Diet Therapy: Self-Instructional Modules, Second Edition, Stanfield

Pediatric Emergency Nursing Procedures, Bernardo/Bove

Perioperative Nursing Care, Fairchild

Perioperative Patient Care, Second Edition, Kneedler/ Dodge

A Practical Guide to Breastfeeding, Riordan

Psychiatric Mental Health Nursing, Second Edition, Janosik/Davies

Ready Reference of Common Emergency and Prehospital Drugs, Cummings

Ready Reference for Critical Care, Strawn

The Research Process in Nursing, Third Edition, Dempsey/Dempsey

Understanding/Responding, Second Edition, Long/Prophit

Writing a Successful Grant Application, Second Edition, Reif-Lehrer

Nursing Research with Basic Statistical Applications

THIRD EDITION

Patricia Ann Dempsey, R.N., Ph.D.
New Mexico State University

Arthur D. Dempsey, Ed.D.
Gadsden (New Mexico) School District

JONES AND BARTLETT PUBLISHERS
BOSTON • LONDON

For the two Gretchens and the two Helens

Editorial, Sales, and Customer Service Offices

Jones and Bartlett Publishers
One Exeter Plaza
Boston, MA 02116

Jones and Bartlett Publishers International
PO Box 1498
London W6 7RS
England

Library of Congress Cataloging-in-Publication Data

Dempsey, Patricia Ann.
  Nursing research with basic statistical applications / Patricia Ann Dempsey.
  Arthur D. Dempsey. —3rd ed.
    p. cm.
  Rev. ed. of: The research process in nursing. 2nd ed. 1986.
  Includes bibliographical references and index.
  ISBN 0–86720–449–4
  1. Nursing—Research—Methodology. 2. Nursing—Research—
Statistical methods. I. Dempsey, Arthur D. II. Dempsey Patricia
Ann. Research process in nursing. III. Title.
  [DNLM: 1. Nursing Research. WY 20.5 D389r]
  RT81.5.D46 1992
  610.73'072—dc20
  DNLM/DLC
  for Library of Congress   91–35386
                                                                   CIP

Printed in the United States of America
95 94 93 92   10 9 8 7 6 5 4 3 2

Contents

APPENDIX A
Example of a Historical Research Proposal

APPENDIX B
Example of a Descriptive Research Proposal

APPENDIX C
Example of a Research Report

Preface

LIKE THE TWO PREVIOUS EDITIONS, the third edition of this text provides basic nursing research principles and techniques for education in research at the undergraduate and beginning graduate levels. Its learning activities are designed to prepare nurses to identify researchable problems, evaluate research reports critically, and use research to refine and extend the practice of nursing. It continues to be our conviction that students exposed to the research process for the first time find that their learning is facilitated (and their anxiety is reduced) when they are guided through the research process in a systematic, step-by-step manner.

The book includes basic nursing research activities designed to help the beginning student to read research reports critically and to understand the components of a nursing research report. The book also will help beginning researchers to understand the process of developing a research proposal and to develop their own research proposals. To this end, research proposals developed by students are again included and reflect the performance expected of a beginning researcher. The written report of a research study implementing a proposal by one of these beginning research students is also included.

We have updated all chapters of the previous edition. Because of the vital importance of the rights of human subjects in research, information on ethical considerations has been included as a separate chapter early in the book, rather than in an appendix as in the previous editions. The material in the previous editions has been expanded to include qualitative as well as quantitative approaches to research. To this end, a comprehensive discussion of the quantitative and qualitative research traditions has been added. In addition, the chapters on data collection and analysis have been expanded to include qualitative approaches. Discussion of the guidelines for writing a research proposal has been expanded to include the writing of a qualitative proposal, and a qualitative proposal developed by a student has been included.

No background in statistics is required for the beginning researcher. In the event that knowledge of statistics should be desired, however, an appendix entitled "A Statistical Primer" has been included. Methods for computing many of the statistical tests discussed in the data analysis chapter are included in this appendix, along with tables for determining levels of significance.

ACKNOWLEDGMENTS

Dr. Theresa Gesse and Dr. Lydia DeSantis, associate professors at the University of Miami School of Nursing, deserve special acknowledgment and our deepest gratitude for their contributions to this edition. We also wish to express our appreciation to Jean A. Newsome and Jan Riordan for their critical reviews and constructive recommendations that have helped to shape this new edition.

Part One

Becoming Acquainted
with Nursing Research

THE MATERIAL IN PART ONE is designed to acquaint you with the nature of research and nursing research. Chapter 1 introduces basic concepts related to the what and why of research in general and nursing research in particular. It also provides a brief overview of the historical development and future trends in nursing research in the United States. Chapter 2 is an overview of the stages of the research process. Chapter 3 presents the traditions of the quantitative and qualitative strategies used by nursing researchers, and Chapter 4 discusses the critical area of ethical behavior that is required of all researchers dealing with human subjects.

1

The Nature of Research
and Nursing Research

WHAT IS RESEARCH?

Now that you are beginning your experience with research—particularly nursing research—it is important that you understand what research *is* and what research *is not*.

[3]

If you are like many people, you probably associate the word *research* with experiments conducted in the laboratory on various animals, or with the discovery of new drugs or treatment methods in medical science. You may also associate research with the scientific experiments being conducted in space during the past several years. In reality, however, the word *research* has many different meanings and broad applications.

What Research Is

There are as many different views of what research is as there are writers who offer such views. We have attempted to synthesize these views and offer the following description of what research is:

> **Research is a scientific process of inquiry and/or experimentation that involves purposeful, systematic, and rigorous collection of data. Analysis and interpretation of the data are then made in order to gain new knowledge or add to existing knowledge. Research has the ultimate aim of developing an organized body of scientific knowledge.**

What Research Is Not

Before we look further at what research is, let us take some time to look at what it is not. Research is not going to the library to collect existing information on a specific topic and then writing a review of the material, such as in a term paper or research project. This activity, involving the reorganization or restatement of knowledge that is already known, is sometimes referred to as *search* rather than *research*. In order to consider a work as "scientific research," we must use present and past knowledge to answer new questions and to add new knowledge to the fund of already existing knowledge. Research activity is intended to find answers to questions or solutions for problems. Communicating knowledge that already exists, therefore, is not considered research activity unless new questions are answered or new problems solved. Research is conducted only after an extensive examination of materials related to the proposed question or problem has been carried out. This examination determines if the answer to the question or problem is available in present knowledge. If correct answers are readily available, there is no need for new research unless the researcher suspects an error or seeks an alternative solution.

Now that we have taken a look at some of the things research is not, let's return to our previous description of what research is. Again, research can be described as a scientific process of inquiry and/or experimentation that involves purposeful, systematic, and rigorous collection of data. Analysis and interpretation of the data are then made in order to gain new knowledge or add to existing knowledge, with the ultimate aim of developing a body of scientific knowledge.

RESEARCH AS A SCIENTIFIC PROCESS OF INQUIRY

Science is a branch of knowledge or study concerned with deriving systematized knowledge by establishing and organizing facts, principles, and methods. The goal of science is to develop theories in order to explain, predict, and/or control phenomena.

The Scientific Method

In research, the *scientific method,* an orderly process that uses the principles of science, is used. The scientific method requires the use of certain sequential steps to acquire dependable information in solving problems. The scientific method is characterized by (1) order, (2) control, (3) empiricism, and (4) generalization and theoretical formulation.[1]

Order

The scientific approach to problem solving requires the application of *order* and discipline so that confidence in the investigation's results can be assured. This entails the use of the scientific method, in which a series of systematic steps is followed: (1) identification of a problem to be investigated, (2) collection of information according to a previously designed plan (which bears on the solution to the problem), (3) analysis of the information, and (4) formulation of conclusions regarding the problem being investigated.

Control

Control of factors not relevant to the investigation is an essential element of the scientific method. This means that the investigator must try to identify the effects of the factors not directly investigated in connection with the identified problem, and must try to keep them from influencing those factors identified for study. For example, when investigating the relationship between cerebrovascular accidents and the use of oral contraceptives, the investigator must take measures to control such influences as stress, diet, and other factors contributing to the development of atherosclerosis.

Empiricism

The scientific method is also characterized by *empiricism.* That is, the evidence gathered to generate new knowledge must be rooted in objective reality and must be gathered directly or indirectly through the human senses.

Generalization

Generalization, another characteristic of the scientific method, means that the investigator does not use the scientific method merely to understand isolated events, but must also be able to apply the investigation's results to a broader setting. The ultimate aim of the experimental clinical study that investigated the effectiveness of stockinette caps on conservation of body heat in newborn infants (Appendix E) was not merely to analyze the effect of stockinette caps on the specific infants in the study. Rather, the study was designed to draw conclusions about the effect of stockinette caps on newborn infants in general. The kinds of generalizations that result from such research studies assist in the development of scientific theories, thus providing explanations and prediction of future events.

Purposes of Research

Research involves finding answers to questions or solutions to problems, discovering and interpreting new facts, testing theories in order to revise accepted theories and/or laws in the light of new facts, and formulating new theories. Finally, research has as its ultimate aim the development of an organized body of scientific knowledge that is systematized and that can be useful in explaining, predicting, and/or controlling phenomena. An example of the usefulness of theory in predicting phenomena is the use of locus of control theory to predict the preoperative coping behavior of children.[2]

Research in Nursing

Nursing research is research conducted to answer questions or find solutions to problems that fall within the specific orientation defined as nursing—that is, "the diagnosis and treatment of human responses to actual or potential health problems."[3] Nursing research complements biomedical research, which focuses primarily on the causes and treatment of disease, as it examines "the biological, biomedical and behavioral processes that underlie health and the environment in which health care is delivered."[4] Nursing research is done to develop an organized body of scientific knowledge that is unique to nursing:

> Nursing research develops knowledge about health and the promotion of health over the full life span, care of persons with health problems and disabilities, and nursing actions to enhance the ability of individuals to respond effectively to actual or potential health problems. . . . Research conducted by nurses includes various types of studies in order to derive clinical interventions to assist those who require nursing care. The complexity of nursing research and its broad scope often require scientific underpinning from several disciplines. Hence, nursing research cuts across traditional research lines and draws its methods from several fields.[5]

The goal of nursing research is to add to the scientific knowledge base to improve the practice of nursing for the ultimate improvement of patient care.

Throughout the past several years, nurses conducting research have added to nursing's scientific knowledge base for the improvement of patient care with studies on such topics as the effects of information on postsurgical coping;[6] adherence to health care regimens among elderly women;[7] the effect of medication distribution systems on medication errors;[8] and uncertainty and adjustment during radiotherapy.[9]

LIMITATIONS OF THE SCIENTIFIC RESEARCH PROCESS

Although the scientific research process is usually considered the highest form of attaining human knowledge, it has a number of limitations involving the types of problems that can be investigated. Questions involving morality or value systems cannot be explored with the scientific research approach. Questions dealing with complex social and psychological phenomena, such as anger and anxiety, are also very difficult to investigate because of the problems involved in measuring these phenomena. When human subjects are needed in the study, constraints to protect them often cause additional difficulties. Such constraints have even precluded the application of the scientific method to the investigation of certain problems. This crucial consideration is discussed in detail in later chapters.

CLASSIFICATION OF RESEARCH ACTIVITIES

If you are going to understand research, it will be helpful to know the meaning of some commonly used research terms used to classify research activities.

Classification by Purpose

Research may be classified by *purpose*—that is, as either *basic research* or *applied research*. This classification reflects the degree to which the findings can be applied to practical problems in the everyday world. *Basic research*, also called *pure research*, is primarily concerned with establishing new knowledge and with the development or refinement of theories. The findings of basic research may not be immediately applicable to practical problems, but they do provide basic scientific knowledge for building further research. Basic research is really "knowledge for the sake of knowledge." This is in contrast to *applied research*, which is also concerned with establishing new knowledge but is further concerned with knowledge that can be applied in practical settings without undue delay. Applied research has been referred to as "practical application of the theoretical." In general, basic research in the behavioral sciences serves to discover general laws concerning human behavior, while applied research generates knowledge about the operation of these laws in specific settings. However, the distinction between basic and applied research often may not be as clear-cut as we have described. Sometimes the results of basic research studies can be applied in a practical setting, while findings from applied research studies can have theoretical implications and may serve as the focus for basic research.

The majority of nursing studies are examples of applied research. For example, the studies conducted by Lindeman and Van Aernam,[10] Lindeman,[11] and King and Tarsitano[12] on the value of structured preoperative teaching, deep breathing, coughing, and bed exercises have applications in practical settings. Two basic research studies conducted in nursing are McKinnon-Mullette's study[13] concerned with circulation research and its potential in clinical nursing research, and Raff's study[14] of the relationship of planned prenatal exercise to postnatal growth and development in the offspring of albino rats.

Classification by Approach

Research may also be classified by *approach*. There are three major approaches: descriptive, experimental, and historical. The *descriptive research approach* raises questions based on the ongoing events of the present. The *experimental research approach* raises questions based on the need to manipulate specific conditions in a controlled or laboratory-like setting in order to investigate the effects of different conditions. And in the *historical research approach*, researchers investigate questions based on the past by using procedures designed to determine the accuracy of statements or facts about past events. Each of these approaches is discussed in more detail in the chapters in Part III.

WHY SHOULD NURSES LEARN ABOUT RESEARCH?

One characteristic of a professional group is that it has a unique body of knowledge and skill. It is generally agreeed that nursing is still in the process of defining not only what nursing is, but also what constitutes its unique body of knowledge and skill. In view of this, nursing needs to direct its efforts toward systematic investigation of questions related to the practice and profession of nursing.

The 1985 guidelines for nursing research prepared by the American Nurses' Association Cabinet on Nursing Research recognize the essential nature of research in improving nursing practice into the twenty-first century:

The future of Nursing practice and, ultimately, the future of health care in this country depend on nursing research designed to constantly generate an up-to-date, organized body of nursing knowledge. Society and its approach to health care are experiencing rapid change. . . . Thus, nursing research needs to proceed in orderly directions, generating knowledge built on previous information in order to provide the foundation for nursing education and practice in the twenty-first century.[15]

The 1989 guidelines, *Education for Participation in Nursing Research,* prepared by the American Nurses' Association Cabinet on Nursing Research, define elements of competence in research that are appropriate to nurses prepared in different types of nursing education programs at the associate degree, baccalaureate, master's, and doctoral levels.[16]

If nursing is to develop an organized body of scientific knowledge, there are several ways that you as a nurse can participate. First, you must develop the ability to read nursing literature critically as a means of validating nursing practice, discovering gaps in knowledge, and evaluating the findings of research studies. Then you can decide whether or not the knowledge could be used in caring for your patients. This is such an important goal that we have included throughout this text the principles and techniques of critical evaluation. With a basic research orientation, you will also be able to generate hunches and raise questions on the basis of which research studies can be carried out. Finally, you may want to become involved, either as a principal investigator or as a participant, in a research project that will contribute new knowledge.

Although the emphasis on research in nursing has become a relatively strong movement only within the past thirty to thirty-five years, historically, nursing research has been emerging over a period of more than a hundred years. The next section provides a brief overview of the historical development of aspects of nursing that have significantly affected the development of nursing research.

NURSING RESEARCH OVER THE YEARS

When Florence Nightingale established her system of nursing and nursing education over a hundred years ago, she envisioned the development of a scholarly, humane, and scientific discipline. She utilized the research process and used her detailed records to formulate ideas for improving nursing and health care. She encouraged nurses to develop the habit of sound observation:

In dwelling upon the vital importance of *sound* observation, it must never be lost sight of what observation is for. It is not for the sake of piling up miscellaneous information or curious facts, but for the sake of saving life and increasing health and comfort.[17] [emphasis in original]

If nursing education in the United States had followed the principles to which Florence Nightingale was dedicated, nursing research might have progressed more swiftly. However, the development of hospital schools of nursing, with their primary emphasis on nursing service by students, resulted in the placement of nurses in subservient roles. Nurses cared primarily for ill persons and meticulously carried out the orders of authority figures, usually physicians. Unfortunately for the progress of nursing research, nurses who accepted these subservient roles were hardly able to develop or refine the questioning attitude and abstract thinking associated with the scientific method of inquiry.

From 1900 to 1950, most leaders in nursing had advanced preparation in the field of education. As a result, many research studies focused on education for nursing rather than the practice of nursing. The majority of these studies were concerned with the characteristics of nursing students themselves as well as with their educational preparation.

Articles in the nursing literature from 1900 to 1950 show nurses concerned and writing about the care of patients with communicable diseases, hygiene and sanitation, asepsis, and high maternal and infant death rates. The first case studies appeared in the *American Journal of Nursing* in the 1920s. They were used as teaching tools for students, as well as patient progress records to improve patient care. By 1930, the need to distinguish nursing orders from medical orders and to evaluate the effectiveness of nursing procedures appeared. Articles began to express the need for student nurses to be free to criticize and to be relieved of excessive nursing service duties in order to benefit fully from their educational programs.

In the late 1940s, after World War II, the broader concept of nursing as practiced by public health nurses became accepted. The primary focus on nursing care for the hospitalized patient was expanded to include the patient and family in a variety of settings, in cooperation with physicians and other health professionals, and the prevention of illness and the promotion of health. An awareness grew of the need for nurses to acquire knowledge of the social, behavioral, and natural sciences, as well as the humanities, in order to care for their patients and their families.

In the 1950s, recognition of the need to prepare nurses at the graduate level for leadership positions, advanced practice, and research contributed to the advancement of nursing research.

In order to communicate the growing body of nursing research, the first issue of *Nursing Research* was published in 1952. This journal serves as an important resource devoted to the issues and problems associated with nursing research and to the publication of nursing research studies. In 1955, the American Nurses' Association established the American Nurses' Foundation, which supports and promotes research in nursing.

Nurses writing since the 1950s have reflected ideas about the conceptual development of nursing, nursing as a science, and the educational preparation needed for nurses to conduct research. From 1955 to 1965, researchers focused on student characteristics, selection and retention of students, and the educational process. Articles dealing with the quality of patient care began to appear in the literature. Research studies focused on long-term care and rehabilitation of patients and on problems of patients with chronic diseases such as heart disease, cancer, and strokes. Hospitals began to report experiences with intensive care and automation.

Prior to the 1970s, *Nursing Research* was the only major publication devoted to communicating the results of nursing research reports. Since that time, nursing research reports and articles representing perspectives on the development of nursing as a science have been included in such journals as the *Western Journal of Nursing Research, Research in Nursing and Health, Advances in Nursing Science, Nursing Science Quarterly,* and *Scholarly Inquiry for Nursing Practice.*

In 1970, the National Commission for the Study of Nursing and Nursing Education, funded by the American Nurses' Association and additional private sources, published the findings of its independent investigation of the quality of U.S. nursing.[18] The commission reported that nursing in the United States presented an ''impoverished figure'' in terms of research capacity and support. At that time, there was very little public or private funding for nursing research. Fewer than 500 U.S. nurses held earned doctoral degrees, the generally accepted level for research competence. Many of these individuals had been prepared for educational administration or teaching, as there were almost no doctoral programs with specific preparation for research into clinical nursing practice or nursing intervention.[19] Thus, little research had been done on the actual effects of nursing intervention and care. Nursing had few definitive guides for the improvement of practice:

> Lack of research leaves us without a body of facts or a set of probabilities to guide or assess the nursing care of a patient. Of necessity, nursing practice today consists of stereotyped techniques sprinkled liberally with personal idiosyncrasy. . . . Since we have not developed valid means for assessing the effects of varied interventions, it is almost impossible to define optimum nursing care.[20]

The 1973 report of the National Commission on Nursing emphasized that nursing was still more an art than a science. Nurse–patient interactions continued to be characterized by a combination of individual judgment, concern for the patient, and supportive care, rather than with procedures based on validated scientific knowledge. However, with the increased amount and complexity of knowledge concerning human health and response to illness, the art of nursing was no longer sufficient to ensure optimum patient care. "The aim of research should be to elevate the practice of nursing—not art *or* science, but art *and* science are needed to ensure the highest levels of humane and capable care"[21] [emphasis in original].

In 1981, Lysaught[22] reported on the extent to which the recommendations of the National Commission for the Study of Nursing and Nursing Education had been implemented over a period of eight years. The report optimistically predicted that the increase in the number of doctoral programs in nursing since the initiation of the National Commission's study should provide for a greater supply of nurses with "investigative skills for conceptual and theoretical inquiry into nursing that will extend the scientific base of all nursing practice."[23] The report also pointed out that in the area of federal funding for nursing research, there had been a "dramatic increase" that had been generally related to the levels recommended in the 1970 report of the National Commission. These funds, however, "have often been used as pawns in political maneuvering, and the result is that planning and execution of research have often suffered through the vagaries of administrative and legislative battling."[24]

A recent analysis of publications related to nursing practice research reflects, to some extent, the degree to which the recommendations and predictions of the National Commission have been realized. Moody and colleagues analyzed 720 journal articles published in the decade between 1977 and 1986 that reported results of nursing practice research. Findings showed that 95 percent of research in nursing practice reported during this time was conducted by nurses as first authors, over half of them with doctoral degrees. One-third of the studies focused on nursing intervention, and two-thirds focused on assessment. These published studies also reflected an increase in research funding during this decade.[25]

In 1976 and 1981, and again in 1985, the American Nurses' Association developed a statement of priorities for research in nursing, designed to guide nurse researchers in the study of areas of nursing that are crucial to the scientific advancement of the nursing profession. The 1985 Priorities for Nursing Research, developed by the ANA Cabinet on Nursing Research, are listed in Chapter 5.

With the establishment of the National Center for Nursing Research in 1986, nursing research made a dramatic advance into the mainstream of health care science. Dr. Ada Sue Hinshaw summarized this historical milestone for nursing in remarks at her swearing-in ceremony as its first director:

> The establishment of the National Center for Nursing Research (NCNR) on April 18, 1986, by Secretary Bowen was an historic moment for the nursing profession. It provides a focal point from which

to stimulate and facilitate the generation and testing of scientific knowledge to guide the practice of one of the country's largest health care professions. . . . The National Center's union with the National Institutes of Health is particularly significant for it brings nursing research into the mainstream of health care science. It allows for nursing research to be developed/conducted in collaboration with the other scientific disciplines in a complementary manner. . . . In turn, knowledge from nursing research can and will be incorporated in the broader base of health care science as a result of being developed and tested within this collaborative interdisciplinary environment.[26]

Currently, there have been major expansions in research related to clinical practice, growing concerns about ethical practices, and the protection of human subjects. Nurses are increasingly studying *nursing*. They see an urgent need to investigate the organization and delivery of nursing care to patients. Predictions for the direction of nursing research for the remainder of this century and into the twenty-first century indicate an increased concentration on research designed to investigate clinical nursing practice in all settings, the continued evolution of nursing theories, an increase in utilization of research results in practice, and significant progress toward the ultimate goal of extending the scientific basis for nursing in order to improve the delivery of patient care.

In this chapter we introduced you to some basic concepts related to research and nursing research, as well as providing a brief overview of the historical development and future of the nursing research movement in the United States.

The following Application Activities should help you apply this information.

APPLICATION ACTIVITIES

1. Define nursing research as you now understand it. List at least five patient care problems that you believe deserve further research from a nursing focus.
2. Select two published research studies on topics that interest you. Using the definition of research presented in the chapter, discuss how each study fulfills the definition:
   a. The study is a scientific process of inquiry and/or experimentation.
   b. The study involves systematic and rigorous collection of data.
   c. The study involves analysis and interpretation of data.
   d. The study was designed to gain new knowledge which has the potential to contribute to an organized body of scientific knowledge.

    e. How could this study contribute to improved nursing practice for better patient care?

    f. Classify the study by research purpose. Is it basic or applied research? Why?

    g. Classify the study by research approach. Is it descriptive, experimental, or historical research? Why?

3. It has been stated that nurses should conduct their own research into the practice and profession of nursing. Do you agree or disagree with this statement? Defend your answer.

REFERENCES

1. Polit, D., and B. Hungler. 1987. *Nursing Research: Principles and Methods,* 3rd ed. Philadelphia: J. B. Lippincott, pp. 16–17.

2. LaMontagne, Lynda L. 1984. "Children's Locus of Control Beliefs as Predictors of Preoperative Coping Behavior." *Nursing Research,* 33(March–April): 76–79.

3. American Nurses' Association. 1980. *Nursing: A Social Policy Statement.* Kansas City: American Nurses' Association, p. 3.

4. National Center for Nursing Research. 1987. *Nursing Science: Serving Health through Research,* October. Bethesda, MD: National Institutes of Health.

5. American Nurses' Association Commission on Nursing Research. 1981. *Research Priorities for the 1980s: Generating a Scientific Basis for Nursing Practice.* Code No. D-68 2M. Kansas City: American Nurses' Association.

6. Ziemer, M. 1983. "The Effects of Information on Postsurgical Coping." *Nursing Research,* 32: 282–287.

7. Chang, B., et al. 1985. "Adherence to Health Care Regimens among Elderly Women." *Nursing Research,* 34: 27–31.

8. Long, G. 1982. "The Effect of Medication Distribution Systems on Medication Errors." *Nursing Research,* 31 (May–June): 182–184.

9. Christman, N. J. 1990. "Uncertainty and Adjustment During Radiotherapy." *Nursing Research,* 39 (January–February): 17–20.

10. Lindeman, C. A., and B. Van Aernam. 1971. "Nursing Intervention with the Presurgical Patient—The Effects of Structured and Unstructured Preoperative Teaching." *Nursing Research,* 20 (July–August): 319–332.

11. Lindeman, C. A. 1972. "Nursing Intervention with the Presurgical Patient: Effectiveness and Efficiency of Group and Individual Preoperative Teaching—Phase Two." *Nursing Research,* 21 (May–June): 196–209.

12. King, I., and B. Tarsitano. 1982. "The Effect of Structured and Unstructured Preoperative Teaching: A Replication." *Nursing Research,* 31 (November–December): 324–329.

13. McKinnon-Mullette, E. 1972. "Approaches to the Study of Nursing Questions and the Development of Nursing Science. Circulation Research: Exploring Its Potential in Clinical Nursing Research." *Nursing Research,* 21 (November–December): 494–498.

14. Raff, B. S. 1977. "The Relationship of Planned Prenatal Exercise to Postnatal Growth and Development in the Offspring of Albino Rats." In F. S. Downs and M. A. Newman, Eds., *A Sourcebook of Nursing Research.* Philadelphia: F. A. Davis, pp. 78–85.

15. American Nurses' Association Cabinet on Nursing Research. 1985. *Directions for Nursing Research: Toward the Twenty-first Century.* Kansas City: American Nurses' Association, p. 1.
16. American Nurses' Association Cabinet on Nursing Research. 1989. *Education for Participation in Nursing Research.* Kansas City: American Nurses' Association.
17. Nightingale, F. 1859. *Notes on Nursing.* Philadelphia: J. B. Lippincott, p. 70.
18. National Commission for the Study of Nursing and Nursing Education. 1970. *An Abstract for Action.* New York: McGraw-Hill.
19. Lysaught, J. 1981. *Action in Affirmation: Toward an Unambiguous Profession of Nursing.* New York: McGraw-Hill, p. 59.
20. National Commission for the Study of Nursing, *An Abstract for Action,* p. 84.
21. National Commission for the Study of Nursing and Nursing Education. 1973. *From Abstract into Action.* New York: McGraw-Hill, p. 125.
22. Lysaught, J. 1981. *Action in Affirmation: Toward an Unambiguous Profession of Nursing.* New York: McGraw-Hill.
23. Ibid., p. 64.
24. Ibid., p. 63.
25. Moody, L. E., M. E. Wilson, K. Smyth, R. Schwartz, M. Tittle, and M. L. Van Cott. 1988. "Analysis of a Decade of Nursing Practice Research: 1977–1986." *Nursing Research,* 37 (November–December): 374–379.
26. American Association of Colleges of Nursing. 1987. *AACN Newsletter* (Lester Kip, Ed.), 13 (July): 1.

BIBLIOGRAPHY AND SUGGESTED READINGS

American Association of Colleges of Nursing. 1987. *AACN Newsletter* (Lester Kip, Ed.), 13 (July): 1.
American Nurses' Association. 1980. *Nursing: A Social Policy Statement.* Code No. NP-63 25M 9/83R. Kansas City: American Nurses' Association.
————. 1976. *Preparation of Nurses for Participation in Research.* Code No. D-54 2500. Kansas City: American Nurses' Association.
————. 1976. *Priorities for Research in Nursing.* Code No. D-51 3M, August. Kansas City: American Nurses' Association.
American Nurses' Association Cabinet on Nursing Research. 1985. *Directions for Nursing Research: Toward the Twenty-first Century.* Kansas City: American Nurses' Association.
American Nurses' Association Cabinet on Nursing Research. 1989. *Education for Participation in Nursing Research.* Kansas City: American Nurses' Association.
————. 1981. *Research Priorities for the 1980s: Generating a Scientific Basis for Nursing Practice.* Code No. D-68 2M. Kansas City: American Nurses' Association.
Chang, Betty L., Gwen C. Uman, Lawrence S. Linn, John E. Ware, and Robert L. Kane. 1985. "Adherence to Health Care Regimens among Elderly Women." *Nursing Research,* 34: 27–31.
Christman, N. J. 1990. "Uncertainty and Adjustment During Radiotherapy." *Nursing Research,* 39(January–February): 17–20.
Dempsey, P., and T. Gesse. 1983. "The Childbearing Haitian Refugee—Cultural Applications to Clinical Nursing." *Public Health Reports,* 98(May–June): 261–267.
————. 1985. "The Childbearing Cuban Refugee: A Cultural Profile." *Urban Health,* 14(May): 32–37.

Dempsey, P., and P. Hippo. 1990. "Beliefs and Practices of Spanish Speaking Child-bearing Women from Mexico." Unpublished manuscript.

Downs, F. S., and M. A. Newman. 1977. *A Sourcebook of Nursing Research*. Philadelphia: F. A. Davis.

Fawcett, J. 1984. "Hallmarks of Success in Nursing Research." *Advances in Nursing Science*, 7(October): 1–11.

———. 1986. "A Typology of Nursing Research Activities According to Educational Preparation." *Journal of Professional Nursing*, 1: 75–78.

Fitzpatrick, J. J. 1988. "How Can We Enhance Nursing Knowledge and Nursing Practice?" *Nursing and Health Care*, 9 (November/December): 516–521.

Gortner, S. 1980. "Generating a Scientific Basis for Nursing Practice: Research Priorities for the 1980s." *Nursing Research*, 29(July–August): 219.

———. 1983. "The History and Philosophy of Nursing Science and Research." *Advances in Nursing Science*, 5 (January): 1–8.

Gortner, S., and H. Nahm. 1977. "An Overview of Nursing Research in the United States." *Nursing Research*, 26(January–February): 10–30.

Hopkins, C. D. 1976. *Educational Research: A Structure for Inquiry*. Columbus, OH: Charles E. Merrill.

King, I., and B. Tarsitano. 1982. "The Effect of Structured and Unstructured Preoperative Teaching: A Replication." *Nursing Research*, 31(November–December): 324–329.

LaMontagne, Lynda L. 1984. "Children's Locus of Control Beliefs as Predictors of Preoperative Coping Behavior." *Nursing Research*, 33(March–April): 76–79, 85.

Lindeman, C. A. 1972. "Nursing Intervention with the Pre-surgical Patient: Effectiveness and Efficiency of Group and Individual Preoperative Teaching—Phase Two." *Nursing Research*, 21(May–June): 196–209.

———. 1973. "Nursing Research: A Visible, Viable Component of Nursing Practice." *Journal of Nursing Administration*, 3(March–April): 18–21.

Lindeman, C. A., and B. Van Aernam. 1971. "Nursing Intervention with the Presurgical Patient—The Effects of Structured and Unstructured Preoperative Teaching." *Nursing Research*, 20(July–August): 319–332.

Long, G. 1982. "The Effect of Medication Distribution Systems on Medication Errors." *Nursing Research*, 31(May–June): 182–184.

Lysaught, J. 1981. *Action in Affirmation: Toward an Unambiguous Profession of Nursing*. New York: McGraw-Hill.

McKinnon-Mullette, E. 1972. "Approaches to the Study of Nursing Questions and the Development of Nursing Science: Circulation Research: Exploring Its Potential in Clinical Nursing Research." *Nursing Research*, 21(November–December): 494–498.

McMurrey, P. H. 1982. "Toward a Unique Knowledge Base in Nursing." *Image*, 14: 86–88.

Moody, L. E., M. E. Wilson, K. Smyth, R. Schwartz, M. Tittle, and M. L. Van Cott. 1988. "Analysis of a Decade of Nursing Practice Research: 1977–1986." *Nursing Research*, 37(November–December): 374–379.

National Center for Nursing Research. 1987. *Nursing Science: Serving Health through Research*, October. Bethesda, MD: National Institutes of Health.

National Commission for the Study of Nursing and Nursing Education. 1970. *An Abstract for Action*. New York: McGraw-Hill.

———. 1973. *From Abstract into Action*. New York: McGraw-Hill.

National League for Nursing. 1978. *Theory Development: What, Why, How?* Publication Code No. 15-1708. New York: National League for Nursing.

Nightingale, F. 1859. *Notes on Nursing*. Philadelphia: J. B. Lippincott.

Peplau, H. E. 1988. ''The Art and Science of Nursing.'' *Nursing Science Quarterly* 1(February): 8–15.

Polit, D., and B. Hungler. 1987. *Nursing Research: Principles and Methods,* 3rd ed. Philadelphia: J. B. Lippincott.

Raff, B. S. 1977. ''The Relationship of Planned Prenatal Exercise to Postnatal Growth and Development in the Offspring of Albino Rats.'' In F. S. Downs and M. A. Newman, Eds., *A Sourcebook of Nursing Research,* 2nd ed. Philadelphia: F. A. Davis, pp. 78–85.

Tinkle, M. B., and J. L. Beaton. 1983. ''Toward a New Science: Implications for Nursing Research.'' *Advances in Nursing Science,* 5: 32–38.

Wysocki, A. B. 1983. ''Basic vs. Applied Research.'' *Western Journal of Nursing Research,* 5: 217–224.

Ziemer, M. 1983. ''The Effects of Information on Postsurgical Coping.'' *Nursing Research,* 32: 282–287.

2

Stages of the Research Process

OVERVIEW OF THE RESEARCH PROCESS
STAGES OF THE RESEARCH PROCESS
    Stage I: Planning the Study
    Stage II: Implementing the Research Proposal
    Stage III: Communicating the Results of the Study
    Stage IV: Utilizing the Results of the Study
RELATIONSHIP OF THE RESEARCH PROCESS TO THE
  PROBLEM-SOLVING PROCESS
    Comparison between Research and Problem Solving
    Which Approach Is ''Better''?
SUMMARY
APPLICATION ACTIVITIES
REFERENCES
BIBLIOGRAPHY AND SUGGESTED READINGS

In Chapter 1 we discussed the nature of research in general and nursing research in particular. This chapter will acquaint you with the nature of the research process and its relationship to the problem-solving process. It describes the four stages of the research process that are used in conducting a research study.

OVERVIEW OF THE RESEARCH PROCESS

As you become acquainted with research terminology, you will see the term *research process* used to refer to the systematic steps, or ongoing phases, in-

[18]

volved in conducting a research study. Although the number and order of these steps may vary, the following outline contains those commonly used:

1. Statement of the research problem
2. Review of related literature
3. Statement of the purpose of the study
4. Collection of the data
5. Analysis and interpretation of data
6. Formulation of conclusions and implications
7. Communication of the results of the study
8. Utilization of the results of the study

Remember, conducting a study using the research process is a systematic, planned activity that can be thought of as a chain of reasoning. It begins with a statement of the problem and proceeds systematically to the communication and utilization of the study's results: "The total process from problem isolation to the addition of new knowledge is a logically structured inquiry into some well-defined problem."[1]

STAGES OF THE RESEARCH PROCESS

It is helpful to consider the systematic steps of the research process as consisting of four sequential stages that should answer the research question or solve the research problem: (1) planning, (2) implementation, (3) communication, and (4) utilization.

Stage I: Planning the Study

The initial stage of the research process is the planning stage. Here the problem question, which the research will answer, is selected and refined into a problem statement, and the methodology for the study is formulated. The problem must be researchable and the answer not already known. The research should contribute to new knowledge. Appropriate methods must be available to investigate the problem. Consideration must be given to the availability of subjects expected to participate in the study, as well as to the ethical implications of the research, such as the protection of the study participants' rights. The constraints of time and money imposed by the study are also important considerations in selecting the problems to be studied. Examples of general problem areas in nursing might include preoperative teaching of hysterectomy patients, compliance of diabetic patients with prescribed treatment regimens, and family caregivers' ways of coping with the home-bound elderly.

To place the problem in the context of what is already known, the researcher then reviews the literature related to the problem, citing references to significant publications and journal articles pertaining to that problem. Because the objective of nursing research is to contribute to scientific knowledge, the problem may be placed within a theory or based on concepts to which the study's results can be related. The literature review summarizes existing knowledge in relation to the problem and helps the investigator to learn more about the problem area. Next, the researcher may use the information gained so far to predict the outcome of the study. This is done by formulating a *hypothesis*—an educated guess—that will be used to guide the rest of the study. Testing the hypothesis then becomes the purpose for conducting the study. Not all research studies are conducted to test hypotheses; some studies are designed to answer questions or describe phenomena.

All of the terms relating to the study must be carefully defined so there will be no question about what the researcher means when using the terms.

The methodology for the study defines the way pertinent information will be gathered in order to answer the research question or analyze the research problem. This includes detailed discussion on the selection of subjects who will participate in the study, and description of the data collection procedures and techniques. Also included is a plan for analyzing the data after they have been collected in a form that facilitates analysis. Limitations of the study are included to identify particular aspects of the study over which the researcher has no control.

Thus, the planning stage of the research process consists of the first five steps in the research process: (1) statement of the problem, (2) review of related literature, (3) statement of the purpose of the study, (4) plans for collection of the data, and (5) plans for analysis of the data.

In order to structure the planning stage of a research study, the researcher formulates a *research proposal:* a detailed written description of the proposed study. Sometimes called a prospectus, the research proposal serves as a blueprint for the research project and *must* be completed *prior* to conducting either a quantitative or a qualitative research study. The written proposal communicates the problem being investigated and the procedures that will be used in the investigation.

A research proposal is written for several purposes. Having to sit down and write a proposal for the research study forces the researcher to think through various aspects of the study that might not otherwise have been considered. The plan can then be evaluated by others, who may improve it by suggesting something that has been left out or by considering whether or not the ideas would be workable in the actual study setting. The written proposal provides a step-by-step guide to follow in carrying out the research project. It saves the researcher from having to remember the many details already considered and the anticipated problems already solved. A well-thought-out proposal saves time, helps avoid mistakes, and should result in a higher quality research study.

Written research proposals are required for all academic research studies, such as theses and dissertations, and for all research submitted for funding by various government agencies and private organizations. Although you are not now in a position to develop such a sophisticated proposal, writing your own proposal will help you to learn more about the research process by actually applying it to a nursing problem of your choice. Remember, research is a learned activity. All those who are now capable of writing sophisticated research proposals were once beginning research students like yourselves.

In developing a research proposal (step 1 of the planning stage of the research process), information related to the first five steps of the research process is included. It is generally agreed that the information to be outlined here should be included in a research proposal. Each of these components will be discussed in more detail in subsequent chapters. Step-by-step guidelines for the development of a research proposal are included in Appendix H.

1. *Statement of the problem:* This section should include the background of the problem and a brief statement of what is being investigated. The significance of the study should also be stated.
2. *Review of related literature:* This section presents summaries of other studies and articles that are related to the problem. It may also include the concepts or theory on which the research is based.
3. *Statement of the purpose of the study:* This section contains a clear statement of the purpose for conducting the research. It may be stated as a hypothesis to be tested, a question to be answered, or a phenomenon to be described or analyzed.
4. *Definitions of the terms used in the study*
5. *Plan for data collection:* This section should include detailed descriptions of the study subjects to be selected, and should describe the data collection techniques and procedures. Assumptions and limitations of the study may also be included here.
6. *Plan for data analysis:* This section contains procedures for analyzing the study data, including the kinds of tables to be used. If you plan to carry out a study requiring the use of statistics but do not have a statistical background, you will need help with this section of your proposal.
7. *Bibliography*
8. *Appendixes* (optional): This section may include materials developed especially for the study (cover letters, consent forms, questionnaires, interview schedules, and so forth).

Stage II: Implementing the Research Proposal

After the completed research proposal has been evaluated by those who can offer suggestions and, perhaps, revised to incorporate their suggestions, it must be approved by the appropriate institutional committees. This is very important, for it assures the protection of the rights of the study subjects as well as conformity to the policies and procedures of the institution. Once this approval is given, the researcher is then ready to implement the written proposal. It is in the implementation stage of the research process that the actual collection and analysis of data for the research study take place. In this stage, the researcher follows the written proposal by systematically gathering data for analysis. If unexpected problems arise in the research situation, the researcher may decide to alter the procedures while still implementing the written proposal as closely as possible.

Stage III: Communicating the Results of the Study

After analyzing the data in relation to the research problem, the researcher formulates conclusions, discusses them, and relates these conclusions to relevant present knowledge. The researcher should cite implications of the research and formulate recommendations for further study. The researcher then writes a report of the complete study to communicate its findings so that others have access to the knowledge. Research reports vary from formal reports to abridged reports for publication. A formal research report usually contains the following information and will be discussed further in Chapter 8.

The research report is divided into three major parts: (1) preliminary materials, (2) main body (text) of the report, and (3) reference materials. Each main part consists of several sections, as follows.

1. *Preliminary materials:* This section includes the title page, table of contents, list of illustrations or figures, list of tables, an abstract, and a preface or acknowledgment, if any.
2. *Main body* (text) of the report:
   a. The *introduction* section includes the statement of the problem, a review of related literature, the conceptual or theoretical framework, the purposes of the study, and a definition of terms.
   b. The *methodology* section includes the research approach, a description of the study subjects, the techniques used for data collection, the procedures, the assumptions, and the limitations of the study.
   c. The *findings* section includes the presentation of the data that have been collected for the study.
   d. The *discussion* section includes interpretation of the findings by the investigator, implications for nursing, and recommendations for further study.

  e. The *summary* section includes a brief restatement of the problem, pur-
      pose, major findings, conclusions, and recommendations.
3. *Reference materials:* This section includes the bibliography and appendices.

Comparing these components of the research report with those of a research proposal, you will see that the completed research report has the added
components of data analysis and interpretation, as well as conclusions and recommendations for further study. This is logical when you recall that the proposal is written in the planning stage of the research process and describes
what the researcher proposes to do. The completed research report represents
the implementation stage and describes what the researcher actually did and
found.

The research proposal is written in the future tense; much of its content
may be used in writing the research report by changing the tense from future
to past.

Stage IV: Utilizing the Results of the Study

The ultimate aim of conducting research into the practice and profession of
nursing and communicating the results is to use the knowledge for the improvement of patient care and of the nursing profession. Nursing research has
become a valued activity as nursing strives to identify and construct its scientific knowledge base. But there is a time lag between the reporting of nursing
research knowledge and its utilization in practice. Although nurses are expected to know the research that has been conducted and to use the findings
as a basis for scientific practice, the majority of nurses are not prepared to read
research journals critically and do not attend research conferences. Thus, *research utilization* may be more practically viewed ''as an organizational process
to be carried out by and for the total staff in a department of nursing.''[2]

Research utilization is discussed further in Chapter 9.

RELATIONSHIP OF THE RESEARCH PROCESS TO THE
PROBLEM-SOLVING PROCESS

Even though research and problem solving are often compared, it is important
to understand that the research process and the problem-solving process are
not the same. The two processes differ in their purpose. Problem solving is
simpler: Its purpose is to find an immediate solution to a practical problem in
an actual setting. The basic purpose of research, on the other hand, goes beyond solving the immediate problem: It provides new knowledge that can be
generalized to a broader setting and can be used to benefit a larger number of
people. For example, the nurse may decide that the application of a stockinette

cap to a newborn infant would be an effective way to conserve body heat. In contrast, a systematic research study (such as the study reported in Appendix E), conducted in relation to the same patient care problem, would be expected to benefit a large number of patients (provided that the design of the study permits its results to be generalized).

Comparison between Research and Problem Solving

Table 2.1 compares the research process with the problem-solving process and summarizes the stages of the research process.

Which Approach Is "Better"?

Once you understand that the research process and the problem-solving process have different purposes, it follows that the use of one process rather than the other to investigate a problem should not be considered better or more valuable. The value lies in correctly using the process that is most appropriate for the investigation.

SUMMARY

In this chapter, we considered the nature and components of the research process and its relation to the problem-solving process. The research process was presented as comprising four sequential stages: (1) the planning stage, in which a research proposal is written to describe the study problem and methodology; (2) the implementation stage, in which the completed research proposal is implemented to collect and analyze the data; (3) the communication stage, in which the researcher formulates conclusions and implications for the study, and writes up the report of the study in order to communicate the new knowledge; and (4) the utilization stage, in which new practices are derived from the research base. In order to apply the principles presented, you should complete the Application Activities listed in the next section.

APPLICATION ACTIVITIES

1. Read the research proposal in Appendix B, which was written by a beginning researcher. This proposal represents the planning stage of the research process and should help you understand the type of information a research proposal contains and what a completed proposal looks like. This researcher planned to use the descriptive research approach. You may also want to read the research proposals in Appendixes A, D, and E, which were also written by beginning research students. They represent,

TABLE 2.1
Comparison of the Stages of the Research Process with the Problem-Solving Process

Research Process	Problem-Solving Process
I. Planning Stage	
Written proposal includes specific problem statement; literature review to place research problem within existing knowledge and within theoretical or conceptual framework if indicated, precise statement of purpose of study; definition of terms; detailed plan for collection and analysis of data.	Detailed written plan not indicated.
II. Implementation Stage	
Institutional assurance of rights of study subjects and conformity to institutional requirements; systematic collection of data according to written proposal; detailed data analysis with appropriate descriptive and inferential statistical technique used.	No formal institutional review indicated. Data collection procedures may not be as rigorous. Simple analytical, statistical, or other method used.
III. Communication Stage	
Written findings should be published so others have access to the new knowledge. Report should be detailed enough to permit replication of the study.	Results and recommendations may be shared with persons in immediate setting.
IV. Utilization Stage	
Research base is derived from replication and verification of scientific research in a common conceptual area.	Information derived by problem-solving process cannot be verified by replication.

respectively, the historical research approach, the descriptive research approach using qualitative methodology, and the experimental research approach.

2. The student who wrote the research proposal in Appendix B was able to implement her proposal and conduct the study. Reading her research re-

port in Appendix C should help you understand the relationship between a research proposal and a completed research report. Notice how the research proposal is used in the research report by changing the tense used from future to past. Use Table 2.1 to systematically analyze the investigator's use of the research process rather than the problem-solving process.

REFERENCES

1. Hopkins, Charles D. 1976. *Educational Research: A Structure for Inquiry.* Columbus: Charles E. Merrill, p. 13.
2. Horsley, J. A., et al. 1983. *Using Research to Improve Nursing Practice: A Guide.* New York: Grune and Stratton, p. 2.

BIBLIOGRAPHY AND SELECTED READINGS

Brink, P. J., and M. Wood. 1983. *Basic Steps in Planning Nursing Research.* Belmont, CA: Wadsworth.

————. 1988. *Basic Steps in Planning Nursing Research,* 3rd ed. Boston: Jones and Bartlett.

Fox, D. J. 1982. *Fundamentals of Research in Nursing,* 4th ed. Norwalk, CT: Appleton-Century-Crofts.

Hopkins, C. D. 1976. *Educational Research: A Structure for Inquiry.* Columbus, OH: Charles E. Merrill.

Horsley, J. A., J. Crane, M. K. Crabtree, and D. J. Wood. 1983. *Using Research to Improve Nursing Practice: A Guide.* New York: Grune and Stratton.

Kidder, L. H., C. M. Judd, and E. R. Smith. 1986. *Research Methods in Social Relations,* 5th ed. New York: Holt, Rinehart and Winston.

Polit, D., and B. Hungler. 1987. *Nursing Research: Principles and Methods,* 3rd ed. Philadelphia: J. B. Lippincott.

Van Dalen, D. B. 1973. *Understanding Educational Research.* New York: McGraw-Hill.

Wandelt, Mabel. 1970. *Guide for the Beginning Researcher.* New York: Appleton-Century-Crofts.

3

The Quantitative and Qualitative Traditions of Inquiry

The material in this chapter will introduce you to two major traditions of scientific inquiry—the quantitative approach and the qualitative approach—and to the use of each approach in investigating nursing problems.

THE NATURE OF QUANTITATIVE AND QUALITATIVE METHODOLOGY

Traditionally, the scientific method of inquiry has been equated with the use of *quantitative research methods* to investigate the variables selected for study. (A *variable* is something that can have more than one value. Height, weight, hair color, and blood pressure all could be variables.) In quantitative research, the variables are preselected and defined by the investigator, and the data are col-

[27]

lected and quantified—translated into numbers—and statistically analyzed with a view to establishing cause-and-effect relationships among the variables. The quantitative approach to research has its roots in the tradition of the "hard" or mathematically based sciences and reflects the rigor of the scientific research approach most often associated with such fields as physics and chemistry. The use of quantitative methodology for investigating human behavior has been associated most often with the disciplines of psychology and sociology.

In the *qualitative research method*, the investigator seeks to identify the qualitative (nonnumerical) aspects of the phenomenon under study from the subjects' viewpoint in order to interpret the totality of the phenomenon. "The qualitative type of research refers to the methods and techniques of observing, documenting, analyzing and interpreting attributes, patterns, characteristics, and meanings of specific, contextual or gestaltic features of phenomena under study."[1]

Qualitative research is often considered "soft" because it does not deal with precise numbers and does not have the apparent "objective reality" that is characteristic of the quantitative approach. The qualitative approach has been associated with the social sciences and humanities, primarily the fields of history and philosophy. The use of qualitative methodology for investigating human behavior is frequently associated with the discipline of social anthropology.

Until very recently, the quantitative methodologies for scientific research have been the only methods legitimized by the scientific community. "Even when these methods have failed to be as valid and reliable in nursing and other human sciences as they have been in the natural sciences, researchers in nursing have clung to them, feeling that their only claim to the title of scientist lay in the quantitative methods."[2] There is no doubt that the quantitative methods used in nursing research have resulted in significant contributions to understanding many of the phenomena of nursing. A growing number of nurse researchers, however, in their conviction that the traditional scientific method imposes constraints on the study of human individuals, are using qualitative methodologies in their belief that "the [scientific] method's inherent nature . . . reduces the human being under study to an object with many small quantitative units . . . [and] gives no clue as to how to fit these small units back into the dynamic whole that is the living human being with whom the nurse interacts in practice."[3]

QUANTITATIVE RESEARCH

Quantitative research methodology rests on the basic assumption that all of the traits or characteristics that make up the units of both human and nonhuman organisms, as well as nonliving objects, exist in some degree and can be measured objectively. In some cases there is no trace of the trait or characteristic; in other cases there is a small trace of the characteristic; in still other cases, there is a moderate amount of the characteristic. Finally, in some cases there is a great deal of the characteristic present. Since terms like *small, moderate,* and *great deal* are too scientifically imprecise to be particularly useful in the quantification of data, the quantitative scientist must establish a numerical scale in order to determine the amount of the trait or characteristic that is present. For example, a researcher wishing to measure the amount of nicotine in a person's blood serum might draw a sample of blood and subject the blood to analysis. There should be no nicotine in the blood of a nonsmoker; this level can be called the zero level. As the presence of nicotine is measured in moderate and heavy smokers, the researcher would then be able to establish a strict numerical scale that would quantify the amount of nicotine in the blood.

Similarly, the blood alcohol tests used by law enforcement agencies provide numerical methods for determining if an individual is intoxicated as defined by the laws of a state. A more positive example of such measuring scales is the numerical measurement of blood sugar in individuals to determine if they suffer from diabetes. This information can be used to enhance the quality of life of individuals suffering from diabetes, and continued testing allows such persons to prolong their lives by stabilizing their blood sugar and insulin levels.

Using numerical scales allows the researcher to be "objective" about the research that is being carried out. Such objectivity allows the researcher to be "outside" of the research; that is, the researcher is not emotionally involved with the subject(s) of the research and is unbiased in the interpretation of the results.

Because nursing research deals with human beings, it is often difficult for the researcher to remain emotionally uninvolved with the subjects. Measuring physiological changes in patients as a result of an experimental technique often can provide such objective data. For example, Callow and Pieper found that a 30-degree backrest elevation had no significant impact on the central venous pressure of children who had had cardiac surgery when compared to the central venous pressure taken while the children were in a supine position.[4] They concluded that this elevation might enhance the children's comfort and safety.

The quantitative method requires that the problem statement and the design of the research be quite specific and detailed prior to conducting the investigation. Attention is paid to identifying factors not being investigated directly in the study and attempting to control their influence on the outcome of the study. Because of the need for control, quantitative researchers often establish a "context-free" environment. The research then takes place in a laboratory or other setting that gives each subject an equal opportunity to be assessed when measured by the data-gathering instrument.

As we have discussed in Chapter 1, one of the characteristics of the scientific method is generalization. Much quantitative research is designed and conducted with the purpose of predicting from the sample(s) measured to the whole population from which the sample was drawn. This requires that the design of the study and statistical analysis of the data conform to the strict requirements for generalization, which will be discussed later in this book.

The quantitative researcher also wants to understand the how and why of events and may seek to establish cause-and-effect relationships between the study variables. The structure of the process becomes an *if . . . then* statement: If *x* (*the independent variable*) happens, then *y* (*the dependent variable*) will happen. For example, *if* a person is a heavy cigarette smoker (*x*), *then* can we predict that this individual has a higher risk of developing lung cancer (*y*) than a person who is not a heavy cigarette smoker? If this is indeed a cause-and-effect relationship, lung cancer should then be controlled by stopping or significantly reducing smoking behavior. The determination of cause-and-effect relationships among study variables requires manipulation of the variables through experimentation, with careful attention to control of *confounding variables* (variables that may interfere with the direct causal relationship between independent and dependent variables) and *extraneous variables* (variables that are uncontrolled and outside the purpose of the study, which might influence the study's results). These ideas are discussed in greater detail in Chapter 12.

Although experimentation is a characteristic of quantitative research, quantitative research is not limited only to experimentation. Precisely defined and developed data collection instruments can be used to measure predefined variables. These include questionnaires, surveys, structured interviews, and other data-gathering instruments.

A major concern of quantitative researchers is replicability or reproducibility. When a researcher obtains certain results, can another researcher use the same procedures and obtain the same or similar results? True quantitative research demands that the research be able to be replicated by other researchers and that such replication will yield the same or very similar results. Achieving this can be extremely difficult when the researcher is investigating the complex world of human behavior.

QUALITATIVE RESEARCH

Qualitative research has several distinct characteristics which can be contrasted with quantitative methods. Whereas quantitative researchers generally have only minimal contact with the subjects of the study, qualitative researchers frequently use themselves as the data-gathering instrument. Rather than using precisely developed data-gathering tools and instruments to gather data about their subjects' knowledge, interests, and backgrounds, many qualitative researchers spend long periods of time with the study's subjects, observing their behaviors and interactions. The researcher keeps detailed notes about the events that have been observed, the interviews that have been carried out, and any other salient facts that might have a bearing on the purpose of the study. Because of the nature of qualitative research, the investigator gathers data in the setting where the activities are taking place.

Because of the mass of data that can be gathered, the qualitative researcher often deals with only a few members of the group being studied. This allows the researcher to focus intently on the subjects and to gather a great deal of information, which must be analyzed very carefully. For example, if a researcher is interested in the activities of student nurses as they learn and practice appropriate patient care, much of the research would take place in a clinical setting. The questions that students ask each other, as well as the questions asked by and of instructors, staff nurses, supervisors, physicians, patients, and any other individuals in the setting, would all be a part of the data gathered by the researcher. In addition to verbal interactions, which the researcher should transcribe if at all possible, nonverbal cues would also be noted. As the study of proxemics has demonstrated, much information can be gathered from a person's posture or stance.

While gathering data, the researcher must attempt to suspend value judgments. This can be difficult if activities are taking place that the researcher considers objectionable. Qualitative researchers can experience feelings of conflict on this point because their nonintervention may be considered a positive acceptance of the subjects' activity. Clearly, in the hospital study mentioned earlier, the researcher would have to intervene if a nursing student was about to make a mistake in patient care that would endanger the patient's well-being.

In planning their research, qualitative researchers often use essentially the same systematic series of steps in their research as quantitative researchers use. The statement of the problem may not be as rigorously defined as in quantitative research, but few qualitative researchers go into the study setting without some notion of the general area they plan to investigate. Qualitative researchers also establish a plan for the process of data collection. Because they are often their own data-collecting instrument, the data collection plan may include only the development and use of field notes. With the data collection devices available today, however, qualitative researchers may also choose to use such instruments as tape recorders and videotapes.

Qualitative researchers also establish a plan to analyze the data and formulate conclusions concerning the data collected. Because the data are qualitative rather than quantitative (numerical), the data analysis method usually do not depend on statistical tests.

Control (the elimination or reduction of confounding or extraneous variables) is difficult but not impossible to achieve. Qualitative researchers can use several methods to ensure that control is provided. The first is the use of multiple informants. If an investigator uses only one informant concerning certain activities, that informant may not really know about the activities under investigation or may choose to be deceptive concerning the activities. Multiple informants reduce the chances of this loss of control. Second, careful rechecking of the researcher's data is essential. Researchers must be careful to report accurately and completely on the data they have gathered and to gather enough data to warrant the conclusions that are formulated.

As we have seen, the scientific method depends on empiricism—the evidence gathered to gain new knowledge must be rooted in objective reality and gathered through the use of the human senses. The root source of knowledge in qualitative research can be described as ''cultural (ethnography), social, environmental, and philosophical phenomena to obtain patterned human interactions, symbols, values, world views, historical and general ethnographic lifeways.''[5]

Generalization, the ability to use the findings of research on a sample to anticipate the actions of larger populations, is a major goal of scientific inquiry. Because the primary purpose of qualitative research is to elicit meaning, qualitative researchers are often unable to generalize from their findings to larger populations. ''Remember, generalizability is not the purpose of qualitative research but the purpose is rather to elicit meaning in a given situation and to develop reality-based theory.''[6] However, given that any population, no matter how small, is a part of a larger population, some valid generalizations concerning the larger population may be formulated. That is to say, the nurses in one hospital are a part of a larger health care system which includes the community, the state, and the nation. ''As each level is explored, greater strength and depth will be added to the explanation of the social phenomenon under consideration.''[7]

QUALITATIVE RESEARCH STRATEGIES

Qualitative researchers employ a variety of strategies to generate useful data related to the phenomena they are investigating. These methods include *phenomenology, ethnography,* and *grounded theory.*

Phenomenology

Phenomenological research is based on the philosophy of phenomenology, which proposes to understand the response of the whole human being to a situation or situations. When this philosophy is translated into a research setting, several processes must occur:

1. A person must communicate an experience or series of experiences to the researcher.
2. The researcher attempts to translate the communicated experience into an understanding of the person's experience.

3. The researcher then breaks this understanding into the underlying concepts that are the themes of the experience.
4. The researcher communicates his or her understandings to an audience in writing so that the members of this audience can then relate their understanding of this information to past and future experiences.

Because of the potentially large amount of data to be gathered and analyzed, phenomenological research is usually based on data gathered from a very small number of individuals. Note that phenomenological research is based on the intuitive analysis of other persons' experiences and that this necessitates special training before the researcher can make valid analyses.

Ethnography

Ethnographic research, often described as "participant observation," has long been the domain of the cultural anthropologist. Such research requires that the researcher be physically present among the subjects during the data-gathering phase of the research process. The ethnographer attempts to describe the culture of a group through in-depth study, involving systematic observation of the group's activities, language, and customs.

Systematic observation requires that the researcher be in the field long enough to see deeply into the group being studied. The procedures for observing and recording data are reported so that other field workers can attempt to replicate the study. Systematic observation is methodical; that is, strategies for observation are carefully laid out prior to the study. Even with such strategies in place, the researcher must be flexible enough to change methods of observation (and document such change) if the study setting requires it.

Ethnographic research has been further divided into a series of subresearch strategies, which have been called *ethnomethodology.* Ethnomethodology is similar to phenomenology in that it involves an attempt to understand how people see, describe, and explain the world in which they live. Ethnomethodologists base their explanatory systems on analysis of the speech and activities of groups rather than attempting to understand the perceptions of individuals, as is done in phenomenology. This kind of data analysis leads to explanations of the commonsense understandings that groups of individuals hold.

Grounded Theory

Grounded theory is a research strategy that generates the theoretical underpinnings of the research being done by "grounding" or basing the theory on the data being collected. The grounded theorist determines the research question by observing how people solve problems in a social setting.

Grounded theory can be used in situations or areas where there has been little previous research, making it extremely difficult to test a previously developed theoretical position. Consequently, the grounded theorist uses the *inductive method* of developing theory while in the process of collecting data. This is in contrast to the *deductive method* of developing theory, in which theory is used to guide data collection and analysis.

As the researcher collects data, using a variety of data collection techniques such as observation, interviews, and questionnaires, each datum (a unit of data) is reviewed and compared to all of the other data. By using this comparative strategy, the researcher begins intuitively to develop concepts concerning the data. That is, the data are placed in categories; certain data fit into one category and other data fit into other categories.

After the data are categorized and concepts emerge, the researcher begins to analyze the data deductively. Theories are developed, and hypotheses based on these theories can be tested either quantitatively or qualitatively. As hypotheses are rejected, the concept that is the most important to theory development emerges. Finally, the data are again compared to the emergent theory so that the theory can be tested and modified to conform with known data.

SUMMARY

In this chapter, we have considered selected aspects of the quantitative and qualitative traditions of scientific inquiry. Both have provided—and will continue to provide—valuable strategies for investigating nursing problems. Neither approach is better than the other. The important point is that the researcher should use the approach that is the most appropriate for the particular purpose of the investigation.

APPLICATION ACTIVITIES

1. For each published research study you selected for the Application Activities in Chapter 1, identify whether the investigator(s) used a qualitative or quantitative strategy.
2. Explain your answers.

REFERENCES

1. Leininger, M. L., Ed. 1985. *Qualitative Research Methods in Nursing.* Orlando, FL: Grune and Stratton.
2. Omery, A. 1983. "Phenomenology: A Method for Nursing Research." *Advances in Nursing Science,* January, p. 62.

3. Ibid., p. 49.
4. Callow, L. B., and B. Pieper. 1989. ''Effect of Backrest on Central Venous Pressure in Pediatric Cardiac Surgery.'' *Nursing Research,* 38 (November–December): 336–338.
5. Leininger, *Qualitative Research Methods,* p. 14.
6. Field, P. A., and J. Morse. 1985. *Nursing Research: The Application of Qualitative Approaches.* Rockville, MD: Aspen, p. 122.
7. Dobbert, M. L. 1982. *Ethnographic Research.* New York: Praeger, p. 180.

BIBLIOGRAPHY AND SUGGESTED READINGS

Aamodt, A. 1982. ''Examining Ethnography for Nurse Researchers.'' *Western Journal of Nursing Research,* 4 (Spring): 209–221.

Berry, J. W. 1980. ''Introduction to Methodology.'' In H. C. Triandis and J. W. Berry, Eds., *Handbook of Cross-Cultural Psychology, Volume 2: Methodology.* Boston: Allyn and Bacon, pp. 1–28.

Callow, L. B., and B. Pieper. 1989. ''Effect of Backrest on Central Venous Pressure in Pediatric Cardiac Surgery.'' *Nursing Research,* 38 (November–December): 336–338.

Dobbert, M. L. 1982. *Ethnographic Research.* New York: Praeger.

Field, P. A., and J. M. Morse. 1985. *Nursing Research: The Application of Qualitative Approaches.* Rockville, MD: Aspen.

Leininger, M., Ed. 1985. *Qualitative Research Methods in Nursing.* Orlando, FL: Grune and Stratton.

Lincoln, Y. S., and E. G. Guba. 1985. *Naturalistic Inquiry.* Beverly Hills, CA: Sage.

Lindzey, G., and E. Aronson, Eds. 1985. *Handbook of Social Psychology,* 3rd ed. New York: Random House.

Morse, J. M., Ed. 1989. *Qualitative Nursing Research: A Contemporary Dialogue.* Rockville, MD: Aspen.

Omery, A. 1983. ''Phenomenology: A Method for Nursing Research.'' *Advances in Nursing Science,* January: 49–63.

Pelto, J. P., and G. Pelto. 1978. *Anthropological Research,* 2nd ed. Cambridge: Cambridge University Press.

Porter, E. J. 1989. ''The Qualitative-Quantitative Dualism.'' *Image,* 21 (Summer): 98–102.

Triandis, H. C., and J. W. Berry, Eds. 1980. *Handbook of Cross-Cultural Psychology, Volume 2: Methodology.* Boston: Allyn and Bacon.

Tripp-Reimer, T., and M. C. Dougherty. 1985. ''Cross Cultural Nursing Research.'' In H. H. Werley and J. J. Fitzpatrick, Eds., *Annual Review of Nursing Research.* New York: Springer.

Werner, O., and G. M. Schoepfle, Eds. 1987. *Systematic Fieldwork.* Beverly Hills, CA: Sage.

Werley, H. H., and J. J. Fitzpatrick, Eds. 1985. *Annual Review of Nursing Research.* New York: Springer.

4

Ethical Considerations for Protection of Human Subjects in Research

---

DEVELOPMENT OF ETHICAL CODES
INSTITUTIONAL REVIEW BOARDS
INFORMED CONSENT
APPLICATION ACTIVITIES
REFERENCES
BIBLIOGRAPHY AND SUGGESTED READINGS

In Chapter 1 we discussed the basic tenets of the scientific method and presented a brief history of nursing research. Chapter 2 provided an overview of the research process. In Chapter 3, quantitative and qualitative methodologies were compared and discussed. The purpose of this chapter is to acquaint you with one of the most important considerations of research that involves human subjects. This is the field of ethics in research.

DEVELOPMENT OF ETHICAL CODES

Researchers working with human subjects must always remember that their subjects are real people with their own needs and wants, not just numbers on a piece of paper. To this end, codes of ethics for human subject research have been developed to ensure the protection of the subjects' dignity and safety and the worthiness of research involving human subjects. These ethical codes are based on the Articles of the Nuremberg Tribunal, which were drawn up after the trials of the Nazi doctors accused of war crimes during the ''doctor trials'' following World War II. The defense that these individuals brought forward was that they were engaged in important research regardless of the pain and suffering they caused in their helpless subjects. The Articles serve as a standard against which to measure the individual rights of subjects participating in experimental and clinical research.

The Nuremberg Code includes the following points:

1. The voluntary consent of the human subject is absolutely essential.
2. The experiment should be such as to yield fruitful results . . . and not random or unnecessary. . . .
3. The experiment should be based on . . . [prior knowledge] and the anticipated results should justify . . . the experiment.
4. The experiment should . . . avoid all unnecessary physical and mental suffering and injury.
5. No experiment should be conducted where there is an a priori reason to believe that death or disabling injury will occur; except . . . where the experimental physicians also serve as subjects.
6. The degree of risk should never exceed . . . the importance of the problem to be solved. . . .
7. Proper preparations should be made and adequate facilities provided to protect . . . subject(s) against . . . possibilities of injury, disability, or death.
8. The experiment should be conducted only by scientifically qualified persons.
9. During the course of the experiment, the human subject should be able to bring the experiment to an end. . . .
10. During the course of the experiment the scientist must be prepared to terminate the experiment if he has probable cause . . . that a continuation of the experiment is likely to result in injury, disability or death to the experimental subject.[1]

The U.S. Department of Health and Human Services has provided a set of guidelines that researchers who are funded by the department must follow when using human subjects.[2] These guidelines require that an institutional review board (IRB) be established to ensure that the following conditions are met:

1. Risks to subjects are minimized by sound research procedures that do not expose subjects to risk unnecessarily. That is, projects using human subjects should be so well thought out that the potential for unforeseen harm, either physical or psychological, should be minimized.

2. The anticipated benefits to subjects should outweigh the risks to the subjects, and knowledge to be gained should be of sufficient importance to merit any risks to which subjects might be subjected.

3. The rights and welfare of the subjects are adequately protected. That is, the researcher must terminate the research if subjects are being deprived of a procedure that might benefit them or are being subjected to one that is causing more harm than was anticipated.

An example of researchers terminating an experimental study in order to allow all subjects in the study to benefit would be the case in which it was determined that significantly lower doses of an expensive drug were just as effective and caused fewer side effects in patients who tested positive for a disease but who had not shown any symptoms. An example of researchers terminating a project because of unanticipated negative consequences would be the case of a social-psychological experiment in which subjects were placed in an uncomfortable situation and the experimenters noticed increasingly negative behaviors in the subjects that could be directly attributed to the experimental treatment.

4. The activity will be periodically reviewed by the institutional review board.

5. Informed consent has been obtained and appropriately documented. This is such an important area of concern that it will be discussed in greater detail in a later section of this chapter.

The 1985 *Human Rights Guidelines for Nurses in Clinical and Other Research*,[3] published by the American Nurses' Association, outlines the responsibilities of nurses in practice, education, and research for safeguarding the rights of human subjects in research. This document details three basic rights:

1. *The right to freedom from intrinsic risk of injury:* As mentioned in the previous discussion, subjects must be protected from physical, social or emotional injury.

2. *The right to privacy and dignity:* Researchers should make every attempt to avoid invading their subjects' privacy and/or placing them in demeaning or dehumanizing situations.

The right to privacy also carries over to a patient's records. The Privacy Act of 1974 specifically denies the opening of records to unauthorized individuals. At times, however, a bona fide researcher needs to have access to existing records. Some states have established laws to protect the privacy of individuals which include access to medical records; other states have not developed such statutes.

Many agencies have developed a prior consent or release of information form, which the potential subject signs as a routine part of obtaining whatever care is being provided. Without such prior consent, however, in many cases, the institutional review board may grant access to records when the board is certain that patient confidentiality will be respected and that only authorized investigators will have access to the records.

3. *The right to anonymity:* The identity of subjects participating in a study must not be disclosed, nor should the identity of individuals be recognizable through discussion or publication of the researchers' results, including photographs of the subject(s). If a subject's identity can be determined from the research, the researcher must have consent from the subject in order to include the information gained from that subject's participation.

The subjects of research include patients and outpatients, persons who are donors of organs and tissues, research volunteers, and volunteers with limited freedom—members of groups vulnerable to exploitation. This last category includes prisoners, residents of institutions for the mentally ill and mentally retarded, military personnel, and students.[4]

INSTITUTIONAL REVIEW BOARDS

As a result of the increasing awareness of ethical decision making in human research over the years, as well as the need to conform to the federal guidelines previously cited, most institutions sponsoring human subject research have a review group or committee whose responsibility is to ensure that researchers do not engage in unethical behavior or conduct poorly designed research. Membership on an institutional review board (IRB) should include professionals who represent the discipline(s) from which the research framework is drawn, as well as representatives from the community at large. This means that the IRB in a hospital should include nurses as well as other health professionals and that the nursing representatives should have an equal voice in the deliberations of the committee.

INFORMED CONSENT

The greatest concern in human subject research is the protection of the subject's right of self-determination by the assurance of informed consent. This means that the subject must be made fully aware of the study and agree to participate in it. The need for this type of agreement may seem self-evident, but a large number of studies have been carried out without the participants' consent. A glaring and tragic example of such research in the United States is the study of black males with syphilis initiated in 1932 by the U.S. Public Health Service. This research project was designed to study the long-term effects of untreated syphilis in a sample of semiliterate black men in Macon County, Alabama. Specific treatment for the disease was withheld from a sample of 399 black males who had been diagnosed as having syphilis. The research subjects thought they were receiving treatment for ''bad blood,'' which the researchers mistakenly thought was a term recognized by the subjects as meaning syphilis. Their progress was compared to that of a control group of 201 black males who did not have the disease. The so-called researchers then intended to follow the subjects through the rest of their lives to determine the long-term effects of untreated syphilis so that the ''natural course'' of the disease could be observed. Even though mortality rates were twice as high for the syphilitic subjects by the mid-1940s and continued to be higher than mortality rates for the control group, the U.S. Public Health Service did not provide treatment for the syphilitic subjects until the research was exposed in 1972— forty years after the experiment began.[5] In 1980, when the first edition of this book was written, the survivors were still being sought, and large amounts of monetary compensation were being given to them and their survivors. In this case, there was no excuse for not obtaining informed consent from the subjects of the study; the cost in suffering and disability can never be justified.

Essentially, the informed consent of subjects consists of the following six elements:

1. An understandable explanation of the purpose of the study and the procedures and techniques to be followed is required, along with the identification of experimental procedures and techniques. Fulfilling this requirement may be difficult. As we point out in Chapter 10, subjects' awareness of the nature of the research or experiment may affect the experiment. There are those who suggest that a researcher cannot get a true random sample of a population, in fact, because the fact of their consenting to be part of an experiment automatically means that the subjects in the experimental study are different from those subjects who refused to participate.

2. An explanation is required of the potential risks and discomforts to the subject as a result of the study. Will the subject be exposed to a potentially harmful situation? Withholding medication or treatment may cause physical or psychological distress to the subject. Further, withholding treatment may actually expose the subject to physical risk. Each subject must know what the potential hazards are. Additionally, the right of personal privacy and dignity for each subject must be assured.

3. Subjects should be told what benefits are to be expected. This can be a broad explanation; it may be the basis for an appeal to the subject's altruism, or it may be merely a simple explanation. The intent of many experiments is to improve the human condition. Providing different treatments to research subjects may mean that treatment modalities will improve. Each time a new treatment is tried, it is usually believed to be more effective than existing treatment modalities.

4. Subjects must be told of alternative procedures that would be advantageous to the subject. For example, in the case of the use of an experimental

drug, subjects should be aware that other, already proven drugs may aid in the treatment, while the experimental drug may do nothing at all. Subjects must also be informed if benefits are to be withheld from them.

5. Researchers must be willing to answer any question that the subjects may have about the experimental procedures. Most subjects want to know what is happening and why it is happening. In a research situation, subjects must be informed of what is happening if they request such information.

6. Subjects must be made aware that they can withdraw from the research investigation at any time without prejudice to their care. Researchers cannot compel or coerce subjects to remain in any investigation against their will.

Unfortunately, the doctrine of informed consent cannot be followed to its fullest in many kinds of research. In the case of qualitative research, much of the research is done in such a way that there is no simple way to explain the nature of the research project, or the explanations may become so broad as to be meaningless. A researcher who simply states to the research subjects that he or she would find it interesting to see how people live their daily lives is not giving those subjects a great deal of information.

Also, it is not uncommon for researchers to be deceptive in their research strategy. This is especially true in psychological studies, where informing subjects of the true nature of the study could bias the results of the study. A classic example of such deception was a study conducted by Milgram.[6] In this study, subjects were told that they were involved in an experiment that proposed to measure the impact of punishment on a person's ability to learn. The subjects were to read a list of words to another person who, unbeknownst to the subjects, was the experimenter's confederate. If the confederate gave a wrong response, the subject was to "punish" the mistake by delivering an increasingly higher level of electric shock. The subject believed, incorrectly, that the confederate could receive a shock as high as 450 volts. Each subject was assured that no "permanent" damage would be done to the "learner." The confederate, however, who did not receive any shock at any time, feigned great pain as the administered shocks increased in strength. When the subject protested about admistering pain, he was told to continue by the experimenter—the voice of authority. A very high degree of obedience to authority was obtained, and the study demonstrated how ordinary individuals might engage in harmful activities if urged to do so by those perceived to have authority over them. It is important to note that each subject was debriefed after the experiment was conducted and was shown that the confederate—the "victim"—was not actually harmed and had, in fact, received no shocks.

When this study was first published, it created an ethical controversy concerning the use of deception with study subjects, and the Milgram study still remains controversial. As a consequence of this and other studies requiring deception, many institutional review boards now demand that if the research design involves any form of deception, the researcher must provide a strong rationale for such deception and present a plan that allows for adequate debriefing of the study's subjects after the conclusion of the experiment.

Another example of deception in research that has generated a great deal of ethical controversy is contained in the work of Humphreys.[7] In this study, published in 1970, Humphreys observed a number of homosexual acts in public restrooms, known as "tearooms" to the participants. He assumed the role of "watchqueen" or lookout, with the responsibility for warning of danger while others performed homosexual acts. Later, by using names and addresses obtained from records of license plate numbers, Humphreys, who altered his appearance and claimed to be a health inspector, interviewed a number of his subjects in their homes. The results of the study showed that only a few of the individuals interviewed were members of the recognized homosexual community; many were married and did not consider themselves either homosexual or bisexual. They did, however, consider their marriages to be marked by tension.

Although Humphreys received the C. Wright Mills Award for outstanding research on a critical social issue, his work generated bitter controversy at the institution that awarded his Ph.D. degree. In fact, some members of the faculty attempted to void his degree because of the controversial nature of his research. Humphreys's work also created a stir in various newspaper columns throughout the country—an almost unheard-of event in the annals of academe.

The controversy generated by this study still lingers. A key issue is the right to privacy demanded when conducting a research study. Did Humphreys adhere to this concept when he obtained the names and addresses of the individuals involved from the license plates of their automobiles parked outside the "tearooms," or did he increase the possibility that they would be arrested? Another important consideration was his active participation as lookout in an illegal activity. Can the study of illegal behaviors be conducted as a value-free enterprise, and does the researcher thereby lend credibility to the activities?

In all research studies it is essential that the researcher be able to document that he or she has obtained the informed consent of the subject(s). Such consent is best obtained on a written form stating that the subject has willingly entered into the research project and is aware of the risks, procedures, and benefits involved. The following form might be used:

I _____ [subject] do agree to participate in a research/experimental study concerning _____.
This project may expose me to _____ risks and attendant discomforts.
    I am aware that _____ might be advantageous

to me in the treatment of my condition instead of the experimental treatment.

I may ask any questions about the procedures and treatments taking place and my questions must be answered honestly and fully.

I am free to withdraw this consent and discontinue participation in this research study at any time without this decision affecting me in any way.

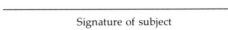

Signature of subject

Oral consent is also valid but should be witnessed by a third party for the protection of both the researcher and the subject. In the event that the potential subjects are not able to give informed consent because of mental or physical disabilities, or because they are below the legal age of consent, the researcher must gain the consent of a legally authorized guardian or next of kin.

Upon completion of a research investigation involving human subjects, the researcher has the obligation to remove any harmful aftereffects, debrief the subjects if necessary, and follow through on any commitments made to the subject. This also includes the provision of any study results that have been promised.

Nurses have a professional obligation to become knowledgeable participants in health care practice and research, and to be sure that they involve themselves in institutional policymaking and review activities:

> Knowledge about the changing scope of nursing responsibility and the emerging ethical issues affecting all practitioners in health care today is necessary for a professional nursing practice that accepts accountability for the protection of the human rights of consumers.[8]

APPLICATION ACTIVITIES

1. Read the informed consent at the end of the qualitative research proposal in Appendix D. Note how the researcher included the six elements of informed consent discussed in this chapter.
2. Read the informed consents included in the experimental and quasi-experimental research proposals in Appendixes E and F, and discuss the extent to which each of the informed consents includes the six elements necessary to ensure the informed consent of the subjects participating in an experimental study.
3. For each of the published studies you read for the Application Activities in Chapters 1 and 3, discuss the extent to which the author reported procedures for the protection of the subjects in the study.

REFERENCES

1. *Trials of War Criminals Before the Nuremberg Military Tribunals, Volumes I and II: The Medical Case.* 1948. As cited in J. Katz. 1972. *Experimentation with Human Beings.* New York: Russell Sage Foundation, pp. 305–306.
2. U.S. Department of Health and Human Services. 1981. "Basic HHS Policy for the Protection of Human Research Subjects." *Federal Register,* 46: 8366–8392.
3. American Nurses' Association. 1985. *Human Rights Guidelines for Nurses in Clinical and Other Research.* Code No. D-46 5M 2/85. Kansas City: American Nurses' Association, pp. 6–7.
4. Ibid., p. 7.
5. Jones, J. H. 1981. *Bad Blood.* New York: Free Press.
6. Milgram, S. 1974. *Obedience to Authority.* New York: Harper & Row.
7. Humphreys, L. 1970. *The Tearoom Trade.* Chicago: Aldine.
8. American Nurses' Association. *Human Rights Guidelines,* p. 16.

BIBLIOGRAPHY AND SUGGESTED READINGS

American Nurses' Association. 1985. *Human Rights Guidelines for Nurses in Clinical and Other Research,* Code No. D-46 5M 2/85. Kansas City: American Nurses' Association.

Anderson, G., and V. Anderson. 1987. *Health Care Ethics.* Germantown, MD: Aspen.

Applebaum, P. S., L. H. Roth, and T. Detre. 1984. "Researchers' Access to Patient Records: An Analysis of the Ethical Problems." *Clinical Research,* 32(October): 399–403.

Cassell, J. 1980. "Ethical Principles for Conducting Fieldwork." *American Anthropologist,* 82: 28–41.

Department of Health and Human Services. 1981. "Basic HHS Policy for the Protection of Human Research Subjects." *Federal Register,* pp. 8366–8392.

Gortner, S. R. 1985. "Ethical Inquiry." In H. H. Werley and J. J. Fitzpatrick, Eds., *Annual Review of Nursing Research.* New York: Springer.

Humphreys, L. 1970. *The Tearoom Trade.* Chicago: Aldine.

Jones, J. H. 1981. *Bad Blood.* New York: Free Press.

Katz, J. 1972. *Experimentation with Human Beings.* New York: Russell Sage Foundation.

Milgram, S. 1974. *Obedience to Authority.* New York: Harper & Row.

Murray, J. C., and R. A. Pagon. 1984. "Informed Consent to Research Publication of Patient-Related Data." *Clinical Research,* 32(October): 404–408.

Ramos, M. C. 1989. "Some Ethical Implications of Qualitative Research." *Research in Nursing and Health,* 12(February): 57–63.

Trials of War Criminals Before the Nuremberg Military Tribunals, Volume I and II: The Medical Case. 1948. Washington, DC: U.S. Government Printing Office.

Werley, H. H., and J. J. Fitzpatrick, Eds. 1985. *Annual Review of Nursing Research.* New York: Springer.

Part Two

Applying the Scientific Process of Inquiry to Nursing Problems

THE MATERIAL IN PART II, designed to acquaint you with the application of the scientific process of inquiry to nursing problems, presents principles and activities for applying the research process to nursing problems using both quantitative and qualitative methodologies.

Chapter 5 focuses on the selection and statement of the research problem, including a review of related literature, the formulation of a conceptual or theoretical framework, and a statement of the purpose of the study. Chapter 6 deals with data collection principles and techniques. Chapter 7 discusses data analysis. Chapter 8 focuses on the communication of research results. Chapter 9 presents a discussion of the final stage of the research process: utilizing the research results.

5

Problem Selection and Statement

In Chapter 2, the research process was described as a chain of reasoning that begins with a statement of the problem and systematically proceeds through the communication and utilization of the study's results.

The material in this chapter is designed to acquaint you with the initial step of the research process: selection and statement of the research problem. This is an extremely important component of the research process. It begins with the identification of a general problem area of interest and involves the subsequent narrowing down of the topic to a very specific problem to be investigated. Although the researcher is not usually expected to identify a research problem until after he or she has done some relevant reading, it is important to become familiar with the sources of research problems and with the criteria for evaluating them.

SELECTION OF A RESEARCHABLE PROBLEM

The selection of the problem to be investigated is an extremely important step and determines to a large extent the nature and quality of the research. Think of the problem as a question needing to be answered or as a situation needing a solution. First, look at your professional experiences. Describe a situation that aroused your interest—even one that annoyed you—and led you to think that something ought to be done about it. Examples of general problem areas in nursing might include preoperative teaching for mastectomy patients, discharge planning for premature infants, successful breast feeding in primiparas, or medication errors made by posthospitalized geriatric patients. If you find that your own experience fails to generate a problem area, use the library for locating literature related to your area of professional interest.

Once you have identified a general problem area related to your interests and experience, narrow it down to one specific problem that is manageable within the research process. A problem that is too broad can result in a study that is too general or too difficult to conduct; the results may be hard to interpret. It is often helpful to state the problem as a question. For example, the general problem area of successful breast feeding in primiparas could be narrowed down by asking, "What is the effect of teaching about breast feeding to primiparas?" This might then generate more specific problems: "Are there differences in comparable success with breast feeding in primiparas taught specific concepts and techniques related to breast feeding versus primiparas not exposed to such teaching?" or "What is the effect of individualized versus group instruction on successful breast-feeding practices in primiparas?"

It is well worth the time and effort it takes to select a problem specific enough to result in a manageable study. In your efforts to narrow down a general problem area, however, be careful not to end up with a question so trivial that it is not worth the time and effort involved in researching it.

SOURCES OF RESEARCH PROBLEMS

There are several major sources of problems that need to be researched. An obvious source is the researcher's own background and personal experiences. As a nurse, you are in an excellent position to identify researchable problems unique to nursing. For example, the research problem identified by the student who wrote the research proposal in Appendix E was a result of her own clinical observation that not only did some nurses routinely place stockinette caps on newborns while others did not, but their reasons for doing this varied.

Another important source of researchable topics is the literature. Research studies reported in various nursing and related journals provide many kinds of problems observed by other researchers. Many studies raise additional questions or include recommendations for further study that can form the basis of new studies. A study that has already been conducted can be replicated in a different setting to see if its findings can be generalized. For example, King and Tarsitano[1] conducted an approximate replication of the Lindeman and Van Aernam study,[2] which investigated the effectiveness of structured and unstructured preoperative teaching in improving the ability of surgical patients to deep-breathe and cough postoperatively.

Investigation of problems derived from theory, a third source, can provide a meaningful contribution to scientific knowledge. Theory is not merely a body of facts; it provides an explanation of facts that is then used to explain or predict certain phenomena. A good theory can guide research by pointing to areas that need to be investigated. Research can also contribute to the related theory by confirming or failing to confirm some aspect of the theory:

> The more research is directed by scientific theory, the more likely are its results to contribute directly to the development and further organization of a scientific body of knowledge in nursing.[3]

It is necessary to be aware of both the sources of research problems and the importance of designing nursing research studies that contribute to nursing's scientific knowledge base.

PROBLEM SELECTION CRITERIA

A researcher should evaluate the proposed problem and decide if it should be pursued through the research process by asking the following questions:

1. Is the topic of interest?
2. Is it researchable?
3. Is it practicable?

4. Is it significant?
5. Is it ethical to conduct research on this problem?

Is the Topic Interesting?

Because the researcher must become deeply involved in planning and implementing the research study, the topic should be one that will sustain interest over a prolonged period of time.

Is the Problem Researchable?

A researchable problem is one that can be investigated through the collection and analysis of data that exist in the real world. The meanings of the concepts must be clear and you must be able to present them through tangible, observable evidence—that is, evidence obtained through direct observation or through other activities that will provide similar evidence relating to the concept.

Is the Problem Practicable?

A research problem is practicable if it is possible to carry out the necessary related activities. Once you have found a topic of interest to you and within your area of expertise, you will still need to consider the following:

1. Are appropriate methodology and resources available in terms of suitable measuring instruments or equipment?
2. Are subjects available?
3. Will you have cooperation from others?

You also need to consider the length of time needed to complete the study and the cost involved.

Is the Problem Significant?

Even though your topic may be interesting in itself, you need to consider if it is sufficiently significant to warrant a study. A good nursing research problem should have practical and/or theoretical significance. Its solution should contribute to the improvement of nursing care or to the advancement of nursing as a profession by providing scientific knowledge and theoretical formulations.

The 1985 Priorities for Nursing Research developed by the American Nurses' Association Cabinet on Nursing Research could serve as guidelines for selecting research problems. These priorities are listed in Table 5.1.

TABLE 5.1
ANA Priorities for Nursing Research (1985)

1. Promote health, well-being, and ability to care for oneself among all age, social, and cultural groups.
2. Minimize or prevent behaviorally and environmentally induced health problems that compromise the quality of life and reduce productivity.
3. Minimize the negative effects of new health technologies on the adaptive abilities of individuals and families experiencing acute or chronic health problems.
4. Ensure that the care needs of particularly vulnerable groups, such as the elderly, children with congenital health problems, individuals from diverse cultures, the mentally ill, and the poor, are met in effective and acceptable ways.
5. Classify nursing practice phenomena.
6. Ensure that principles of ethics guide nursing research.
7. Develop instruments to measure nursing outcomes.
8. Develop integrative methodologies for the holistic study of human beings as they relate to their families and life-styles.
9. Design and evaluate alternative models for delivering health care and for administering health care systems so that nurses will be able to balance high quality and cost-effectiveness in meeting the nursing needs of identified populations.
10. Evaluate the effectiveness of alternative approaches to nursing education for the kind of practice that requires broad knowledge and a wide repertoire of skills, and for the kind of practice that requires specialized knowledge and a focused set of skills.
11. Identify and analyze historical and contemporary factors that influence the shaping of nursing professionals' involvement in national health policy development.[4]

Source: Reprinted with permission of the American Nurses' Association from *Directions for Nursing Research: Toward the Twenty-first Century.* Copyright © 1985 American Nurses' Association Cabinet on Nursing Research, Kansas City, Missouri.

Is the Research Ethical?

Finally, you must evaluate the ethical implications of your problem in order to protect the rights of the subjects who would participate in the study. Obtaining informed consent from participants, protecting them from harm, and maintaining anonymity and confidentiality are major considerations, as we pointed out in Chapter 4.

In summary, the selection of the research problem—the initial step in the research process—is extremely important and determines the nature and quality of the research study.

Beginning researchers usually need to seek help in evaluating their problem selection and in deciding if they should pursue it through the research process.

REVIEW OF RELATED LITERATURE

The initial review of the literature should help you identify and state a research problem. The second review, involving the systematic identification and analysis of information pertaining to the specific problem you selected for study, should be done during the initial stages of the research process. Unfortunately, beginning researchers often fail to appreciate the importance of conducting the literature review at this point in the process. In their enthusiasm to proceed with the rest of the study, they fail to put the problem in the perspective of what has already been done.

Why Review the Literature?

There are four primary reasons for conducting a literature review. The first is to determine what has already been done that relates to your problem. This helps avoid the duplication of previous studies and helps you develop a framework for the problem that relates it to completed studies. Because one of the aims of research in nursing is to develop theories of nursing, the literature search may provide a theoretical framework within which to investigate the problem. For example, theory related to learning might form the theoretical framework within which the problem of group versus individual instruction for breast feeding could be investigated. Beginning researchers may not be expected to include a theoretical framework in their studies.

Second, the literature review provides ideas about the kinds of studies that need to be done. Previous investigators and writers often make suggestions regarding problems that need further investigation. Reviewing the literature may stimulate the researcher to develop new insights into reported research or devise new problems to be investigated.

Third, the literature review serves to point out research strategies, specific research procedures, and information regarding measuring instruments that have been found to be productive as well as nonproductive for the problem. Capitalizing on the successes as well as the errors of other researchers helps the researcher to profit from and build upon the experiences of other researchers.

Finally, the literature review can help you interpret the results of the study after it has been conducted by allowing you to discuss the findings in terms of agreement or nonagreement with other studies. Results that contradict the findings of other studies can suggest further studies to resolve such contradictions.

Recommendations for Locating Pertinent Materials

It is very important to become familiar with the available library resources before beginning the literature review. The time you spend initially in familiarizing yourself with these resources ultimately will save you much valuable time. Try to get a written guide explaining the resources and services of the library and the procedures that need to be followed. It is often helpful to participate in a guided tour of the library so you can learn to use the library to its fullest extent. Ask the librarian for help when you need it.

You should become familiar with the use of the card catalogue and locate pertinent encyclopedias and dictionaries, government publications, and other audiovisual resources. Ask about interlibrary loans, which are designed to help you obtain references not available in your own library. If your library has computerized literature searches such as MEDLARS or MEDLINE, you should investigate them with your librarian to see how they can help you. MEDLARS (*Medical Literature Analysis and Retrieval System*) is the computerized literature retrieval service of the National Library of Medicine in Bethesda, Maryland. MEDLARS contains millions of references to journal articles and books in the health sciences published after 1965. MEDLINE (MEDLARS on-line), the retrieval capability of MEDLARS, contains citations and selected abstracts from approximately 3,000 journals published in the United States and foreign countries. It has hundreds of thousands of references to biomedical journal articles published in the current year and the three preceding years.

Table 5.2 provides a list of some, but not all, of the available computerized literature searches. These data bases are valuable sources for locating pertinent references.

Indexes and abstracts are most helpful in identifying relevant references. Indexes are lists of books and articles, or the contents of a book, whereas abstracts present the main ideas of articles and books.

The following indexes are most helpful:

1. The *Cumulative Index to Nursing and Allied Health Literature,* published continuously since 1956, indexes approximately 250 English-language journals in nursing and allied health sciences, as well as selected articles from popular magazines and some biomedical journals from *Index Medicus.*

2. *Hospital Literature Index,* published quarterly by the American Hospital Association, selectively indexes approximately 600 English-language journals on health care administration and planning.

3. *Index Medicus,* a government publication under the auspices of the National Library of Medicine, surveys over 2,600 international biomedical journals, of which several are nursing journals.

4. *International Nursing Index,* published quarterly by the American Journal of Nursing Company in cooperation with the National Library of Medicine, surveys approximately 200 domestic and foreign journals, in addition to nursing articles from over 2,600 nonnursing journals.

TABLE 5.2
Computerized Literature Searches

Data Base	Content
AVLINE, CATLINE	Audiovisuals and books in the biomedical sciences
BIOETHICS	Ethics
BIOSIS	Biological research
CANCERLIT	Cancer literature
CANCERPROJ	Cancer-related research projects
CHEMLINE	Dictionary of chemicals
CLINPROT	Clinical cancer protocols
DIOGENES	FDA and drug information
DIRLINE	Directory of information resources
EMBASE	Formerly *Excerpta Medica*
ERIC	Educational Resources Information Center, U.S. Office of Education
HEALTH	Health care aspects, such as planning
HEALTH INSTRUMENT FILE	Describes behavioral instruments used by nurse researchers
HISTLINE	History of medicine and related sciences
PSYCINFO	Psychology and related literature, including nursing
SOCABS	*Sociological Abstracts,* American Sociological Association
TOXLINE	Toxicological information

The following abstracts are most helpful:

5. *Dissertation Abstracts International* contains abstracts of doctoral dissertations in the humanities and social sciences, the sciences, engineering, and nursing.

6. *Psychological Abstracts,* published by the American Psychological Association, abstracts the international literature on psychology and related disciplines and contains categories related to nursing and nursing education.

7. *Sociological Abstracts* contains abstracts of the international literature in sociology and has sections on nursing.

The following indexes and abstracts are the other major sources commonly used by nurse researchers:

Abstracts of Health Care Management Studies
American Journal of Nursing: Annual and Cumulative Indexes
Biological Abstracts
Bioresearch Abstracts

Child Development Abstracts
Education Index
ERIC
Excerpta Medica
International Index
Nursing Outlook: Annual and Cumulative Indexes
Nursing Research: Annual and Cumulative Indexes
Nutrition Abstracts
Public Health, Social Medicine and Hygiene
Readers' Guide to Periodical Literature
Research Grants Index
Science Citation Index

In addition to indexes and abstracts, compilations of measuring instruments can be very helpful in identifying relevant references and locating appropriate measuring instruments. The following compilations are specifically related to nursing research:

Clayton, Gloria M., and Marion Broom. 1989. *Instruments for Use in Nursing Education Research.* No. 15-2248. New York: National League for Nursing.
Ward, Mary Jane, and Carol Lindeman, Ed. 1978. *Instruments for Measuring Nursing Practice and Other Care Variables.* 2 vols. DHEW Publication No. HRA 78-53. Washington, DC: U.S. Government Printing Office.
Ward, Mary Jane, and Mark Fetter. 1979. *Instruments for Use in Nursing Education Research.* Boulder, CO: Western Interstate Commission for Higher Education.

Following is a list of selected sources for locating measuring instruments that are not specifically related to nursing research but might relate to your research topic:

Buros, Oscar K., Ed. 1970, 1975. *Personality Tests and Review.* 2 vols. Highland Park, NJ: Gryphon Press.
Chun, KiTaek, Sidney Cobb, and John French, Jr. 1975. *Measures for Psychological Assessment.* Ann Arbor: University of Michigan Institute for Social Research.
Goldman, Bert, and John Saunders. 1974. *Directory of Unpublished Experimental Measures.* 2 vols. New York: Behavioral Publications.
Johnson, Orval. 1976. *Tests and Measurements in Child Development: Handbook II.* 2 vols. San Francisco: Jossey-Bass.
Keyser, D. J., and R. C. Sweetland, Eds. 1984. *Test Critiques.* Kansas City: Test Corporation of America.
Miller, Delbert, Ed. 1977. *Handbook of Research Design and Social Measurement,* 3rd ed. New York: McKay.
Mitchell, J. V., Jr., Ed. 1985. *Mental Measurements Yearbook,* 9th ed. Lincoln: University of Nebraska Press.
———. 1983. *Tests in Print III.* Lincoln: University of Nebraska Press.
Reeder, Leo, Linda Ramacher, and S. Gorelnik. 1976. *Handbook of Scales and Indices of Health Behavior.* Santa Monica, CA: Goodyear Publishing Company.

Shaw, Marvin E., and Jack M. Wright. 1967. *Scales for the Measurement of Attitudes.* New York: McGraw-Hill.

Strauss, Murray, and Bruce W. Brown. 1978. *Family Measurement Techniques: Abstracts of Published Instruments, 1935 to 1974,* revised. Minneapolis: University of Minnesota Press.

Sweetland, R. C., and D. J. Keyser, Eds. 1986. *Tests: A Comprehensive Reference for Assessments in Psychology, Education and Business,* 2nd ed. Kansas City: Test Corporation of America.

It is extremely helpful to make a list of key words to guide you in the literature search. For example, key words related to the topic of breast feeding might include *nutrition, infant nutrition, newborn, neonatal, nursing, lactation, pregnancy, bottle feeding, mothering,* and *feminism.*

It is preferable to obtain reference material from primary (original) sources rather than secondary (not original) sources. This minimizes error and allows the researcher to analyze the material. Articles you plan to quote directly should be photocopied to reduce citation errors. You should also plan to photocopy all tables and charts that you cite so that you have the complete information when writing the report.

Of concern to the beginning researcher is the amount of time spent on the literature review for writing a research proposal. We concur with Verhonick and Seamen that for a circumscribed study of one semester, two weeks should be appropriate to review literature with the objective of the research kept clearly in mind.[5] The library search application activity at the end of the chapter is designed to familiarize you with a large variety of reference sources.

Abstracting the Reference

After locating references that are pertinent to your topic, you should begin with the latest one since it may contain additional references from previous research. Read the abstract of the article and/or the summary to see if the article is pertinent to your topic. Then scan the article, noting the important points. Plan to use separate index cards (4 × 6 is a convenient size) to record useful information. A separate index card for each reference helps organize the materials when you are ready to write up the literature review. The card should contain the following information:

1. Record the complete bibliographic reference in the format of the style manual required by your department. Doing this will save you time when you are ready to write the bibliography for your proposal.

2. Record the complete call number for a source in case you need to recheck it.

3. Develop your own coding system for each reference. Mark such factors as relevance to your study, type of article, and whatever else would be helpful

for your research. For example, information on the relevance of references could be coded as R + (very relevant), R (relevant), or R − (less relevant). Information concerning the type of reference could be coded as RS (research study) or V (an article expressing the author's viewpoint).

4. Summarize the reference on the card by listing its essential points and noting the important or unusual aspects of the article that will contribute to your study. If you quote directly from the article, you must copy the quotation word for word, being careful to note if it is a direct quotation.

5. Note if the reference is a primary or secondary source. Primary sources are first-hand information, not interpretations. Secondary sources are interpretations of or references to primary sources.

Writing the Literature Review

After thoroughly investigating the relevant references, you will need to organize them in order to write the literature review. To refresh your memory, review the notes on each card, discarding irrelevant references. Include only those references that you used to substantiate your research. Next, make a tentative outline showing the relationships among the topics. Then analyze your cards, putting them into the appropriate categories of the outline. For each category, analyze the similarities and differences between the references. Summarize those references that state essentially the same thing—for example, "Smith (1987), Brown (1988), and Green (1990) report that . . . " Include studies that show results contradictory to those you expect to find from your study. When organizing the literature review, first discuss the references that are least related to the problem, progressing to the most relevant references. Conclude the review with a brief summary of the main points, general conclusions, and implications.

PLACING THE PROBLEM WITHIN A THEORETICAL OR CONCEPTUAL FRAMEWORK

Beginning researchers are usually unnecessarily frightened or confused by the terms *theoretical framework* or *conceptual framework*. Several basic definitions should help. A *concept* is a single idea (often one word) that represents several related component ideas. Examples of concepts are *grief, alienation,* and *happiness*. Concepts are the basic ingredients of a *theory*, which in turn consists of a set of statements called *propositions*, which link the concepts. These are stated in such a way as to form a logically interrelated deductive system. Such a system allows for the logical production of new statements from the original set of propositions. A theory can be used to explain and/or predict events (phenomena). Examples of theories include Rotter's social learning theory, Festinger's cognitive dissonance theory, Selye's adaptation theory, and systems theory.

Theoretical Framework

The term *theoretical framework* simply means the use of one theory or interrelated theories to support the rationale (reason) for conducting the study and provide a guide to analyzing the results. For example, Stillman investigated women's health beliefs about breast cancer and breast self-examination within the theoretical framework of cognitive dissonance.[6] Ketefian investigated moral reasoning and moral behavior among practicing nurses within the theoretical framework of moral development formulated by Kohlberg.[7]

Conceptual Framework

The term *conceptual framework* means the use of one or more related concepts that underlie the study problem and support the rationale (reason) for conducting the study. When one concept is used, it is the discussion of the component ideas within it that forms the basis for the conceptual framework. The concepts should also be discussed in relationship to the variables being investigated in the study. As described in Chapter 2, a *variable* is an observation or measurement that can assume a range of values along some dimension.

The student who wrote the research proposal investigating the variations in third-stage blood loss and placental trapping associated with the administration of synthetic oxytocics (Appendix F) identified and discussed the relationship of the major concepts of the purposeful action of synthetic oxytocics and their relationship to placental separation and control of blood loss as the conceptual framework for the study.

At this time in its development, nursing does not have well-defined and tested theories of nursing but, rather, various conceptual frameworks, which are also referred to as conceptual schemes or models, depending on the level of their development toward nursing theory. Examples of these formulations are Sister Callista Roy's model of adaptation, Dorothea Orem's model of self-care, and Martha Roger's framework based on the principle of homeodynamics. The student who wrote the research proposal in Appendix E planned to use Roy's conceptual framework for her study. The student who wrote the report of her research reprinted in Appendix C used Orem's framework to guide her data analysis.

If nursing research is to make an essential contribution to the scientific knowledge base, quantitative researchers should place each study within a theoretical or conceptual framework so that new findings can be placed in the broader areas of already existing knowledge:

> Any one research project provides only a small bit of information, but these bits of information can eventually be brought together to form larger generalizations and conclusions, provided they are all conducted within the same frame of reference and directed toward the same end.[8]

STATEMENT OF THE PURPOSE OF THE STUDY

The purpose of the study is the single statement that identifies the focus of the research. The purpose should state what you intend to do to answer the research question that generated the problem you are studying. Brink and Wood suggest that the statement of the research study's purpose can be written in three ways: (1) as a declarative statement, (2) as a question, or (3) as a hypothesis. The form depends on the way the research question is asked and the extent of the researcher's knowledge about the problem. The statement of the purpose should include information about what the researcher intends to do to collect data (such as observe, describe, or measure some variable), information about the setting of the study (where the researcher plans to collect the data), and information about who the study subjects will be.[9]

The Purpose as a Declarative Statement

In our previously formulated question designed to describe the relationship between the type of teaching and success in breast feeding by primiparas, the purpose of the study written as a declarative statement could read: ''The purpose of this study is to describe the effect of structured individualized versus structured group instruction on successful breast feeding by primiparas in their home setting.'' Note that the statement includes information about what the researcher intends to do (to describe), the setting of the study (home setting), and the subjects of the study (primiparas).

The Purpose as a Question

The purpose of the study, written as a question, could read: ''The purpose of this study is to answer the question: Is there a significant relationship between a method of teaching about breast feeding and successful breast feeding by primiparas in their home setting?'' Methods of teaching might include structured individual teaching, structured group teaching, and unstructured (incidental) teaching. The primiparas in the study could be interviewed regarding their perceptions of their own success with breast feeding and their satisfaction with the method of teaching to prepare them for breast feeding.

The Purpose as a Hypothesis

The purpose of the study, written as a hypothesis, could read: ''The purpose of the study is to test the following hypothesis: Primiparas who receive individualized instruction in breast feeding will have a significantly more successful breast-feeding experience in their home setting than primiparas who receive structured group instruction in breast feeding.''

MORE ABOUT HYPOTHESES

A *hypothesis* is simply a statement of predicted relationships between the variables being studied. It is often referred to as the researcher's "educated or calculated guess" as to the study question's answer. It should be supported by existing theory and previous research findings. A study may have more than one hypothesis (which are then referred to as *hypotheses*). In the statement of a hypothesis, an antecedent condition—called the *independent variable*—is related to the occurrence of another condition or effect, called the *dependent variable*. This can be shown as follows:

Condition X is related to the occurrence of *Condition Y*

Independent variable (antecedent condition)—Dependent variable (effect)
or
Method of instruction on breast feeding—Degree of success on breast feeding

To test the hypothesis, the researcher purposely manipulates the independent variable and attempts to control all the other conditions. The effect on the dependent variable, which occurs presumably as a result of the manipulation of the independent variable, is then noted. Thus, the independent variable comes first in time and is manipulated by the researcher. The dependent variable is the phenomenon that occurs as the researcher alters the independent variable.

Functions of the Hypothesis

Prior to the systematic review of the literature relevant to the research problem, researchers often have a tentative hypothesis or hypotheses that express an expectation of the outcome of their study. At this point in the research process, it is necessary to refine and finalize this hypothesis, since the hypothesis serves to narrow down the field of the research study and forces the researcher to be precise in stating the specific situation being studied. In addition, the hypothesis guides the methodology for the remainder of the study—that is, the collection of relevant data and the plan for analysis of the data. The hypothesis also serves as a framework for stating conclusions of the study as a direct answer to the purpose of the study. A good hypothesis will not only be consistent with theory and previous research, it will also be a reasonable explanation or prediction of the situation being studied. Finally, the hypothesis will be testable; that is, the researcher will be able to collect data that can then be analyzed statistically to determine if the hypothesis can be supported. A hypothesis is not proved; it is either supported or not supported (rejected).

Is a Hypothesis Always Necessary?

A hypothesis can be formulated only if the researcher has enough information to predict the study's outcome and intends to test the significance of the prediction. Although a hypothesis may specify a cause-and-effect relationship, most hypotheses specify a relationship between two or more variables. These variables may exist together, or a change in one will be associated with a change in the other. A hypothesis must be theoretically or conceptually based and is necessary in an experimental study that is designed to predict the relationship between variables. It is optional in a descriptive study in which the investigator describes what is, or may use the data to raise questions and/or generate hypotheses for further studies. Many historical research studies have hypotheses to examine the occurrence of events and conditions.

Classification of Hypotheses

You will hear the terms research hypothesis and statistical hypothesis used as classifications. A *research hypothesis* states the expected relationship between the variables that the researcher expects as the study's outcome. It is stated in the declarative form. The *statistical hypothesis* is also referred to as the *null hypothesis* because it is stated in the null form—that is, a statement of no difference or no relationship between the variables. This statement may not reflect the outcome expected by the researcher and thus may confuse the beginning researcher. It is used as a part of the decision-making procedures, which are statistically based. The null hypothesis exists because present statistical procedures generally cannot test the research hypothesis directly. For example, in the following research hypothesis, the researcher predicts the outcome of the study: ''Primiparas who receive individualized instruction on breast feeding will have a more successful breast-feeding experience in their home setting than primiparas who receive group instruction on breast feeding.'' The following statistical hypothesis, stated in the null (no difference) form, does not reflect the outcome that is really expected by the researcher: ''There will be no significant difference in the breast-feeding experience in their home setting between primiparas who receive individualized instruction on breast feeding and primiparas who receive group instruction on breast feeding.''

Many researchers prefer to state the hypothesis in the null form because to them it reflects a more objective and scientific statement of the relationship between the variables. Also, the statistical procedures they plan to use to test the hypotheses may require the null form in order to determine whether an observed relationship is probably a chance relationship (due to sampling error, for example) or is probably a true relationship. The null form of the hypothesis, however, often does not reflect the researcher's true prediction of the study's outcome. And statements in the null form make it difficult to tie the hypothesis back to the background and theory of the research. Other researchers, therefore, prefer to use the research hypothesis, in which case the underlying null hypothesis is usually assumed without being explicitly stated.

Stating the Hypothesis

Brink and Wood provide guidelines for writing a hypothesis.[10] The hypothesis to test the relationship between method of instruction about breast feeding and a successful breast-feeding experience was stated as: "Primiparas who received structured individualized instruction in breast feeding will have a significantly more successful breast-feeding experience in their home setting than primiparas who receive structured group instruction in breast feeding." The first clause of the hypothesis identifies both the sample (primiparas) and one position of the independent variable (method of instruction on breast feeding, specified here as "structured individualized instruction"). The next clause specifies the expected direction of the dependent variable (degree of success on breast feeding, specified here as "more successful"). The final clause of the hypothesis specifies the other portion of the independent variable (specified here as "structured group instruction in breast feeding").

Gay suggests a general paradigm or model for stating research hypotheses (predictions of differences between variables) for experimental studies.[11]

X's who get Y do better on Z than X's who do not get Y (or get some other Y).
In this model X's are the subjects.
Y is the treatment (independent variable).
Z is the outcome (dependent variable).

For example, "Primiparas (X's, subjects) who receive individualized instruction on breast feeding (Y, the treatment) will have a more successful breast-feeding experience in their home setting (Z, observed outcome) than primiparas who receive group instruction (get some other Y, treatment)."

When this model is applied to the null hypothesis previously stated, it looks like this: "There will be no significant difference in the breast-feeding experience in their home setting (Z, expected outcome) between primiparas (X's, subjects) who receive individualized instruction on breast feeding (Y, the treatment) and primiparas who receive group instruction on breast feeding (some other Y, treatment)."

Another form for a research hypothesis is the "If . . . then" form: "*If* primiparas receive individualized instruction on breast feeding, *then* they will have a more successful breast-feeding experience in their home than primiparas who receive group instruction." Any of these formats should help you write a statement that is truly a hypothesis.

In summary, although a hypothesis may be stated in different ways, the hypothesis statement should be in the form of an answer to the question(s) proposed by the study. It should state an expressed relationship, should be stated clearly and concisely, and should be based on an accepted theory and/or valid research findings when possible. It must also be testable; that is, the researcher formulates a hypothesis for a research study in order to accept or to reject it statistically. The researcher must be able to collect and analyze data in such a way as to determine the validity of the hypothesis. Remember, a hypothesis is either *supported* or *rejected*, it is never proved or not proved.

The success of a research study does not depend on the hypothesis being supported by the data. A well-designed and well-executed research study in which the hypothesis is not supported can add just as much to the knowledge base, and to the theory from which it was derived, as a well-designed and well-executed study where the hypothesis was supported.

DEFINITION OF TERMS

Just as the conceptual or theoretical framework and the hypothesis stem from the literature review, so do the definitions of the terms used in the study. The words in the statement of the study's purpose pertaining to the variables of the study should be defined either directly, operationally, or theoretically. A direct definition is the definition found in a dictionary. The other two types of definition are discussed in this section.

Operational Definitions

An *operational definition* provides a full description of the method by which the concept will be studied. This is stated in behavioral, observable, demonstrable terms by citing the *operations* (the manipulations and observations) necessary to produce the phenomenon. For example, in the previously described statement of the purpose of the study, ''the purpose of this study is to describe the effect of structured individualized versus structured group instruction on successful breast feeding by primiparas in their home setting,'' the variables to be defined include structured individualized instruction, structured group instruction, successful breast feeding in a home setting, and primiparas. ''Structured individualized instruction'' might be defined as a one-to-one instructional relationship between the professional nurse and the primipara, where a planned teaching protocol is consistently used. ''Structured group instruction'' might be defined as instruction of several primiparas by the nurse, where a planned teaching protocol is consistently used. ''Successful breast feeding in a home setting'' might be defined as the duration of breast feeding (weeks or months) or as the degree to which difficulties with home breast feeding were identified as problematic on a questionnaire administered to the mother six weeks after delivery. These are all operational definitions. ''Primipara'' can be defined directly by the definition found in a dictionary.

Theoretical Definitions

A *theoretical definition* of a variable uses the definition found in the specific language of the theory or theories being used in the study. For example, in cognitive dissonance theory, anxiety is defined as "the component of dissonance related to a state of drive or need or tension."[12]

WRITING THE PROBLEM STATEMENT SECTION OF A RESEARCH PROPOSAL

In this chapter we discussed the initial step in the research process—the selection and statement of the research problem. The introductory phase of a research proposal entails a discussion of the following elements of research:

1. Background and rationale for selecting the study problem, including the significance of the problem and the relevance of the problem to nursing
2. Review of related literature
3. Placement of the problem within a conceptual or theoretical framework
4. Statement of the purpose of the study, followed by definitions of all the terms used in the statement of the purpose

In this initial section of the research proposal, the study's general subject area is discussed and then narrowed down to the focus of the study. It concludes with the research question, which should be stated in declarative form. Enough background material should be presented to acquaint the reader with the problem's importance. The rationale for selecting the problem should be discussed, as well as the study's significance and its contributions to nursing's scientific knowledge base. If appropriate, the problem should be placed in a theoretical or conceptual framework and a review of the relevant literature should be presented. The study's purpose should be stated in a clearly defined statement as a declarative sentence, a question, or a hypothesis (hypotheses) to be tested. All terms used should be defined either directly, operationally, or theoretically. "Guidelines for Writing a Research Proposal" (Appendix H) should help you to write the problem statement section of your proposal.

A NOTE ON CRITICAL ANALYSIS OF PUBLISHED RESEARCH

The Commission on Nursing Research of the American Nurses' Association has recommended that education in research at the undergraduate level should prepare the nurse to be a critical consumer of research. This entails the reading, understanding, and interpretation of published research studies to determine their scientific merit and application to nursing theory and practice.

In order to give you a systematic experience in learning the skills to become a critical consumer, you will be repeatedly reading four published research reports dealing with the same research topic. You may wish to select four of the published research reports on the topic of preoperative instruction listed in the Bibliography and Suggested Readings section at the end of this chapter. Or you may wish to select your own research topic and locate four studies that are related to your topic (e.g., sleep deprivation, stress, pain).

As you learn each step in the research process, the Application Activities at the end of this and the following chapters will direct you to read and evaluate the corresponding section of each of the research studies. Eventually, you will have read all the sections of all the reports and will have evaluated their adequacy, both individually and in comparison with the other studies.[13] This process is designed to enable you to develop your skills as a competent consumer of published research.

The following Application Activities are designed to help develop your skills in evaluating published research, as well as to help you evaluate your understanding of the selection and statement of a research problem.

APPLICATION ACTIVITIES

 I. Critical evaluation of research studies
 1. Locate four of the studies on preoperative instruction listed in the Bibliography and Suggested Readings at the end of this chapter, or locate four studies related to a topic of your choice. The studies should interest you enough to use them to learn the process of critical evaluation.
 2. Use the "Guidelines for Evaluating a Research Report" provided in Appendix I (Sections A through E) to evaluate the problem selection and statement sections of each of the four studies you have selected.
 3. In which study was
 a. the research problem most clearly identified?
 b. the conceptual or theoretical framework most clearly explained?
 c. the purpose of the study most clearly stated?
 II. Problem selection
 1. Make a list of at least three general problem areas in nursing that interest you enough to conduct a research study on them.
 2. Narrow each of these general problem areas to a specific research problem stated in the form of a question.
 3. Select two of these research problems and evaluate them in terms of the problem selection criteria presented in this chapter.

III. Review of related literature

Complete the following exercise, designed to familiarize you with a variety of library sources on the research topic you finally decide to investigate.*

1. List as many key words as you can that might relate to your nursing research topic. For example, for the topic "breast feeding," the following key words could be related:

Infants: feeding
Nutrition: infant nutrition
Newborn
Neonatal
Nursing
Lactation
Milk
Pregnancy
Bottle feeding
Mothering
Feminism

2. List three complete references from the *Cumulative Index to Nursing Literature* concerning your topic.

3. Go to the *Index Medicus* and list two complete references related to your topic.

4. Using *Excerpta Medica*, list two complete references related to your topic.

5. List one complete reference from *Dissertation Abstracts* related to your topic.

6. Using *Psychological Abstracts* to locate psychological studies related to your topic, list at least two complete references from this source.

7. List at least three books that relate to your topic (include author, title, publication date, and library call number).

8. Look in *Child Development Abstracts* to determine pediatric applications of your topic.

9. Are there any geriatric implications for your topic?

10. List at least two references from *Nursing Research* related to your topic.

11. Are there references related to your topic in:
    a. *Hospital Literature Index?*
    b. *International Nursing Index?*
    c. *Readers' Guide to Periodical Literature?*

12. List at least three references from government documents related to your topic.

*Adapted from "Improving Basic Library Skills" by P. Dempsey. Copyright © 1977, American Journal of Nursing Company. Reproduced with permission from *Nursing Research*, September–October, Vol. 26, No. 5, p. 390.

13. There are many other abstracts and indexes available that might provide additional reference citations related to your topic.
    a. List at least four abstracts and indexes related to your topic in addition to those you have already used.
    b. Cite one reference from each of the abstracts or indexes you have listed above related to your topic.
14. Investigate your media center regarding audiovisual holdings concerning the broad area of nursing.
    a. List the names of three films.
    b. List the names of three videotapes.
    c. List the names of three film loops.
    d. List the names of three audiotapes.
    e. List the names of three filmstrips.
15. Investigate a computerized literature search available to you through your library or through other sources.

IV. Formulation of hypotheses
    1. Three hypotheses follow. State the independent and dependent variable for each hypothesis.
       a. Patients with slightly elevated blood pressure will have lower blood pressure after training in stress reduction techniques.
       b. Nurses working with AIDS patients have a higher level of anxiety than nurses working with oncology patients.
       c. Primiparas whose husbands have received instruction in neonatal care have fewer adjustment problems with their baby than those whose husbands have not received such instruction.
    2. State each hypothesis in the null form.
    3. Provide an operational definition for each term used in one of the null hypotheses.

V. Writing the problem statement section of your research proposal
    1. Reread the proposals written by beginning researchers (Appendixes A, B, D, E), paying special attention to the problem statement sections, which include all the material down to the plan for data collection (or methodology) section of their proposals.
    2. Using the information and procedures presented in the chapter and the guidelines in Appendix H, write a tentative first draft of the problem statement section of your own proposal that includes:
       a. statement of the problem, including background and significance to nursing.
       b. review of related literature.
       c. placement of the problem within a conceptual or theoretical framework, if appropriate.
       d. statement of the purpose of the study.
       e. definition of terms.

Although you will no doubt revise this material later, much of it will be the initial section of your final research proposal.

REFERENCES

1. King, I., and B. Tarsitano. 1982. "The Effect of Structured and Unstructured Pre-Operative Teaching: A Replication," *Nursing Research*, 31(November–December): 324–329.
2. Lindeman, C., and B. Van Aernam. 1971. "Nursing Intervention with the Pre-surgical Patient—The Effects of Structured and Unstructured Preoperative Teaching," *Nursing Research*, 20(July–August 1971): 319–332.
3. Abdellah, F., and E. Levine. 1979. *Better Patient Care through Nursing Research* (2nd ed). New York: Macmillan, p. 75.
4. American Nurses' Association Cabinet on Nursing Research. 1985. *Directions for Nursing Research: Toward the Twenty-first Century*. Kansas City: American Nurses' Association, pp. 2–3.
5. Verhonick, P., and C. Seamen. 1978. *Research Methods for Undergraduate Students in Nursing*. New York: Appleton-Century-Crofts, p. 24.
6. Stillman, M. J. 1977. "Women's Beliefs about Breast Cancer and Breast Self-Examination." *Nursing Research*, 26(March–April), pp. 121–127.
7. Ketefian, S. 1981. "Moral Reasoning and Moral Behavior among Selected Groups of Practicing Nurses," *Nursing Research*, 30(May–June): 171–176.
8. Fox, D. J. 1982. *Fundamentals of Research in Nursing*. Norwalk, CT: Appleton-Century-Crofts, p. 32.
9. Brink, P. J., and M. J. Wood. 1988. *Basic Steps in Planning Nursing Research*. Boston: Jones and Bartlett, p. 68.
10. Ibid., p. 78.
11. Gay, L. R. 1987. *Educational Research: Competencies for Analysis and Application*, 3rd ed. Columbus, OH: Charles E. Merrill, p. 57.
12. Silva, M. C. 1981. "Selection of a Theoretical Framework." In S. Krampitz and N. Pavlovich, Eds., *Readings for Nursing Research*. St. Louis: C. V. Mosby, p. 19.
13. Mallick, M. J. 1983. "A Constant Comparative Method for Teaching Research to Baccalaureate Nursing Students," *Image* 15 (Fall): 120–123.

BIBLIOGRAPHY AND SUGGESTED READINGS

Note: Research studies on preoperative instruction are preceded by an asterisk (*).

Abdellah, F., and E. Eugene, 1979. *Better Patient Care through Nursing Research*, 2nd ed. New York: Macmillan.
American Nurses' Association. 1975. *Human Rights Guidelines for Nurses in Clinical and Other Research*. Code No. D-465M. Kansas City: American Nurses' Association.
————. 1981. *Guidelines for the Investigative Function of Nurses*. Code No. D-69 3M. Kansas City: American Nurses' Association.
————. Cabinet on Nursing Research. 1985. *Directions for Nursing Research: Towards the Twenty-First Century*. Kansas City: American Nurses' Association.

Barnard, R., and J. Fawcett. 1981. "A Guide to Research Instruments." *Image,* 13(October): 28.

Benoliel, J. Q. 1977. "The Interaction between Theory and Research." *Nursing Outlook,* 25(February): 108–113.

Brink, P. J., and M. Wood. 1988. *Basic Steps in Planning Nursing Research.* Boston: Jones and Bartlett.

Dempsey, P. 1977. "Improving Basic Library Skills." *Nursing Research,* 26(September–October): 390.

Dickson, G., and H. Lee-Villasenon. 1982. "Nursing Theory and Practice: A Self-Care Approach." *Advances in Nursing Science,* 5(October): 29–40.

*Felton, G., K. Huss, et al. 1976. "Preoperative Nursing Intervention with the Patient for Surgery: Outcome of Three Alternative Approaches" (experimental study). *International Journal of Nursing Studies,* 13: 83–96.

Field, P. A., and J. M. Morse. 1985. *Nursing Research: The Application of Qualitative Approaches.* Rockville, MD: Aspen Systems.

Fitzpatrick, J., and A. Whall. 1989. *Conceptual Models of Nursing: Analysis and Application,* 2nd ed. Norwalk, CT: Appleton and Lange.

*Fortin, F., and S. Kirouac. 1976. "A Randomized Controlled Trial of Preoperative Patient Education" (experimental study). *International Journal of Nursing Studies,* 13: 11–24.

Fox, D. J. 1982. *Fundamentals of Research in Nursing,* 4th ed. New York: Appleton-Century-Crofts.

Gay, L. R. 1987. *Educational Research: Competencies for Analysis and Application,* 3rd ed. Columbus, OH: Charles E. Merrill.

*Johnson, J., V. Rice, S. Fuller, et al. 1978. "Sensory Information, Instruction in a Coping Strategy, and Recovery from Surgery" (experimental study). *Research in Nursing and Health,* 1: 4–17.

Ketefian, S. 1981. "Moral Reasoning and Moral Behavior among Selected Groups of Practicing Nurses." *Nursing Research,* 30(May–June): 171–176.

Kim, H. 1983. "Use of Rogers' Conceptual System in Research." *Nursing Research,* 32(March–April): 89–91.

*King, I., and B. Tarsitano. 1982. "The Effect of Structured and Unstructured Preoperative Teaching: A Replication" (experimental study). *Nursing Research,* 31 (November–December): 324–329.

*Klos, D., M. Cummings, J. Joyce, et al. 1980. "A Comparison of Two Methods of Delivering Presurgical Instructions" (experimental study). *Patient Counselling and Health Education,* 1st quarter: 6–13.

Krampitz, S., and N. Pavlovich. 1981. *Readings for Nursing Research.* St. Louis: C. V. Mosby.

*Lindeman, C. 1972. "Nursing Intervention with the Presurgical Patient" (experimental study). *Nursing Research,* 21(May–June): 196–209.

*Lindeman, C., and B. Van Aernam. 1971. "Nursing Intervention with the Presurgical Patient—The Effects of Structured and Unstructured Preoperative Teaching" (experimental study). *Nursing Research,* 20(July–August): 319–332.

Mallick, M. 1983. "A Constant Comparative Method for Teaching Research to Baccalaureate Nursing Students." *Image,* 15(Fall): 120–123.

*Morgan, J., et al. 1985. "Effects of Preoperative Teaching on Postoperative Pain: A Replication and Expansion" (experimental study). *International Journal of Nursing Studies,* 22:267–280.

National League for Nursing. 1978. *Theory Development: What, Why, How?* NLN Publication No. 15-1708. New York: National League for Nursing.

Polit, D., and B. Hungler. 1987. *Nursing Research: Principles and Methods,* 3rd ed. Philadelphia: J. B. Lippincott.

*Shimko, C. 1981. "The Effect of Preoperative Instruction on State Anxiety" (descriptive study). *Journal of Neurosurgical Nursing,* 13(December): 318–322.

Silva, M. C. 1981. "Selection of a Theoretical Framework." In S. Krampitz and N. Pavlovich, Eds., *Readings for Nursing Research.* St. Louis: C. V. Mosby.

Stillman, M. J. 1977. "Women's Health Beliefs about Breast Cancer and Breast Self-Examination." *Nursing Research,* 26(March–April): 121–127.

Verhonick, P., and C. Seaman. 1978. *Research Methods for Undergraduate Students in Nursing.* New York: Appleton-Century-Crofts.

*Williams, P. D., et al. 1988. "Effects of Preparation for Mastectomy/Hysterectomy on Women's Post-operative Self-Care Behaviors" (experimental study). *International Journal of Nursing Studies,* 25: 191–206.

*Ziemer, M. 1983. "Effects of Information on Postsurgical Coping" (experimental study). *Nursing Research,* 32 (September–October): 282–287.

6

Data Collection

In the previous chapters, we have presented material on the application of the research process to nursing problems. In the problem selection and statement step of the research process, a researchable problem is selected for study. The material in this chapter acquaints you with the next step in the research process: development of the overall plan to collect the information directly related to the study problem.

THE NATURE OF DATA

Data are the raw materials from which all research reports are generated. The data collected may be gathered in quantitative (numerical) forms or in qualitative (verbal/descriptive) forms. In either case, the investigator's job is to be sure that the data gathered are accurate and amenable to appropriate analysis.

THE RESEARCH APPROACH

In Chapter 1, we stated that the research approaches most commonly used can be classified as (1) descriptive (which includes surveys and qualitative strategies), (2) experimental (also termed explanatory), and (3) historical (also termed documentary).

Differences between Research Approaches

These approaches are differentiated by their time orientation and the extent to which the investigator has control over manipulating the independent variable. The *historical* approach is past-oriented in that it examines what has already occurred; the investigator has no control over manipulating the independent variable. The *descriptive* approach is present-oriented, describing what is. The investigator has no control over manipulating the independent variable. The *experimental* approach is future-oriented; it predicts what will occur. Here the investigator has control in manipulating the independent variable in the experimental setting, and subjects are randomly assigned (each individual is assigned a place in a group based on chance alone) to the treatment (experimental) condition specified in the study. The term *quasi-experimental* refers to a modification of the experimental approach in which the investigator may have control in manipulating the independent variable, although subjects are not randomly assigned to the treatment condition. Table 6.1 summarizes these differences between the approaches.

Selecting the Research Approach

You will also see the research approaches referred to as *research methods* or *research designs*. All these terms refer to the overall plan for eliciting information

TABLE 6.1
Differences between Research Approaches

Research Approach	Time Orientation	Control of Independent Variable by Investigator	Random Assignment to Treatment Condition
Historical	Past (examines "what was")	No	No
Descriptive	Present (describes "what is")	No	No
Experimental	Future (predicts "what will be")	Yes	Yes

about the study problem. You remember that the research process has been described as a chain of reasoning beginning with the statement of the problem and proceeding systematically through the communication and utilization of the study results. From this it is evident that the statement of the problem section of the research plan guides the choice of the study's research approach. An important consideration in quantitative research is the extent to which the research problem fits the framework of existing knowledge and theory. Use of the experimental approach requires more extensive knowledge, a problem that is formulated within a theoretical base and the ability to predict the action of the variables.

The form in which the purpose of the study is stated also guides the choice of the research approach. In general, the declarative statement and question indicate a descriptive or historical approach, whereas the hypothesis indicates an experimental approach because the investigator has control in manipulating the independent variable. Although it is possible to have a hypothesis in the historical or descriptive approach, such a hypothesis is not tested by direct manipulation of the variables, as in the experimental setting, but by statistical manipulation of the existing data.

Thus, in the step-by-step chain of reasoning that characterizes the research process, the components of the statement of the problem and the form of the statement of the purpose guide the selection of the research approach. The proposal printed in Appendix E can be used to illustrate these principles. The investigator planned to study the effect of stockinette caps (the independent variable) on heat regulation (dependent variable) in newborn infants. The main components of the problem statement and the literature review, which included a fairly extensive discussion of knowledge related to the variables of the study and an elaboration of the conceptual framework of Roy's adaptation model, guided her choice of the experimental research approach. The investigator predicts the action of the variables (that is, the relationship between the variables that the investigator expects as the study's outcome) in the purpose of the study, stated here as a research hypothesis: "The purpose of the study is to test the following hypothesis: The amount of heat loss in newborns wearing stockinette caps for 30 minutes after birth is significantly less than the amount of heat loss in newborns not wearing stockinette caps for 30 minutes after birth." Notice that the investigator has control over manipulating the independent variable (stockinette caps).

DATA-GATHERING TECHNIQUES

We have seen that the research approach refers to the overall method for obtaining the study's data. Choice of the techniques for gathering the data depends on the nature and sources of the data to be collected. Many research studies use more than one technique for gathering data. For example, in a study designed to describe the learning achieved by student nurses when caring for terminally ill patients, learning could be measured in the cognitive, affective, and psychomotor domains. A paper-and-pencil test could be used to gather data measuring cognitive learning (knowledge); an interview schedule could be used to ascertain attitudes on the affective domain; and an observational checklist might be used to gather data on the student's technical proficiency in performing psychomotor skills (procedures).

The terms *continuous data* and *discrete data* are used to refer to quantitative variables. Continuous data can be located at some point along a continuum or scale and are characterized by fractional values of a whole unit. For example, 98.6°F, body temperature, is a point on the Fahrenheit scale used to measure body temperature. Discrete data, on the other hand, exist only in distinct units expressed as whole numbers that are precise and definite: 6 patients, 5 hospitals, 6 beds (not $6\frac{1}{2}$ patients, $5\frac{1}{4}$ hospitals, or $6\frac{2}{3}$ beds).

The decision as to which form to use to collect data depends on the nature of the study's research approach, the need for precision, and the availability of appropriate data collection instruments. One problem with quantification is the lack of instruments for collecting appropriate quantitative data. Nursing research is often concerned with such areas of study as wellness, illness, and reactions to various situations, which are not easily amenable to quantified measurements.

CHARACTERISTICS OF QUANTITATIVE RESEARCH INSTRUMENTS

When we refer to research instruments or research tools, we are talking about devices or equipment used to gather the research data. Research instruments must possess certain basic attributes, which assure us that they will provide dependable measurements of the variables under investigation. The most important attributes are (1) validity, (2) reliability, and (3) usability.

Validity

Validity refers to the ability of a data-gathering instrument to measure what it is supposed to measure, to obtain data relevant to what is being measured. Validity is an extremely important characteristic of a measuring instrument. A clinical thermometer is a valid instrument for measuring an individual's body temperature, but a sphygmomanometer is not valid for this purpose. A yardstick is a valid instrument for measuring cloth, but a baby scale is not. In estimating the validity of a measuring instrument, the questions ''Valid for what?'' and ''Valid for whom?'' must be answered. In the case of measuring body temperature, the clinical thermometer is valid for measuring body temperature (what?) on human beings (whom?).

There are three main approaches for estimating the validity of a measuring instrument designed to collect quantitative data: content validity, construct validity, and criterion-related validity.

The *content validity* of a measuring instrument is the extent to which the instrument represents the factors under study. Each content area must be defined, and representative behaviors are then identified. A number of experts in the field of the specific study topic are then asked to examine each item and to make judgments regarding how well the items and the entire instrument reflect the previously defined content area(s). No statistical procedures are involved in determining the content validity of a measurement instrument. A subtype of content validity is *face validity*, which is determined by inspecting the items to see if the instrument contains important items that measure the variables in the content area. Face validity is the least time-consuming and least rigorous method for determining validity because it is based entirely on the subjective judgment of the investigator.

Construct validity is the degree to which a measuring instrument measures a specific hypothetical trait or *construct*, such as intelligence, grief, or prejudice. Establishing construct validity is a complicated and time-consuming process that requires the measuring instrument to be used in a succession of different studies that use various methods for testing construct validity. A basic approach to establishing construct validity is the *known-groups technique*, in which the instrument is administered to several groups known to differ on a certain construct. If the results obtained demonstrate statistically significant differences, as expected, then the instrument is said to have a degree of construct validity. For example, in establishing the construct validity of an instrument for measuring preoperative anxiety, it would be expected that the preoperative anxiety reported by a group of patients having minor surgery in an ambulatory care unit would differ from the preoperative anxiety reported by patients admitted to the hospital for major surgery. Other procedures for demonstrating construct validity (such as factor analysis) are discussed in more advanced research and statistics textbooks. Although construct validity is considerably more difficult to establish than content validity, it is important to establish construct validity when complex concepts are being measured.

Criterion-related validity refers to the relationship of the measuring instrument to some already known external criterion or other valid instrument. *Predictive validity* predicts how well a person will do in the future. For example, the scores received on the Graduate Record Examination are supposed to predict a student's potential for success in graduate work in a college or university. *Concurrent validity* is a measure of how well an instrument correlates with another instrument that is known to be valid. For example, an individual's score on the Stanford-Binet IQ test should be very similar to that individual's score on the Wechsler intelligence test.

Reliability

The *reliability* of a measuring instrument refers to its ability to obtain consistent results when reused. An instrument is reliable when it consistently does whatever it is supposed to do in the same way. For example, when a paper-and-pencil test of intelligence is administered to a person, the test should produce approximately the same result if it is readministered as a retest. The more reliable a measuring instrument is, the more confidence we can have that the scores obtained would not fluctuate too greatly from administration time to administration time.

Reliability is usually expressed as a number, called a *coefficient*. A high coefficient indicates a high reliability. A measuring instrument that has a perfect reliability would have a coefficient of 1.00. Rarely, however, is a measuring instrument perfectly reliable. Reliability is more often reported as less than 1.00—that is, .80, .70, or .50. Less than perfect reliability of an instrument can be due to errors in measurement, such as the conditions under which the instrument was administered (e.g., improper directions); problems with the instrument itself (e.g., poorly constructed items); or characteristics of the persons responding to the instrument (e.g., illness or fatigue).

There are several main types of reliability that may be determined through *correlation:* (1) test–retest reliability, (2) alternate forms reliability, (3) split-half reliability, and (4) interrater reliability.

Test–retest reliability indicates variation in scores from one administration of the instrument to the next, resulting from measurement errors. The procedure for determining test–retest reliability is to administer the instrument to individuals similar to the ones you plan to study, let some period of time elapse (say a week) to allow for some loss of memory of the items, then give the instrument to the same individuals again. The scores on the two instruments are then correlated statistically to yield a coefficient referred to as the *coefficient of stability*. If the results are the same or similar, the coefficient will be high—say .90—and the instrument is said to have high test–retest reliability. One of the major problems with this method of estimating reliability is that of deciding realistically how long the time interval between the test and the retest should be. If the interval is too short, the individuals tend to remember their responses to the items on the first administration. This results in an artificially high coefficient of reliability. If the time interval is too long, some individuals may do better on a retest because of their own learning and maturation during the interval between the test and the retest.

Alternate forms reliability is also called ''equivalent forms reliability.'' To establish this type of reliability, at least two different forms of the instrument are constructed. Although the actual items on the instruments are not the same, each form has the same number of total test items, is designed to measure the same variable or variables, and has the same level of difficulty. Both use the same procedures for administration, scoring, and interpreting results. At least two different forms of the instrument must be available. The procedure for determining alternate forms reliability is to administer one form of the test to a group of individuals and then, at the same session or very shortly thereafter, administer a second form to the same individuals. The two sets of scores are then statistically correlated, and the instrument has good alternate forms reliability if the correlation coefficient is high. There are two major problems with this method. One is the difficulty involved in constructing two forms that are equivalent; this can result in measurement errors. The second is the difficulty in administering two different instruments to the same individuals within a relatively short time period.

Split-half reliability, also called ''odd–even reliability,'' yields the coefficient of internal consistency. This estimate of reliability requires only one administration of an instrument in order to estimate its reliability. The entire instrument is administered to a group of individuals, and then the responses for each individual are divided into two comparable halves: all the responses to even items in one half and all the responses to odd items in the other. The response score for each individual is then computed separately for the two halves, resulting in a response score for the even items and a response score for the odd items. The two sets of scores are then correlated statistically to yield a correlation coefficient. If this is high, the instrument is said to have good split-half reliability. This method is more effective for longer instruments. For an instrument consisting of a limited number of items, a correlation formula such as the Spearman-Brown prophecy formula must be applied. The split-half method of estimating reliability has the advantage of requiring only one administration and one form of the instrument; it also eliminates the problems associated with more than one administration of the instrument to the same individuals. Other common reliability coefficients are Cronbach's alpha and the Kuder-Richardson formula (K-R 20).

Interrater reliability is also called "interobserver reliability." Two or more different observers independently observe and record their observations using the same recording format. The strength of the agreement between the two sets of observations may be computed as a correlation.

Usability

The usability of a measuring instrument refers to the practical aspects of using it. These include ease of administration, scoring, and interpretation as well as financial, time, and energy considerations. It is important to an instrument's usability that these practical aspects be considered.

In summary, the three basic attributes of dependable quantitative research instruments or tools are (1) validity, (2) reliability, and (3) usability. Because the outcome of a research study depends on the instrument(s) used to collect the data, research instruments that meet these criteria increase the potential for high-quality research.

CONSIDERATIONS IN SELECTING A MEASURING INSTRUMENT

Given that it takes a great deal of time and skill to develop your own instrument, it is better to select an appropriate instrument that has already been developed. If you are fortunate enough to locate an instrument that appears to measure what you want, keep looking and try to compare more than one tool. The sources of instrument compilations listed in Chapter 5 may help you locate instruments appropriate for your study.

If you must use a self-developed measuring instrument, you can take parts of one or more instruments for use in developing it. Do not plan to use a self-developed instrument unless you can pretest the instrument on a group similar to the one to be used in your study. A *pretest* is the process of testing the effectiveness of the instrument in gathering the appropriate data by administering the instrument to subjects who meet the criteria for study subjects, and then evaluating the instrument's strengths and weaknesses and revising it as necessary.

VALIDITY AND RELIABILITY IN QUALITATIVE RESEARCH

Qualitative researchers are also concerned with establishing validity and reliability during their data collection. However, the meanings of the terms differ for qualitative and quantitative research because the selection of the sample, the data collection, and the data analysis are carried out differently.

In qualitative research, *validity* refers to the extent to which the research findings represent reality.[1] The investigator must thoroughly check the information gathered to determine whether it makes sense when compared to other information that has been gathered. In a qualitative research study that uses multiple informants and accurate observation by the researcher, if all of the informants state that something is the case and the researcher observes that what the informants have stated either is not true or is somehow in conflict with observed behaviors, then the researcher must include this information in the research report and attempt to reconcile the differences. For example, if a researcher interviews nurses in a hospital setting and is told that they always perform certain activities, but then observes that these activities are either omitted or overelaborated, the researcher must attempt to determine why the differences between the reported and actual behavior occurred.

Reliability in qualitative research has two specific concerns. The first is that the information gathered from the research's informant(s) is accurate. This concern can cause problems because an informant either may not have sufficient information or may be lying. In order to reduce or eliminate these possibilities, the researcher must use a variety of informants, if possible, and must ask the questions crucial to the research in several different ways in order to determine whether the responses garnered are consistent.

Since the data-gathering instrument for a qualitative research study is often an interviewer or observer, the second concern related to reliability in qualitative research is the reliability of the data collector. If the data collector is careless or biased, the reliability of the study will be either substantially diminished or completely absent. One way to determine the reliability of a qualitative research study is to see if the research report gives enough documentation of the questions asked and the responses obtained so that another researcher could go to the same or a similar setting and obtain similar responses by asking the same questions.

SELECTING THE STUDY SUBJECTS FOR QUANTITATIVE RESEARCH

An essential part of the data collection plan is the selection of the study subjects who will provide the necessary data in relation to the purpose of the study.

The Target Population

The investigator must delineate a *target population*, consisting of individual people or things that meet the designated set of criteria of interest to the researcher. In nursing research, the target population usually consists of human beings. However, it can also consist of human characteristics (e.g., personality, job activities), inanimate objects (e.g., hospitals), or abstract concepts (e.g., professional ethics, community attitudes).[2]

The Sample

Because size, cost, time, or lack of accessibility often make it impossible to study the whole population directly, a study is usually done on a smaller part of a target population, called a *sample.* The term *sampling* refers to the process of selecting a number of individuals from the delineated target population in such a way that the individuals in the sample represent as nearly as possible the characteristics of the whole target population. The sample can be thought of as a miniature of the larger target population. A single unit or member of the target population is referred to as a *population element* or a *sampling unit.*

For example, a study proposes to investigate the effect of educational preparation on the political perceptions of all licensed nurses in the state of Florida. Because it would probably not be feasible to study such a large number of individuals, a sample of these nurses would be selected for inclusion in the study. This would be done in such a way that they would be representative of all the licensed nurses in Florida. Such a selection could be accomplished by first obtaining a computer listing of all the licensed nurses in the state from the Florida Board of Nursing. The investigator would then select a fraction of the licensed nurses on the list in such a way that those selected for inclusion in the study would be representative of all licensed nurses in Florida. Each licensed nurse in the sample would then be a population element and a sampling unit.

Purpose of Sampling

A basic purpose of sampling is to be able to use the sample's findings to generalize or extrapolate beyond the actual sampling units without having to study each element of the target population. The extent of this ability to generalize beyond the actual sampling units to the target population depends on the sampling approach used.

Quantitative Sampling Approaches

Sampling theory distinguishes between two main approaches to sampling in quantitative research: *probability sampling* and *nonprobability sampling.*

Probability Sampling.   Here the investigator is able to specify, for each element of the population, the probability that it will be included in the sample. Usually each element has the *same* probability of being included in the sample, but the basic requirement is that there exists a *known* probability that a given element will be included. The sampling units are selected by chance, and neither the investigator nor the population elements have any conscious influence on what is included in the sampling.

Nonprobability Sampling. Here the investigator has no ability to estimate the probability that each element of the population will be included in the sample or even that it has some chance of being included.

The importance of the ability to estimate probability lies in the interpretation of the study findings to the target population with a given degree of certainty. Probability sampling has the advantage of permitting the investigator to generalize from the sample's findings to the target population with a given degree of certainty. That is, these sample findings do not differ by more than a specific amount from the expected findings if the investigator were using the total population. Nonprobability samples do not permit generalization of the study findings from the sample to the population.

Choice of the sampling approach depends on the research problem and the purpose of the study. Not all studies are conducted with the purpose of being able to generalize to the entire population. The important point is that the sampling approach must be consistent with the purpose of the study.

Probability Sampling Methods

Major methods of probability sampling include (1) simple random sampling, (2) stratified random sampling, and (3) cluster sampling. The following discussion of each is intended to provide you with an overview of the sampling methods. You will need to refer to sources on more advanced research methodology for detailed procedures.

Simple Random Sampling. In this method, the required number of sampling units is selected at random from the population in such a manner that each population element has an equal chance (probability) of being selected for the sample. Each choice of a sampling unit must be independent of all other choices. One of the most acceptable methods for selecting a simple random sample is to use a table of random numbers, which can be found in a statistics textbook. The numbers in a random-number table have been generated in such a way that there is no sequencing pattern. The same probability exists that any digit will follow any other digit, and each selection was an independent choice.

To obtain a simple random sample, first list each of the population elements, then assign consecutive numbers to each of these elements. Then, referring to a table of random numbers (Table 6.2), arbitrarily start at any point in the table and proceed in any direction to identify enough tabled numbers to

TABLE 6.2
Excerpt from a Table of Random Numbers

57	87	89	93	27	86	05	14	21	98
04	67	95	16	47	11	37	31	34	21
87	22	50	14	55	00	34	33	21	24
47	14	30	62	50	67	96	51	49	40
43	80	44	48	62	90	52	60	28	86
51	92	99	77	98	26	64	77	32	29
20	34	47	55	69	81	45	58	72	83
83	80	73	19	77	80	33	14	76	93
40	93	76	82	83	55	52	48	67	21
15	87	46	87	92	06	03	21	27	71
07	68	15	05	64	84	59	73	39	87

associate with the population elements until the desired sample has been selected.

Rather than using a table of random numbers, it is also possible to select a
simple random sample by drawing numbers from a box. The names of the target population elements are written on pieces of paper which are then folded,
placed in a container, and mixed well. The first name chosen is assigned to the
sample, but because the probability associated with subsequent choices is not
constant, the slip should be replaced in the container each time a name is selected in order to approach random selection more fully. This procedure,
called *sampling with replacement,* is not as rigorous as using a table of random
numbers in that each choice of a sampling unit is not independent of all other
choices; once a unit is chosen, it will not be included in the sample again.

One of the problems in using simple random sampling is the difficulty of
obtaining or compiling a list of each of the population elements, either because
they are not known or because, for a large population, the listing proves pro-
hibitively long.

Stratified Random Sampling.   This method of sampling is a variation of the
simple random sample. The population is divided into two or more strata or
groups with different categories of a characteristic. A simple random sample is
then taken from each group. This procedure is used when the composition of
the population is known with respect to some characteristic or characteristics.
The variables (characteristics) chosen to stratify the population must be important to the study. For example, a population of 500 human elements may be
stratified on the basis of sex. Then one-half of the sampling units may be cho-

sen from the female category and the other half from the male category by simple random sampling. This assures that the sample will consist of equal allocations from each population stratum. A population may be divided into other strata or categories, such as age, educational background, occupation, and so on.

The purpose of selecting random samples—either simple or stratified—is to permit the investigator to use appropriate inferential statistical procedures. These depend on random selection and allow the investigator to make generalizations from the sample results to the study population.

Cluster Sampling. This method, also known as multistage sampling, is used in large-scale studies in which the population is geographically spread out. The primary sampling unit is the cluster, which consists of groups, rather than individuals, all of whom have the same characteristic. A cluster could consist of nursing homes, hospitals, or schools of nursing as the primary sampling units. For example, if the primary sampling unit is a group of hospitals, in subsequent sampling stages a random sample of the various nursing units in each hospital could be taken; then the next (cluster) stage could sample the patients on whom the actual measurements are needed for the study.[3] Cluster sampling has the advantage of convenience and involves less time and money than large-scale studies while retaining the advantages of probability sampling.

The term *systematic sampling* is used to refer to the selection of sampling units by taking every *k*th name on a population list, such as every fourth name listed on a hospital census sheet. Systematic sampling is considered a method of probability sampling *only if* the population list is randomly ordered (no pattern in the listing) and each population element has a known probability of being included in the sample.

Nonprobability Sampling Methods

In nonprobability sampling, the investigator has no ability to estimate the probability that each element of the population will be included in the sample. Major methods of nonprobability sampling include (1) *accidental sampling,* (2) *purposive sampling,* and (3) *quota sampling.*

Accidental Sampling. This method of sampling is also called *convenience sampling.* The sampling units are selected simply because they are available: They are in the right place at the right time for the investigator's purposes. For example, in the investigation of an emergency care facility during the night hours (Appendixes B and C), the investigator selected an accidental sample consisting of any veteran presenting himself to the emergency facility for medical problems between the hours of midnight and 6:00 A.M. during a one-month period. Many nursing studies use accidental sampling because of the availability of already existing population groups.

Purposive Sampling.   This method of sampling is also called *judgment sampling.* The investigator establishes certain criteria felt to be representative of the target population and deliberately selects sampling units according to those criteria. For example, in investigating the characteristics of undergraduate nursing students most likely to succeed in graduate programs, the investigator might ask persons who are knowledgeable regarding nursing education to select the actual students for the study.

Quota Sampling.   This method of sampling is much like accidental sampling, but certain controls are established so that the sample size does not become overloaded with subjects having certain characteristics. The investigator specifies a percentage for the inclusion of each characteristic in each group so that it is proportionate to the characteristics of the population. For example, quota sampling may be used to ensure that males and females from certain age, ethnic, and occupational groups are represented in the sample in proportion to these characteristics in the population.

Although it is often difficult to achieve probability sampling in clinical research, both probability and nonprobability sampling have a respected place in research. The important factor in determining which sampling approach to use is consistency with the research problem and the purpose of the study.

Sample Size

In determining how many subjects to include in a quantitative study (the total n for the study), it may be feasible to collect data regarding each element of the population. More often, however, the investigator will need to sample from the target population and must decide how large a sample will produce sufficient data to fulfill the study's purpose. There are no simple rules for determining sample size. Sample size is primarily determined by the degree of precision required, the type of sampling procedure used, the homogeneity of the population, and cost and convenience factors. There are mathematical formulas and computer programs available for calculating adequate sample size. A general rule is to use as large a sample as possible within feasible constraints. The larger the number in the sample, the more likely it is to be representative of the population from which it was selected. Representativeness of the sample is an important concern:

> The question of how large a sample should be is basically unanswerable, other than to say that it should be large enough to achieve repre-

sentativeness. How large this is will, of course, vary from study to study.[4]

In general, the larger the sample, the more generalizable the study results. If the population is homogeneous, a smaller sample size may be adequate.

We have found the following general guidelines helpful in determining sample size:

1. A sample of 10 percent of the population is considered a minimum for descriptive studies. For smaller populations, 20 percent may be required. Fifteen subjects per group is considered minimum for experimental studies.[5] Ten to twenty subjects per group is considered the minimum for simple studies with tight experimental control.[6]
2. Statistical analysis on samples of less than ten is not recommended and samples of thirty or more are more likely to reflect a population accurately.[7]

Even with these general guidelines, the investigator should bear the following in mind:

A large sample cannot correct for a faulty sampling design. The researcher should make decisions about the sample size and designs with the following in mind: the ultimate criterion for assessing a sample is its representativeness, not the quantity of data it produces.[8]

In summary, the method of selecting subjects for a quantitative study must be consistent with the problem and the purpose of the study and involves identification of the target population. If sampling is indicated, the sample should be of sufficient size to be representative of the population and should provide sufficient data for analysis. The sampling approach (probability or nonprobability) must also be consistent with the research design.

SELECTING THE STUDY SUBJECTS IN QUALITATIVE RESEARCH

Researchers may use a number of different ways to obtain a sample for a qualitative investigation. A qualitative researcher may choose to use the same sampling methodologies that a quantitative researcher would use. There are some sampling techniques, however, that qualitative researchers might use but that quantitative researchers might choose to ignore. First, the researcher may be able to use the entire population, which is especially useful when the investigator is working in a restricted area where the population is small or lives or works in a limited setting. For example, all of the staff members or patients in a small community's hospital could be used as informants during a study.

The Nominated Sample.   The *nominated* or *snowball* technique of sampling is used by some researchers. Investigators using this strategy ask their investigative questions of individuals whom they believe to have useful information. They then ask the subjects to name (''nominate'') other individuals who might be able to support or give additional details concerning the research question. In this manner, the initial sample of respondents determines an additional sample of potential respondents. If the investigator does not establish trust among the research subjects, especially if the subjects are engaged in activities that might be socially unacceptable, the investigation may founder on the shoals of false information and inappropriate leads. This technique may also be called ''network sampling.''

Purposive Sampling.   Qualitative investigators may also use *purposive* or *judgmental* sampling strategies. That is, individuals are identified as knowledgeable about the subject under investigation. If the researcher wanted to know about the perceived leadership roles of head nurses in a major hospital, for example, the main group of individuals interviewed and observed would be head nurses. Other individuals might also be interviewed and observed to provide confirmation or validation for the researcher.

Voluntary Sampling.   A researcher may also issue a request for volunteers to give information. Such a request might be given through an organization such as the Red Cross (e.g., for a study of couples in prenatal or neonatal classes) or through solicitation by advertisements in newspapers or other journals. However, the investigator's data may be biased because those individuals who did not choose to volunteer might have provided data that would have either expanded or contradicted the information obtained from the volunteering subjects.

STATING THE ASSUMPTIONS OF THE STUDY

An assumption is a statement whose correctness or validity is taken for granted. Assumptions may be so self-evident as to require no further testing, they may be based on theories applicable to the study topic, or they may be based on previous research findings.[9] In most studies, assumptions are implied by the investigator and need not be stated explicitly. If they are significant enough to affect the study's course or outcome, the investigator should state these assumptions explicitly so that others may evaluate their effect on the study. For example, note the four assumptions of the study included in the proposal in Appendix E. The student who wrote this proposal felt it was necessary to state each of these assumptions for her study on the effect of stockinette caps on the conservation of body heat in newborn infants.

STATING THE LIMITATIONS OF THE STUDY

The limitations of a quantitative study are restrictions that may affect the investigator's ability to generalize the study results but over which the investigator has no control. Although all studies are limited in some way, limitations in quantitative studies are usually related to the use of small, unrepresentative samples and inadequate methodology. Important limitations should be stated, both in the research proposal and in the research report, to allow the reader to judge their effect on the study. Often, qualitative researchers may not be able to state limitations prior to the study. The limitations may not be known until the qualitative researcher is in place and gathering the data.

WRITING THE DATA COLLECTION SECTION OF A QUANTITATIVE OR QUALITATIVE RESEARCH PROPOSAL

In this chapter, we discussed principles and methods for the development of the overall plan to collect the data for the study problem. The data collection section of a research proposal consists of a discussion of the following topics on the plan for collecting the data:

1. The research approach
2. Plans for selecting the study subjects (sampling)
3. Techniques for data collection
4. Procedures for data collection
5. Assumptions of the study
6. Limitations of the study

In writing this section of the research proposal, the research approach is described as either historical, descriptive, or experimental. Plans for selection of the study subjects are specified in terms of the target population, kinds and numbers of study subjects, and the sampling approach and method (if applicable). Techniques for collecting the data are described in relationship to the study's purpose. The measuring instruments for a quantitative study are described and discussed in terms of their reliability, validity, and usability. An experimental study should also include a description of the experimental design. Steps in the procedure for data collection should be listed in chronological order with attention to the protection of human rights. Any explicit assumptions that would significantly affect the study should be stated. Finally, the limitations of the study should be listed. The guidelines for writing a research proposal (Appendix H) should help you write this section of your proposal.

The following Application Activities are designed to help you evaluate your understanding of principles and procedures of data collection.

APPLICATION ACTIVITIES

I. Critical evaluation of research studies
    1. Use the "Guidelines for Evaluating a Research Report" provided in Appendix I (Section F) to evaluate the data collection sections of each of the four studies you have selected to critique.
    2. In which study
        a. were the study subjects most clearly described?
        b. was the sampling most representative?
        c. was the data collection procedure most informative?
        d. was the protection of human rights most evident?
II. Selecting study subjects by simple random sampling
    The desired sample size for a quantitative study is 20 subjects selected from a target population of 40 elements. Select the subjects to be included in the sample by the following procedure:
    a. List the elements (names) of the target population.
    b. Number the names consecutively from 01 to 40.
    c. Arbitrarily select a two-digit column from the excerpt of a table of random numbers in this chapter (Table 6.2).
    d. When a number corresponds to a number assigned to a name on the list of the target population, assign that name to the sample.
    e. Skip any number that is not between 01 and 40, inclusive, and go on to the next number.
    f. Continue to select each two-digit number that corresponds to a list of names until twenty names have been assigned to the sample.
III. Criteria for evaluating quantitative measuring instruments
    Locate at least two measuring instruments which might be helpful in collecting data related to some aspect of a quantitative study. For each instrument:
    a. Describe how the reliability was established and reported.
    b. Describe how the validity was established and reported.
    c. Discuss the usability of the instrument.
IV. Data collection in a qualitative study
    1. Reread the plan for data collection in the qualitative research proposal in Appendix D.

    a. List each of the data collection techniques the researcher planned to use.

    b. Explain how each of these data collection techniques assists the researcher in achieving the purpose of the study.

    c. Are there any additional techniques the researcher could (or should) use to achieve the purpose of her study?

V. Writing the data collection section of your research proposal

    1. Reread the proposals in Appendixes A, B, D, and E. Pay special attention to the data collection section of each proposal.

    2. Using the principles and procedures in this chapter and the guidelines in Appendix H, write a tentative first draft of the plan for the data collection section of your own proposal that includes:

        a. Description of the research approach

        b. Plan for the selection of the study subjects

        c. Techniques for data collection

        d. Procedures for data collection

        e. Assumptions and limitations of the study

Although you will undoubtedly revise some of this material, you should be able to use much of it in your final research proposal.

REFERENCES

1. Field, P. A., and J. M. Morse. 1985. *Nursing Research: The Application of Qualitative Approaches.* Rockville, MD: Aspen, p. 139.
2. Abdellah, Faye, and Eugene Levine. 1979. *Better Patient Care through Nursing Research,* 2nd ed. New York: Macmillan, p. 152.
3. Ibid., p. 329.
4. Fox, David J. 1982. *Fundamentals of Research in Nursing,* 4th ed. New York: Appleton-Century-Crofts, p. 287.
5. Gay, L. R. 1987. *Educational Research: Competencies for Analysis and Application,* 3rd ed. Columbus, OH: Charles E. Merrill, pp. 114–115.
6. Roscoe, J. T. 1975. *Fundamental Research Statistics for the Behavioral Sciences,* 2nd ed. New York: Holt, Rinehart and Winston, p. 184.
7. Ibid., p. 184.
8. Polit, D., and B. Hungler. 1987. *Nursing Research: Principles and Methods,* 3rd ed. Philadelphia: J. B. Lippincott, p. 220.
9. Abdellah and Levine, *Better Patient Care,* p. 145.

BIBLIOGRAPHY AND SUGGESTED READINGS

Abdellah, F., and E. Levine. 1979. *Better Patient Care through Nursing Research,* 2nd ed. New York: Macmillan.
Brink, P. J., and M. Wood. 1988. *Basic Steps in Nursing Research.* Boston: Jones and Bartlett.

Burns, N., and S. Grove. 1987. *The Practice of Nursing Research: Conduct, Critique and Utilization.* Philadelphia: W. B. Saunders.

Dobbert, M. L. 1982. *Ethnographic Research.* New York: Praeger.

Field, P. A., and J. M. Morse. 1985. *Nursing Research: The Application of Qualitative Approaches.* Rockville, MD: Aspen.

Ford, J. 1975. *Paradigms and Fairy Tales.* London: Routledge and Kegan Paul.

Fox, D. 1982. *Fundamentals of Research in Nursing,* 4th ed. New York: Appleton-Century-Crofts.

Gay, L. R. 1987. *Educational Research: Competencies for Analysis and Application,* 3rd ed. Columbus, OH: Charles E. Merrill.

Goetz, J. P., and M. D. LeCompte. 1984. *Ethnography and Qualitative Design in Educational Research.* Orlando, FL: Academic Press.

Hopkins, C. D. 1976. *Educational Research: A Structure for Inquiry.* Columbus, OH: Charles E. Merrill.

Halley, S., and S. Cummings. 1988. *Designing Clinical Research: An Epidemiological Approach.* Baltimore, MD: Williams and Wilkins.

Kidder, L., C. M. Judd, and E. R. Smith. 1986. *Research Methods in Social Relations,* 5th ed. New York: Holt, Rinehart and Winston.

Morse, J. 1989. *Qualitative Nursing Research: A Contemporary Dialogue.* Rockville, MD: Aspen.

Notter, L. 1978. *Essentials of Nursing Research,* 2nd ed. New York: Springer.

Polit, D., and B. Hungler. 1987. *Nursing Research Principles and Methods,* 3rd ed. Philadelphia: J. B. Lippincott.

Roscoe, J. T. 1975. *Fundamental Research Statistics for the Behavioral Sciences,* 2nd ed. New York: Holt, Rinehart and Winston.

Werner W., and G. M. Schoepfle. 1987. *Systematic Fieldwork.* Beverly Hills, CA: Sage.

United Nations. 1973. *A Short Manual on Sampling, Volume II: Computer Programmes for Sampling Design.* New York: United Nations Press.

Verhonick, P., and C. Seaman. 1978. *Research Methods for Undergraduate Students in Nursing.* New York: Appleton-Century-Crofts.

7

Data Analysis

The purpose of this chapter is to acquaint you with some basic information about the analysis and interpretation of data in research studies. It should help you understand and evaluate different methods of treating both quantitative and qualitative data.

Since we do not expect that beginning researchers be statisticians, this chapter contains a simplified overview of statistical techniques and analyses. Researchers who need more help in developing statistical analysis may find additional information in the "Statistical Primer," Appendix J to this book.

If you require more information about either quantitative or qualitative data analysis techniques, we urge you to read more advanced textbooks or to contact your instructors, a statistician or anthropologist, or other individuals qualified to discuss appropriate methods of data analysis.

QUANTITATIVE DATA ANALYSIS

It is highly significant that statistical analysis in nursing research traces its roots back to Florence Nightingale. Although Nightingale lacked the sophisticated techniques available to the nurse researcher today, she did utilize and publish descriptive statistical analyses using graphs and charts concerning the mortality of soldiers during the Crimean War. For a brief review of Nightingale's statistical techniques, you might want to read Cohen's article in the March 1984 issue of *Scientific American.*[1]

THE USE OF STATISTICS IN DATA ANALYSIS

Statistics are ways of measuring things or groups of things. Any time we measure opinions, average numbers of miles per gallon, or the odds in a card game, we are using statistics. Basically, there are two kinds of statistics: descriptive and inferential. *Descriptive statistics* simply describe the population with which we are concerned. Inferential statistics allow us to draw other kinds of conclusions about a population based on a sample or samples, and to predict future happenings. Both quantitative and qualitative researchers may use a variety of statistical techniques to analyze their data. Quantitative researchers usually tend to use more complex statistical analyses than qualitative researchers.

DESCRIPTIVE STATISTICS

Essentially, descriptive statistics describe. This type of statistical analysis is the simple reporting of facts and collective occurrences based on a number of sam-

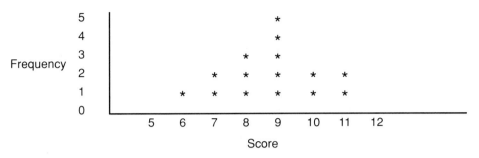

FIGURE 7.1
Histogram

ples. Sometimes the easiest way to describe a set of data is to draw a picture or pictures of the information. For example, suppose we had the following set of scores on a test.

$$7, 6, 8, 9, 10, 9, 7, 11, 11, 9, 9, 9, 10, 8, 8$$

It is very hard to make any sense out of such data. But if the researcher organized the data by making a histogram (graph), the results are much clearer (Figure 7.1).

Another way to organize these data would be to make a bar graph (Figure 7.2). This type of representation clearly shows the number of scores at each level of scoring.

A third way to show these data would be by the use of a frequency polygon. In this instance, the midpoints on the bar graph are connected and the bars are eliminated, so that the scores are as shown in Figure 7.3. As we can see, the corners of a frequency polygon can be smoothed out so that we get a figure resembling a normal curve (Figure 7.4).

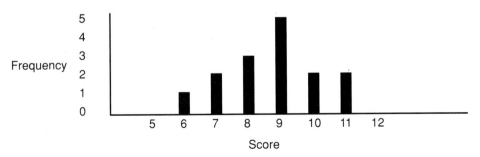

FIGURE 7.2
Bar Graph

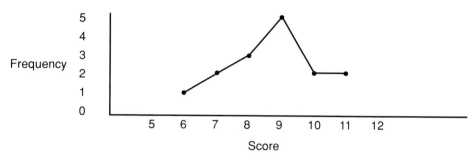

FIGURE 7.3
Frequency Polygon

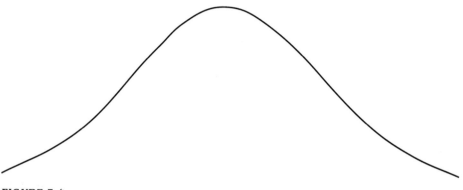

FIGURE 7.4
Normal Curve

When we use descriptive statistics, we are concerned with several types of measures: (1) centrality or central tendency, (2) dispersion, and (3) location or position within the sample or the population.

If you were to measure any large population, you would find that the members of the population would distribute themselves across what is known as the *normal curve*.

The Mean

As you can see, most of the population clusters about the high point or the center of the curve. If the curve is perfectly symmetrical, the center of the normal curve is called the *mean*. Statistically, the mean is shown by the symbol $\overline{X}$. The mean may be thought of as the average. For example, suppose we have seven scores on a simple test:

$$5, 4, 3, 2, 6, 7, 8$$

When we add these scores and then divide the sum by the total number of tests, we find that 5 is the mean, or average, in this case.

Of course, means often describe essentially mythical characteristics. No one owns 1.3 cars or 2.2 television sets, or has 2.5 children. The mean gives us some idea of what a total population may be like, but it is not a measure in which we can put our complete trust. For example, suppose we have seven more scores from a test:

$$6, 7, 8, 5, 4, 10, 23$$

The mean of these seven scores is now 9. Yet only two scores are above 9. Thus, this average implies something that does not accurately reflect what happened with the test scores. The curve is distorted.

The Median

When we have extreme scores that cause distortion of the curve, we can use another measure to show how central the mean really is. This is called the *median*. The median is the number that divides the sample in half, so that 50 percent of the sample falls above the median and 50 percent falls below. In our first example of seven scores, we find that the median is 5, the same as the mean. In the second example, however, the mean is 9, but the median is 7. In this particular instance, 7 is probably more descriptive of what is really happening.

The Mode

Still another measure of central tendency is the *mode*. This statistic tells us where scores tend to cluster. For example, consider these numbers:

$$4, 5, 6, 6, 6, 7, 8$$

The most frequently occurring score or number is 6. Consequently, the mode is 6. In this example the mean and the median also happen to be 6.

Remember, it is fairly unusual and inadvisable to use descriptive statistics exclusively with small samples. Using such techniques distorts the data analysis.

Percentile Rank

Measures that reflect the relative position of a score in a distribution are also descriptive in nature. One the most commonly used statistics is the *percentile rank*. The percentile rank is the point below which a percentage of scores occurs. In percentile rank, the median is always the fiftieth percentile. A person scoring at the sixtieth percentile is above 60 percent of the other test takers and below the other 40 percent.

Other percentage-based statistics commonly found in the literature are the decile (10 percent) and the quartile (25 percent). Means, medians, and modes are used when we want to describe central tendency. They give us an idea of how alike members of a population are. Sometimes, however, we want to know how a population is actually distributed over the curve. Then we must use measures of dispersion. The most frequently used measure of dispersion is the standard deviation.

The Standard Deviation

On all normal curves, certain proportions of the sample cluster around the mean. We can find out how widely distributed the scores are by measuring the *standard deviation*. When a curve is normal, about 68 percent of the population will be within one standard deviation, plus or minus, of the mean. We discuss the ''average'' characteristics of a population when we report the mean, but we usually consider this 68 percent (34 percent above the mean and 34 percent below the mean) to be within the normal or average range. Ninety-five percent of the population will be within two standard deviations from the mean, and 99.7 percent will be within three standard deviations (Figure 7.5).

The important idea is not the percentages of the population that are contained under any portion of a curve but, rather, the shape of the curve. There is one standard (imaginary) bell-shaped curve that we have been using to illustrate the statistical curve. Curves can take many shapes, some with a narrow range and others with a wide range between standard deviations (Figure 7.6).

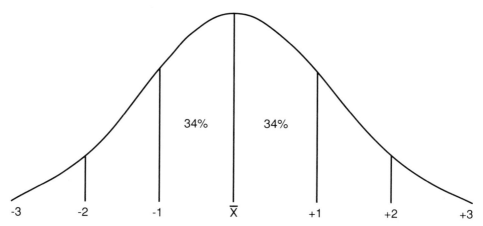

FIGURE 7.5
Normal Curve Showing Standard Deviation

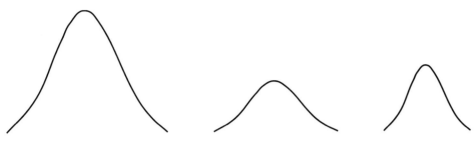

FIGURE 7.6
Three Normal Curves

If a test is given and the standard deviation is found to be 2 and the mean 16, this means that 68 percent of the population will fall between the scores of 14 and 18 on the normal curve. If the standard deviation of the same test is 4, the curve will assume a different shape; if the standard deviation is 8, still another shape will be assumed. Consequently, we can always describe the shape of the curve on the basis of the standard deviation. We can also get some idea of the range of scores and a better feeling for an average individual.

INFERENTIAL STATISTICS

Descriptive statistics give us a quantitative way of viewing the world. They enable us to describe certain factual aspects of a population. Most researchers, however, are concerned with other kinds of judgments as well. This leads us to the use of *inferential statistics*. Inferential statistics do not examine a whole population. Rather, as described in Chapter 6, a sample or samples are drawn from the population and the characteristics of the population are deduced or inferred from the responses of this sample.

In addition to this type of *inference*, the researcher uses inferential statistics to determine whether or not certain experimental treatments or techniques are better, worse, or not significantly different from other types of treatments or techniques. This is called *hypothesis testing* and is based on probability. When reading research, the beginning researcher continually runs across the proposition $H = p < .05$. (Remember that H_0 is called the null hypothesis, as discussed in Chapter 5.) Here, $p < .05$ is called the *level of significance*. That is, the researcher states that the results will probably *not* be significantly different from the standard or common treatment. Most researchers really want to reject the null hypothesis, but research convention has cast this as the most common type of research hypothesis. The symbol p stands for probability. The probability in the statement $p < .05$ means that there will be no conclusion of a significant difference between treatments unless 5 or fewer treatments out of 100 have the same result as the original or standard treatment.

When a level of significance is selected, the experimenter is telling the world that chance has little to do with the results of the experiment. Medically related experiments may set extremely high levels of significance; usually, one chance in a thousand or less ($p < .001$). In cases of life and death, the chance of error must be diminished as much as possible.

LEVELS OF MEASUREMENT

When dealing with inferential statistics, we must be concerned with what are called *levels of measurement*. Often, the researcher works with data represented by responses to questions that can be posed in various ways.

The Nominal Scale

The first level of data measurement is called the *nominal* level or nominal scale. The responses to this scale deal only with mutually exclusive data. There are no qualifiers. For example, we can classify all people in the world as having either blue eyes or brown eyes. If we choose to do this, anyone whose eyes are considered green, grey, or black must be placed in the category blue or brown. Nominal scales deal only with exclusive categories and do not attempt to find gradations between them. The categories are absolute, and the mode is the only measure of central tendency.

In nursing research, the nominal scale might be used to determine if pregnancies and abortions occur statistically more frequently in one of two socially different groups of women. This can be done by simply identifying members of one group or the other and asking each subject if she has ever had an abortion. The responses of each group could then be tallied and analyzed statistically to determine if there was a significant difference in the frequency of abortion between the two groups (Figure 7.7).

The Ordinal Scale

The next highest level of measurement is called *ordinal* measurement. Subjects are asked to rank ideas, items, or other things. The subject can respond that

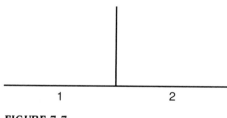

FIGURE 7.7
Nominal Scale

item A is more or less than items B or C, but cannot tell exactly how much more or less. For example, a patient may experience more or less discomfort, depending on certain postures or other physical phenomena that can be adjusted. The amount cannot be quantified by saying, "I am twice as uncomfortable," but the feeling of more or less comfort can be experienced. If eye color is graded with a range from black to blue, we could consider this *ordinal data,* and ordinal statistics such as the median then come into play (Figure 7.8).

The Interval Scale

The third and most commonly used level of statistical measurement is interval measurement. Actually, much ordinal data is treated as if it were *interval data.* There is a great debate in statistical circles as to whether or not this can really be done. Interval measurements are based on absolutely equal distances between measurements, but there is no absolute zero starting point on an interval scale. Because temperatures can be measured in either Fahrenheit or Celsius and neither of these scales has an absolute zero (i.e., no temperature at all), a clinical thermometer is an interval-measuring instrument (Figure 7.9).

The Ratio Scale

The highest level of measurement is the ratio scale (Figure 7.10). This scale has a starting point or base of absolute zero. All subjects start at zero and travel or respond in some manner along this same scale. Length, weight, and volume are examples of ratio measurements because they start with an absolute zero (no length, no weight, or no volume). Practically speaking, nursing research is rarely of a type that deals with ratio scales.

COMMONLY USED STATISTICAL TESTS

Regardless of the scale level used, the researcher must answer the question, "Are the differences I see caused by chance, or are other factors responsible, such as my treatment?" For example, when a researcher sees that two differ-

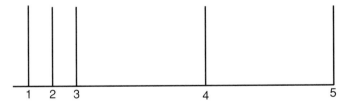

FIGURE 7.8
Ordinal Scale

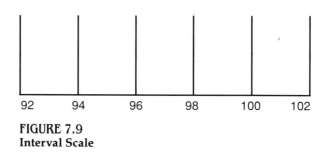

FIGURE 7.9
Interval Scale

ent groups have different means, the next task is to test the differences between the means to determine if they are significantly different statistically.
Based on the level of data, the researcher selects the statistical test that is the
most appropriate to determine if chance is the overriding factor. The terms
parametric statistics and *nonparametric statistics* are associated with level of measurement of the data to be analyzed. Each of these terms refers to a different
group of inferential statistical techniques. Parametric statistical techniques are
intended for use with interval- and ratio-level data; nonparametric statistical
techniques are intended to be used with nominal- and ordinal-level data.

Parametric Statistical Tests

The term *parametric statistics* is used to describe ''a class of inferential statistics
that involves (a) assumptions about the distribution of the variables, (b) the
estimation of a parameter, and (c) the use of interval measures.''[2] The most
frequently used parametric tests include (1) *t*-tests, (2) analysis of variance, and
(3) analysis of covariance.

   t-Tests.   In order to determine whether the differences between the means
of two different sets of scores are statistically significant, the researcher first
determines whether the two samples are independent (such as in the case of
an experimental and a control group) or if they are dependent (using the same
group of individuals and their responses prior to and after a treatment). This

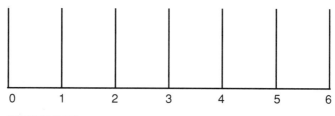

FIGURE 7.10
Ratio Scale

must be done because there are several ways to compute the t statistic. If an inappropriate method is used, the researcher might obtain incorrect results in either accepting or rejecting the hypothesis.

An example of the use of the t statistic can be found in Moss and Craft's 1989 article concerning visual perception.[3] In this instance, the researchers defined two independent samples from a group of 56 student nurses to determine whether or not instruction in estimating volumes of fluids visually would enhance the experimental group's ability to perform this task. The researchers found that instruction did enhance the experimental group's ability to estimate volume visually and concluded that the differences between the experimental and the control groups were statistically significant at the .01 level using the t statistic.

Analysis of Variance (ANOVA). Sometimes the researcher has more than two means to test to determine if there are significant differences between them. In this instance, using the t statistic could be exceedingly tedious because of the number of possible permutations of the t-test. Also, the more individual t-tests conducted, the greater the possibility of what is called a *Type I error* or a *Type II error*. A Type I error means that the investigator has rejected the null hypothesis when it should be accepted. A Type II error occurs when the investigator accepts the null hypothesis when it should be rejected. Consequently, the statistical analysis of variance, or ANOVA, is often used. With this technique, it is possible to determine if there is a significant difference between several means simultaneously. The literature will report these differences as the F-test or the F ratio.

Also, when many means have been tested, the researcher will want to know exactly which means were significantly different from the other means. There are other methods, such as Sheffe's test or the Tukey HSD test, that can be applied in determining which means were significantly different from the other means.

An example of the use of analysis of variance can be found in Rosswurm's study of deficits of visual matching ability and short-term memory recall.[4] In this study, Rosswurm used analysis of variance to compare 60 elderly individuals, 30 of whom were diagnosed as having senile dementia of the Alzheimer's type (SDAT) and 30 who were considered nondemented. The groups were compared on their ability to perform matching tasks by matching patterns on selected cards and their ability to recall patterns on selected cards when the selected card was paired with another card. The researcher found that there was a significant difference between the two groups in their ability to recognize and recall patterns, with those suffering from Alzheimer's disease scoring the most poorly.

Finally, beginning researchers should be aware that analysis of variance may be applied when there is more than one dependent variable to be examined. Statisticians call this *multiple analysis of variance* or MANOVA. This type of statistical analysis can become quite complex, and we urge you to have someone prepared in statistical methodology help you design such an analysis.

An example of the use of MANOVA is Foley and Stone's pilot study of stress inoculation with nursing students.[5] Students who were given training in coping with future stressors were compared with nursing students who were not given such training. The researchers identified multiple dependent variables as indicators of the extent and breadth of the impact of stress inoculation, and they found that such instruction had the potential to reduce stress and to enhance the coping skills of their subjects.

Analysis of Covariance (ANCOVA). Frequently, because of the nature of the research setting, it is impossible for a researcher to place subjects into truly randomly assigned groups. In this case, there may be variables that confound the variable under consideration. This means that the researcher's data may or may not show significant differences unless the confounding variable or variables are accounted for.

In order to account for the confounding variable, the researcher may utilize analysis of covariance, or ANCOVA, which is also reported as an *F* statistic or *F* ratio. This procedure may be used in place of the *t* statistic when two groups are involved and there is no way to achieve the requirements of randomness necessary for appropriate use of the *t* statistic. Analysis of covariance may also be used on more than two sets of subjects or when there is more than one dependent variable.

Nonparametric Statistical Tests

The term *nonparametric statistics* is used to describe ''a general class of inferential statistics that does not involve rigorous assumptions about the distribution of the critical variables; most often used when samples are small or when the data are measured on the nominal or ordinal scales.''[6]

Because there are literally dozens of nonparametric tests available, we will discuss and highlight only a few of the more commonly used statistics: (1) chi-square, (2) Mann-Whitney U, (3) Kruskal-Wallis one-way analysis of variance, and (4) Friedman two-way analysis of variance.

Chi-Square (χ^2). Perhaps the most commonly used nonparametric statistic is the *chi-square* (χ^2) measure. This statistic can be applied to nominal or higher levels of measurement and can be used in one or more samples. Essentially, the chi-square test is used to determine if the observed frequencies of events in certain categories fall within the range of frequencies expected to fall in these categories.

For example, Byers used the chi-square statistic in her study of the relationship between infant crying and bottle feeding during aircraft descent.[7] Byers found that there was a significant difference in the amount of crying as a result of changes of air pressure in infants' ears between infants who were bottle fed during the descent and infants who were not bottle fed during the descent. Bottle-fed infants cried significantly less than their unfed counterparts.

Mann-Whitney U. A very powerful nonparametric alternative to the *t*-test is the Mann-Whitney U test. By using this statistic, a researcher can determine whether or not two groups are significantly different when the scores from two sets of data are ranked. Kalish et al. examined 320 television episodes from 28 series on prime time television from 1950 to 1980 in which nurses and nursing were portrayed.[8] Data on Nielsen ratings were used to rank the programs for level of exposure to the viewing public. A variety of statistics, including the Mann-Whitney U, were used to analyze the data. By ranking the various shows by their Neilsen ratings and applying the Mann-Whitney U, these authors concluded that technical care was the nursing action that received the highest audience exposure and that menial, nonnursing tasks had very low audience exposure.

Kruskal-Wallis One-Way Analysis of Variance. Even as parametric tests provide techniques for the analysis of variance, so do nonparametric tests. The Kruskal-Wallis statistic is one such test which allows for a one-way analysis of variance with ordinal data. Kalish et al. also utilized this statistic when they analyzed the world of nursing as portrayed on television.[9] The results of this study are most interesting:

> The findings showed that nurses were depicted as working in acute care settings, entering nursing for altruistic reasons, predominately acting as a resource to other health professionals, not using problem-solving and evaluation skills, deficient in administrative abilities, and remiss in providing physical comforting, engaging in expanded role activities, patient education and scholarly endeavors. Since the 1960s the trend in the quality of nurse portrayals has been downward. This has created a current crisis in communicating the world of nursing to the public via the most powerful form of mass communication, television.[10]

Friedman Two-Way Analysis of Variance by Ranks. Even as a researcher might need to use a parametric multiple analysis of variance, occasionally there is a need to use a nonparametric ANOVA. Vanbree et al. used the Friedman two-way analysis of variance to determine if there were significant differences in skin bruising as a result of three different subcutaneous injection techniques for administering low-dose heparin.[11] This analysis required the ranking of observations for each subject, which in this case called for ranking of sizes of bruises from the smallest to the largest. After ranking the various bruise sizes, the investigators concluded that there was no significant difference between the three subcutaneous injection techniques for administering low-dose heparin.

Correlations

Researchers are often concerned about the relationship between two variables. The relationship between two variables is measured by correlation statistics, often called measures of association. Correlation statistics range from -1.0 to $+1.0$. It is very important to note that correlations do not imply cause-and-effect relationships. Correlations that report the presence or absence of something else do not necessarily mean that one factor caused the other. For example, the correlation between houses with roofs and houses with basements probably approaches $+1.0$, but this does not mean that the presence of roofs causes basements to be present. Such a correlation would be a spurious correlation: the assumption of relationship where none really exists.

It is also important to note that a correlation of -1 is just as strong as a correlation of $+1$. The closer a correlation coefficient is to either -1 or $+1$, the stronger the relationship is between the variables being studied.

Pearson r. The commonly used parametric statistic for correlation is the Pearson product-moment correlation coefficient, otherwise known as the Pearson r, or more simply as r. In this test, two different sets of interval-level data are compared to determine the degree of relationship between them. Since r's range from -1 through 0 to $+1$, we can say that such sets of items are related either positively or negatively. As the correlation coefficient approaches -1 or $+1$, the items become more highly related. On the other hand, if the correlation coefficient approaches 0, we know that the items have little or no relationship.

Whether or not the degree of association is statistically significant may also be measured. That is, is the correlation coefficient a result of chance, or is the correlation really statistically significant? Jones and Thomas investigated cardiovascular changes in 148 first-time fathers while holding and interacting with their newborn infants.[12] They found that the systolic blood pressure, diastolic blood pressure, and heart rate of new fathers were significantly higher during the new fathers' verbal interaction with their newborn. The researchers also found that the diastolic blood pressure of the new fathers was positively related to the frequency of the infant crying.

Spearman Rho Correlation. As is the case in parametric statistical analysis, there is a host of nonparametric correlation techniques. One of the most common is the Spearman rho correlation (r_s). Researchers utilizing this statistic rank their observations of the two variables under consideration and then determine the level of relationship between them. For example, a researcher might want to test the relationship between patients' perceived level of comfort and their perception of the quality of care provided by the nursing staff in a hospital. In this instance, the patients would be given two attitude evaluation scales (one to measure each variable), and then the two scores would be ranked and a Spearman rho computed.

An example of the use of the Spearman rho can be found in the study of renal transplant patients conducted by Sutton and Murphy.[13] The researchers compared the coping scores of 40 renal transplant patients, 20 of whom had had their transplants within 23 months of measurement of their coping strategies to deal with stress and 20 other renal transplant patients who had had their transplants from 23 to 48 months before being given the same coping scale. Using the Spearman rho correlation, the investigators found that the rank orderings of coping methods according to mean degree of use were significantly correlated between the two study groups (r_s = .87). The findings of their study suggest that renal transplant patients may experience continuing stress as long as four years after transplant surgery.

You may also find a number of other nonparametric statistic correlation coefficients in the studies that you examine, such as Kendall's tau or Cronbach's alpha.

Partial and Multiple Correlation.   Occasionally the researcher has a number of items that might be interrelated. In this instance, partial correlations can be computed. The intent of this method is to eliminate the confounding effects of one or more variables when measuring the relationships between a number of variables. This is shown as $r_{12.3}$, where variables 1 and 2 are correlated and variable 3 is eliminated mathematically.

Conversely, if you want to lump together all of the variables, this can be done by a technique called multiple correlation (symbolized by the letter R). O'Rourke used multiple correlation to investigate a sample of employed women's subjective appraisal of their psychological well-being (PWB), the dependent variable, and the following independent variables: (1) subjective self-reports of menstrual and nonmenstrual symptoms, (2) sociodemographic factors (age, income, ethnicity), and (3) a health factor (represented by self-reports of current health status).[14] Results of the study indicated "a strong positive relationship between the independent variables when analyzed as a set and PWB (R = .86).[15] A major finding of the study was that the presence of specific menstrual symptoms did not negatively affect PWB; rather, these women had a higher PWB than those with nonmenstrual symptoms.

In summary, we have discussed the use of descriptive and inferential statistics in data analysis and have briefly presented a few of the commonly used parametric and nonparametric statistical tests, as well as correlations.

META-ANALYSIS

Meta-analysis is a quantitative data analysis strategy that examines research findings across studies: "It is the statistical analysis of a large collection of results from individual studies for the purpose of integrating the findings into a single, generalizable finding."[16] Meta-analysis is most effective when numerous studies concerning the same variables are available, but the technique can be used when only a few studies have been done.

For example, Broome, Lillis, and Smith conducted a meta-analysis of 27 studies on pain management intervention with children.[17] The authors screened 123 articles in 83 journals and 20 dissertations published since 1979 to find data that would fit a rigorous, predefined set of criteria for inclusion in their study. The researchers found 27 studies in this body of literature that met the criteria. Using meta-analytical techniques, the researchers found that there were significant relationships of a small magnitude between pain management interventions and children's responses on behavioral and physiological measures; that is, the pain management programs helped to reduce children's distress responses.

A NOTE ON COMPUTERS AND CALCULATORS
IN QUANTITATIVE DATA ANALYSIS

With the advent of computers and hand-held calculators, statistical analysis has become increasingly sophisticated. This is because many calculations that required hours or days when worked by hand or on mechanical calculators can now be done in seconds or minutes by the computer or hand calculator, with far greater accuracy and fewer mistakes.

Anyone who is serious about research and statistics should acquire a hand calculator. These range from simple, inexpensive devices to fairly expensive, programmable machines. For ease of computation, there are a number of calculators designed to compute the mean, standard deviation, and variance. We strongly urge that any hand calculator you buy have these features.

Most researchers also have access to one or more computers. These technologically complex machines may be intimidating to a beginning researcher. Remember, the computer is simply a tool that one uses for data analysis.

Computers use a number of "languages." Fortran, BASIC, APL, COBOL, and Pascal are a few of the commonly used languages. Each of these languages enhances human–machine interaction and aids in data analysis. It is not necessary, however, for a researcher to know a specific computer language to use the machine. Usually, there are teams of consultants who are quite willing and able to help researchers program the machine, and many prewritten statistical packages are widely available. One of the easiest and most powerful set of programs to use is Minitab. Another commonly available statistical package is the Statistical Package for the Social Sciences (SPSS). Yet another very useful set of programs is the Biomedical Data Package (BMDP). Finally, the data analysis package Statistical Analysis System (SAS) is also available. Although these statistical packages were written for mainframe or large computers, some have been modified for use on smaller personal computers.

All researchers would do well to remember the saying "garbage in, garbage out." The computer can only act on the data given it. If your research is poorly designed or organized, the finest computer in the world will not give you a valid statistical analysis.

There is a great temptation to subject all data to computer analysis just because of the availability of the machine. Frequently, when the number of subjects is small (some say less than 100) and the statistical computation fairly simple, it is faster and cheaper to do one's calculations with a hand calculator. Just setting up a program and removing flaws (debugging) can take a great deal of time. Do not become so enamored of the computer that you waste time trying to use it for all quantitative data analysis.

QUALITATIVE DATA ANALYSIS

Data for qualitative studies "are usually in the form of narrative text derived from transcribed interviews, written descriptions of observations in field notes and reflections on the dynamics of the setting in the researcher's diary."[18] As a result, qualitative studies have voluminous amounts of data that often makes data analysis more difficult and time-consuming than in quantitative studies. In qualitative research, data collection and analysis occur simultaneously, as the researcher continually interprets data from the outset of the study. Data are coded to facilitate the identification and analysis of meaningful categories inherent in the data. The analysis of qualitative data requires a great deal of mulling over of the data before the researcher can draw conclusions and communicate the findings. The following discussion of published studies that exemplify the major qualitative approaches is intended to give you an idea of how data are collected, analyzed, and interpreted in qualitative studies.

Phenomenology

Phenomenology was previously defined as the study of human experience. A data analysis technique used in phenomenological studies involves data from interviews with study subjects to discover themes or categories of experiences as viewed from the subjects' perspective. For example, McLain used a phenomenological approach to determine nurse–physician interactions between nine family nurse practitioners and their physician partners.[19] Participants were interviewed both separately and together about their practice relationships. An analysis of emergent themes in the data revealed the existence of distorted communication and nonmeaningful interaction. Elements that could contribute to a successful collaborative practice included "a willingness to move beyond basic information exchange in nurse/physician interactions, the willingness and ability to challenge distortions and assumptions in the relationship, and a belief system based on critical self-reflection."[20]

Grounded Theory

Grounded theory uses the steps of the research process simultaneously. The researcher observes, collects data, organizes the data, and develops theory all at the same time. The grounded theory researcher uses the constant comparative method of data analysis in which every piece of data is compared to every other datum (an individual data item). In her study of caregiving of relatives with Alzheimer's dementia, Wilson used the constant comparative method to explore the dilemmas faced by family members trying to cope with a relative with Alzheimer's dementia.[21] She used the computer program *Ethnograph* to analyze the verbal data collected from 20 in-depth face-to-face interviews with family caregivers. Findings indicated that caregivers had only negative choices in caring for their afflicted relative at home; that is, no matter which choice was made, there were undesirable consequences for the caregiver.

Ethnography

Ethnographic research has its roots in the discipline of anthropology. The ethnographer's purpose is to study cultures by using systematic observation. This type of study allows the researcher to gain knowledge and insights concerning the lifeways or patterns of particular cultures. Ethnographic research can prove to be extremely valuable in gaining knowledge of folk medicine practiced by a cultural group in order to understand how to improve health care practices by members of the group. Such a study was done by Cheon-Klessig et al. when they studied the folk medical practices of Hmong refugees residing in the United States.[22] The researchers used a variety of data-gathering techniques including "unstructured interviews, informal conversations, written documents, and participation in events . . . " to gather "data that were used to identify the general health care patterns and folk medicine usage in this group of Hmong refugees. . . ."[23]

The researchers found that the Hmong used a variety of herbal medicines and that householders often grew some of the plants used. The researchers also found that herbalists were called upon to treat ill individuals and that the Hmong called in shamans to diagnose and treat diseases. Further, they found that many Hmong were reluctant to use U.S. health care practices because they felt that surgery and blood tests had the potential for great harm both in the present and in the afterlife. In this instance, there is a great conflict between the beliefs of the Hmong and the U.S. medical system. As a result, many Hmong either do not use the U.S. health care system or may not comply with treatments if the treatments are in conflict with their traditional medical beliefs.

A NOTE ON THE USE OF COMPUTERS IN QUALITATIVE DATA ANALYSIS

It is important to note that qualitative data may also be analyzed using computers. There are a number of programs mentioned in the qualitative data analysis literature, and beginning researchers are urged to explore appropriate programs prior to attempting qualitative analysis. Programs such as *Ethnograph* and *General Inquirer* can analyze verbal data to find themes or problem areas that are shared by subjects. Occasionally, the use of a word-processing program that displays word counts will aid the qualitative researcher in finding common themes or ideas.

WRITING THE DATA ANALYSIS SECTION OF A QUANTITATIVE OR QUALITATIVE RESEARCH PROPOSAL

It may seem strange to you that it is important to formulate a plan for data analysis in the planning stage of the research study and to describe this plan in detail in the research proposal. This ensures that the researcher will collect the data in a form that facilitates analysis. The data analysis plan should be appropriate to the problem being investigated and to the methodology of the study. The method of tabulating and organizing the data for quantitative studies should be clearly presented, along with a description of appropriate statistical procedures to be applied and the rationale for selecting them.

Skeleton outlines or dummy statistical tables, charts, and graphs provide a format for analyzing the variables being investigated and may lead to additional ideas for data analysis. Note that each of the students who wrote the research proposals in the appendixes established her data collection plan as part of the proposal. Although the best plans for analysis may turn out later to be incomplete or somewhat inappropriate, a carefully formulated plan for data analysis established prior to the actual data collection should result in higher quality research studies. It can also eliminate much distress on the part of the researcher.

Qualitative researchers should also establish their data analysis plan before beginning their studies. Because of the nature of qualitative data, the plan for analysis may not be as complete as in a quantitative study. Still, planning ahead can facilitate data analysis later. The guidelines for writing a research proposal (Appendix H) should help you write this section of your proposal.

This chapter presented a few basic ideas about data analysis. Any researcher who wishes to deal in greater depth in either quantitative or qualitative strategies is strongly urged to take one or more courses that feature the appropriate data-gathering and analysis techniques.

APPLICATION ACTIVITIES

I. Critical evaluation of research studies
   1. Use the "Guidelines for Evaluating a Research Report" provided in Appendix I (Section G) to evaluate the data analysis for each of the four studies you have selected to critique.
   2. If the studies were quantitative in nature, in which study:
      a. were the statistics the most clearly discussed in the text?
      b. were the tables the easiest to understand?
   3. If the studies were qualitative in nature, which study provided the most information on how the data were analyzed?
II. Writing the data analysis section of your research proposal
   1. Reread the proposals in the appendixes with special attention to the data analysis sections.
   2. Write a tentative first draft of the plan for the data analysis section of your own proposal, which includes:
      a. a description of the data analysis procedures you plan to use.
      b. dummy charts, graphs, and tables as necessary for either quantitative or qualitative data analysis.

REFERENCES

1. Cohen, B. 1984. "Florence Nightingale." *Scientific American,* 250(March): 128–137.
2. Polit, D. F., and B. P. Hungler. *Nursing Research: Principles and Methods.* Philadelphia: J. B. Lippincott, 1987, p. 534.
3. Moss, J. R., and M. J. Craft. 1989. "Visual Estimation Accuracy." *Western Journal of Nursing Research* 11(June: 352–359).
4. Rosswurm, M. A. 1989. "Assessment of Perceptual Processing Deficits in Persons with Alzheimers's Disease." *Western Journal of Nursing Research,* 11(August: 458–467.
5. Foley, J., and G. L. Stone. 1988. "Stress Inoculation with Nursing Students." *Western Journal of Nursing Research,* 10(August): 435–448.
6. Polit and Hungler, *Nursing Research,* p. 533.
7. Byers, P. H. 1986. "Infant Crying During Aircraft Descent." *Nursing Research,* 35(September–October): 260–262.
8. Kalish, P. A., B. J. Kalish, and J. Clinton. 1982. "The World of Nursing on Prime

Time Television, 1950 to 1980." *Nursing Research,* 31(November–December): 358–363.

9.   Ibid.

10. Ibid, p. 358.

11. Vanbree, N., A. D. Hollerbach, and G. P. Brooks. 1984. "Clinical Evaluation of Three Techniques for Administering Low-Dose Heparin." *Nursing Research,* 33(January–February): 15–19.

12. Jones, L. C., and S. A. Thomas. 1989. "New Fathers' Blood Pressure and Heart Rate: Relationships to Interaction with Their Newborn Infants." *Nursing Research,* 38(July–August): 237–241.

13. Sutton, T. D., and S. P. Murphy. 1989. "Stressors and Patterns of Coping in Renal Transplant Patients." *Nursing Research,* 38(January–February): 46–49.

14. O'Rourke, M. W. 1983. "Subjective Appraisal of Psychological Well Being and Self-Reports of Menstrual and Non-Menstrual Symptomatology in Employed Women." *Nursing Research,* 32(September–October): 288–292.

15. Ibid., p. 288.

16. Lynn, M. R. 1989. "Meta-Analysis: Appropriate Tool for the Integration of Nursing Research?" *Nursing Research,* 38(5): 302.

17. Broome, M. E., P. P. Lillis, and M. C. Smith. 1989. "Pain Interventions with Children: A Meta-Analysis of Research." *Nursing Research,* 38(May–June): 154–158.

18. Field, P. A., and J. M. Morse. 1985. *Nursing Research: The Application of Qualitative Approaches.* Rockville, MD: Aspen, p. 96.

19. McLain, B. R. 1988. "Collaborative Practice: A Critical Theory Perspective." *Research in Nursing and Health,* 11(December): 391–398.

20. Ibid., p. 391.

21. Wilson, H. S. 1989. "Family Caregiving for a Relative with Alzheimer's Dementia: Coping with Negative Choices." *Nursing Research,* 38(March–April): 94–98.

22. Cheon-Klessig, Y., D. Camilleri, B. J. McElmurry, and V. M. Ohlson. 1988. "Folk Medicine in the Health Practice of Hmong Refugees." *Western Journal of Nursing Research,* 10: 647–660.

23. Ibid., p. 650.

BIBLIOGRAPHY AND SUGGESTED READINGS

Brent, E. 1984. "Qualitative Computing: Approaches and Issues." *Qualitative Sociology,* 7(Spring–Summer): 360–365.

Broome, M. E., P. P. Lillis, and M. C. Smith. 1989. "Pain Interventions with Children: A Meta-Analysis of Research." *Nursing Research,* 32(September–October): 154–158.

Byers, P. H. 1986. "Infant Crying During Aircraft Descent." *Nursing Research,* 35(September–October): 260–262.

Cheon-Klessig, Y., D. Camilleri, B. J. McElmurry, and V. M. Ohlson. 1988. "Folk Medicine in the Health Practice of Hmong Refugees." *Western Journal of Nursing Research,* 10: 647–660.

Cochran, S., and J. Holliman. 1974. *Cheat Sheet for Stat.* Commerce, TX: Authors.

Cohen, Bernard. 1984. "Florence Nightingale." *Scientific American,* 250(March): 128–137.

Field, P. A., and J. M. Morse. 1985. *Nursing Research: The Application of Qualitative Approaches.* Rockville, MD: Aspen.

Foley, J., and G. L. Stone. 1988. "Stress Inoculation with Nursing Students." *Western Journal of Nursing Research,* 10(August): 435–448.

Jones, C., and S. A. Thomas. 1989. "New Fathers' Blood Pressure and Heart Rate: Relationships to Interaction with Their Newborn Infants." *Nursing Research,* 38(July–August): 237–241.

Kalish, P. A., B. J. Kalish, and J. Clinton. 1982. "The World of Nursing on Prime Time Television, 1950 to 1980." *Nursing Research,* 31(November–December): 358–363.

Knapp, R. G. 1978. *Basic Statistics for Nurses.* New York: Wiley.

Lynn, M. R. 1989. "Meta-Analysis: Appropriate Tool for the Integration of Nursing Research?" *Nursing Research,* 38(September–October): 302–305.

McLain, B. R. 1988. "Collaborative Practice: A Critical Theory Perspective." *Research in Nursing and Health,* 11(December): 391–398.

Moss, J. R., and M. J. Craft. 1989. "Visual Estimation Accuracy." *Western Journal of Nursing Research,* 10(August): 445–448.

Mullen, B., and R. Rosenthal. 1985. *Basic Meta-Analysis Procedures and Programs.* Hillsdale, NJ: Lawrence Erlbaum Associates.

Munro, B. H., M. A. Visintainer, and E. B. Page. 1986. *Statistical Methods for Health Care Research.* Philadelphia: J. B. Lippincott.

O'Rourke, M. W. 1983. "Subjective Appraisal of Psychological Well Being and Self-Reports of Menstrual and Non-Menstrual Symptomatology in Employed Women." *Nursing Research,* 32(September–October): 288–292.

Polit, D., and B. P. Hungler. 1987. *Nursing Research: Principles and Methods.* Philadelphia: J. B. Lippincott.

Rosswurm, M. A. 1989. "Assessment of Perceptual Processing Deficits in Persons with Alzheimer's Disease." *Western Journal of Nursing Research,* 11(August): 458–467.

Seidel, J. V., and J. A. Clark. 1984. "The Ethnograph: A Computer Program for the Analysis of Qualitative Data." *Qualitative Sociology,* 7(Spring–Summer): 110–125.

Siegal, S. 1956. *Nonparametric Statistics for the Behavioral Sciences.* New York: McGraw-Hill.

Spradley, J. P. 1979. *The Ethnographic Interview.* New York: Holt, Rinehart and Winston.

Stone, P. J., et al. 1966. *The General Inquirer: A Computer Approach to Content Analysis.* Cambridge, MA: MIT Press.

Sutton, T. D., and P. S. Murphy. 1989. "Stressors and Patterns of Coping in Renal Transplant Patients." *Nursing Research,* 38(September–October): 46–49.

Vanbree, N., A. D. Hollerbach, and G. P. Brooks. 1984. "Clinical Evaluation of Three Techniques of Administering Heparin." *Nursing Research,* 33(January–February): 15–19.

Wilson, H. S. 1989. "Family Caregiving for a Relative with Alzheimer's Dementia: Coping with Negative Choices." *Nursing Research,* 38(March–April): 94–98.

8

Communicating the Research Results

In the previous chapters we presented material related to Stage I of a research study, the *planning stage*. The first six steps of the research process were discussed:

1. Statement of the problem
2. Review of related literature
3. Statement of the purpose of the study
4. Definition of the terms
5. Plan for data collection
6. Plan for data analysis

During the planning stage, the investigator develops a research proposal and provides specific information on these six steps in the research process.

In Stage II of the research study, the *implementation stage*, the investigator puts the research plan into action by collecting the data and analyzing them in order to determine the study's results.

In Stage III of the research study, the *communication stage*, the investigator interprets the findings, formulates conclusions for the study, and communicates these in the written report of the completed study so that others may share the knowledge. This is the task we will discuss in Chapter 8.

INTERPRETING THE FINDINGS

The data collected in carrying out the study now need to be given meaning by the investigator, who interprets them in terms of the study's purpose. If the purpose of the study was to describe certain variables, then meaningful descriptions are indicated. If the study asked a question, the findings should be interpreted to answer this question. If a hypothesis was tested, the study findings should be interpreted as support or rejection of the hypothesis.

Data interpretation is a subjective process; the investigator must be extremely careful not to interpret beyond what the data indicate and must relate conclusions to the study purpose.

Researchers are often hesitant to report negative results of their studies. These are results that contradict the theoretical or conceptual framework or fail to support the study's hypothesis. In a well-designed research study, however, such scientifically derived results can add as much to the existing body of scientific knowledge as the results of studies where the results expected by the investigator are produced.

Sometimes a study has important and unexpected findings not related to the original purpose of the study. These are called *serendipitous findings*. The investigator needs to be aware of the possible existence of such findings and the importance of interpreting and reporting them. In order to add to existing knowledge, the investigator should also be prepared to relate the study findings to other studies in the same area. All studies have their own limitations over which the investigator has no control. These limitations and their effect on the interpretation of the data should be discussed.

Finally, because the investigator is the expert on this study, interpretation of the data should result in a discussion of implications for the practice or profession of nursing, and recommendations for further research.

WRITING THE RESEARCH REPORT

As a final step in the research process, the investigator writes a research report to make the results available and known to others.

Purposes and Characteristics

A research report has several purposes. It may communicate the research results to other investigators, in which case the report should communicate the purpose, procedures, and findings in sufficient detail so that another investigator could replicate the study. In addition, consumers of nursing research need to become aware of reported research so that they may critically analyze the findings and use them in practice.

Format

A research report should be objective, concise, and scholarly in spelling, grammar, and punctuation. Use a dictionary and a style manual when writing the report. Individual authors such as Campbell and Turabian and associations such as the American Psychological Association and the Modern Language Association have developed style manuals. Some journals have developed their own style sheets, available upon request; or the required format may be found on the journal's front or back cover.

Research reports vary from detailed reports to abridged versions for publication. The following format is suggested for preparing a detailed report.

Guidelines for Writing a Research Report

The report is divided into three major parts: (1) preliminary materials, (2) main body (text) of the report, and (3) reference materials. Each major part consists of several sections, represented in the following outline:

I. Preliminary materials
    A. Title page
    B. Table of contents
    C. List of illustrations (figures)
    D. List of tables
    E. Preface or acknowledgment (if any)
II. Main body (text) of the report
    A. Introduction
        1. Statement of the problem
        2. Review of related literature, including conceptual or theoretical framework if appropriate
        3. Purpose of the study
        4. Definition of terms
        5. Assumptions of the study
    B. Methodology
        1. Research approach
        2. Study subjects
        3. Techniques for data collection
        4. Procedures
        5. Limitations of the study

    C. Findings
        1. Data are reported and their meaning discussed.
        2. Tables, graphs, figures are included and discussed in the text.
    D. Discussion
        1. Interpretation of findings and conclusions
        2. Comparison of findings with those of other investigations
        3. Implications for nursing
        4. Recommendations for further study
    E. Summary
        1. Brief restatement of problem
        2. Brief review of procedures, major conclusions, and recommendations
III. Reference materials
    A. Bibliography
    B. Appendix(es) (if any)
    C. Glossary (if any)

Note that the main body (text) of the research report in Appendix C uses the research proposal for the study (Appendix B) through the methodology section of the report with few changes.

In the findings section of the report, the investigator reports and analyzes the data objectively. Appropriate statistical information is presented and discussed. Each table, graph, or figure used to summarize the data is discussed in the text and should be placed as close as possible to the first text reference to it.

In the discussion section of the report, data are interpreted according to the study's purpose and the study results are compared with results obtained in other studies. The investigator then formulates implications for nursing and recommendations for further research.

In the summary section, the study's most important aspects are presented in a brief restatement of the problem and the purpose of the study. A brief review of the data collection procedures and a brief summary of the major conclusions and recommendations are also included.

The bibliography section should list all the sources used to write the report. A style manual should be used to write this section. The appendix section includes materials especially designed for the study, such as cover letters or questionnaires. The raw data from the study may be included in this section.

PREPARING AN ABSTRACT OF THE STUDY

An abstract is a concise summary of the study. Although abstracts vary in length, depending on the purpose of the study, they are usually limited to 150 to 200 words.

Researchers write abstracts for several purposes. When placed at the beginning of a research report published as a journal article, an abstract presents an overview of the research problem and the methodology used, and an interpretation of the results of the study. This brief overview permits the reader to decide whether or not to read the complete article. Abstracts are also written in response to a call for papers for professional meetings, primarily to determine if the study topic is relevant to the sessions being planned for the meeting.[1] Examples of abstracts of completed research studies are presented in Appendix G.

A NOTE ON PUBLICATION

If you decide to write an article for a professional journal based on your research, it is advisable to look over current publications in the area of your study to see where it will have the best chances of being accepted. You should then write a query letter to the editor of the publication to which you would like to submit your article. This letter should include a brief statement of your own background relevant to your article, a brief description of the article you plan to write, and an outline of the article if possible. You should also request publication guidelines in your letter.

Although it is permissible to submit query letters to several publication editors at the same time, journal stipulations and professional ethics dictate that the manuscript for the final article be submitted to only one publication at a time.[2] The term *refereed* is used in connection with submitting manuscripts for publication. The referee system is a process of having three or more experts independently review and judge the merits of the manuscript before making a decision about publication:

> The implication is that refereed nursing journals are the source and repository of reliable, valid clinical papers through which the refinement of professional practice occurs—and hence, bring higher prestige to authors appearing in them than nonrefereed journals do.[3]

A final word: Do not become discouraged if your first query letter fails to elicit a positive response. Keep on trying with other journals.

A NOTE ON PRESENTATIONS

Meetings of professional organizations give researchers an opportunity to present their findings before an audience of their peers. These presentations may range from formal to quite informal sessions. In any case, certain basic guidelines should be followed.

Your paper should be prepared well in advance of the presentation. Although organizations usually request an abstract before accepting a paper, the preparation of an abstract does not mean that the entire paper is ready. It is embarrassing for both audience and presenter when it is obvious that the presenter has not mastered the information to be presented.

Be sure that any audiovisual materials that you plan to use are appropriate and that the devices needed to present them are available. If the organization does not indicate whether the necessary equipment is available, you should contact the organizers or bring your own.

Be sure that your audiovisual materials are properly arranged and organized. Slides that must be viewed upside-down or backwards, or overhead projection materials that are too small to read from the back of the room, lead audiences to boredom and presenters to frustration.

Many organizations now provide opportunities for researchers to present at poster sessions. These presentations are more informal than the presentation of a paper, but posters should be well organized and interestingly presented. Remember, the information that you have to give is important, and the amount of time and effort spent in research can be negated or trivialized if the materials are poorly organized.

The following Application Activities are designed to help you evaluate your understanding of principles and procedures related to the material in this chapter.

APPLICATION ACTIVITIES

1. Use the "Guidelines for Evaluating a Research Report" provided in Appendix I (Sections H and I) to evaluate the conclusions, recommendations, and summary sections of each of the four studies you have chosen to critique.
2. In which study:
    a. were the results most clearly described in relation to the study's purpose?
    b. was the conceptual or theoretical framework most effectively used to discuss the results?
    c. were the conclusions most clearly stated and the resulting recommendations the most plausible?
3. Evaluate each of the four studies in Section J of the "Guidelines" ("Other Considerations").
    a. Which study provides the best example of an investigator who pos-

sessed the appropriate qualifications to conduct and report the study?

b. Which study title was most appropriate?

c. Which study had the best organization and logical presentation of material?

4. Discuss your conclusions regarding the general level of acceptability for each of the four studies. You may find it useful to use the method suggested in the introduction to the "Guidelines" at the beginning of Appendix I.

REFERENCES

1. Fuller, E. 1983. "Preparing an Abstract of a Nursing Study." *Nursing Research*, 32(September–October): 316–317.
2. Brosnan, J., and A. Kovalsky. 1980. "Perishing while Publishing." *Nursing Outlook*, 28(November): 688.
3. Clayton, B. C., and K. Boyle. 1981. "The Refereed Journal: Prestige in Professional Publication." *Nursing Outlook*, 29(September): 531.

BIBLIOGRAPHY AND SUGGESTED READINGS

Brosnan, J., and A. Kovalsky. 1980. "Perishing while Publishing." *Nursing Outlook*, 28 (November): 688.

Clayton, B. C., and K. Boyle. 1981. "The Refereed Journal: Prestige in Professional Publication." *Nursing Outlook*, 29(September): 531–534.

Field, P. A., and J. M. Morse. 1985. *Nursing Research: The Application of Qualitative Approaches*. Rockville, MD: Aspen.

Fuller, E. 1983. "Preparing an Abstract of a Nursing Study." *Nursing Research*, 32(September–October): 316–317.

Gay, L. R. 1987. *Educational Research: Competencies for Analysis and Application*, 3rd ed. Columbus, OH: Charles E. Merrill.

Hagemaster, J. N., and K. M. Kerrins. 1984. "Six Easy Steps to Publishing." *Nursing Educator*, 9: 32–34.

Johnson, S. H. 1982. "Selecting a Journal." *Nursing and Health Care*, 3: 258–263.

Mirin, S. 1981. *The Nurses's Guide to Writing for Publication*. Rockville, MD: Aspen.

Notter, L. 1978. *Essentials of Nursing Research*, 2nd ed. New York: Springer.

Styles, M. 1978. "Why Publish?" *Image*, 10 (June): 28–32.

Swanson, E., and J. C. McCloskey. 1982. "The Manuscript Review Process." *Image*, 14: 72–76.

Swanson, E., and J. C. McCloskey. 1986. "Publishing Opportunities for Nurses." *Nursing Outlook*, 34: 227–235.

9

Utilizing the Research Results

RELATIONSHIP OF RESEARCH CONDUCT AND RESEARCH
   UTILIZATION
ISSUES IN RESEARCH UTILIZATION
MAJOR UTILIZATION PROJECTS
   Regional Program for Nursing Research and Development (WICHE)
      Project
   Nursing Child Assessment Satellite Training (NCAST) Projects
   Conduct and Utilization of Research in Nursing (CURN) Project
APPLICATION ACTIVITIES
REFERENCES
BIBLIOGRAPHY AND SUGGESTED READINGS

In previous chapters we have presented material related to the steps involved in the first three stages of the research process. In Stage I, the planning stage, a research proposal developed by the investigator addresses the first six steps of the research process. In Stage II, the implementation stage, the researcher activates the research plan by collecting data and analyzing them in order to determine the study's results. In Stage III, the communication stage, the investigator interprets and communicates the findings, either in a written or verbal report or in publications.

In Stage IV of the research process, the utilization stage, efforts are directed toward using the results to improve nursing practice. The material in this chapter is designed to acquaint you with current issues regarding utilization of research knowledge and the processes involved in translating valid research-based findings into the delivery of improved patient care.

RELATIONSHIP OF RESEARCH CONDUCT
AND RESEARCH UTILIZATION

Research conduct and research utilization are interdependent processes, both of which help to further the development of a scientific basis of practice for nursing: "The purpose of research is to identify and refine solutions to problems through the generation of new knowledge, while the purpose of research utilization is to get the new solutions used for the good of society. Neither process taken alone is sufficient to meet the needs of society."[1]

Research conduct is directed toward producing knowledge that is generalizable beyond the study population, whereas research utilization is directed at transferring this specific research-based knowledge into actual practice. The term *research utilization* has a simple, straightforward meaning: to use the methods and products of research. "In the most general sense, research methods and products are used to expand knowledge and to verify or change practice."[2]

The potential gap between the scientific identification of solutions to problems through research conduct and the utilization of these solutions is exemplified in the following:

> Merely imparting or transmitting the results of research is usually insufficient. For example, as a guide for future planning, one mental hospital undertook to study the effect of the furnishings in dayrooms on patients' socialization patterns. One dayroom was furnished with Swedish Modern furniture and the other with Early American. Observations over a considerable period of time showed that the patients constantly favored the room with Swedish Modern furniture; they found it more congenial and comfortable. However, when the hospital needed new furniture, the staff responsible for requisitioning new supplies paid no attention to the results of this study. They ordered what they had always ordered, Early American furniture. . . . Here was research that was not utilized. Unfortunately, this is not an uncommon kind of occurrence.[3]

As the nursing profession has come to value nursing research, the research base for nursing practice has increased over the past few years. However, there is a major time lag between the knowledge generated by research and its utilization for the improvement of nursing practice.

The 1970 report of the National Commission for the Study of Nursing and Nursing Education encouraged

> the immediate establishment of a national clearinghouse for nursing research to collect, catalogue, and distribute information on investi-

gations completed or in progress. In the case of nursing, with its pro-
found influence on the delivery of optimum health care, we must be
concerned that research findings are translated with speed into application and changed practice.[4]

In a national survey reported by Lindeman in 1975, fifteen priorities were
established that were considered to have the most significant potential for impact on the welfare of patients. "In the decade since those priorities were published, research has made strides in most of these areas. The priority item, 'Determine means for greater utilization research in practice,' however, has not
enjoyed as much success as the other priorities."[5]

Nursing is not alone in its concern with translating research findings into
practice:

> The processes of utilization in agriculture, education, industry, and
> medicine have been closely scrutinized. As a consequence, measures
> have been taken to decrease the time lag and improve the utilization
> of research findings in these fields.[6]

ISSUES IN RESEARCH UTILIZATION

Issues related to the generation of nursing research for utilization in practice
fall into several categories: those associated with the dissemination of valid
findings to receptive users; those related to the varied contexts in which nurse
scientists and nurse clinicians work; and those related to the actual utilization
of the findings in practice, specifically to determining who is expected to assume the responsibility for carrying out the activities necessary to transfer
research-based knowledge into research-based practice.

In 1972 Diers identified three barriers related to the dissemination and utilization of the findings of nursing research: (1) finding the findings; (2) finding
the good findings—that is, those findings that meet the criteria for quality research and significance to nursing practice; and (3) implementing the good
findings.[7]

Krueger et al. described the need for a systematic analysis of research
studies: "Nursing research must be made accessible by systematic identification, evaluation, and collation of generalizations."[8] These authors assert that
this is primarily the responsibility of experts in nursing practice and research—
not the individual nurse—and that the results should be made available
through published indexes and nursing journals.

In 1981 the project staff for the longitudinal study of the impact of the National Commission for the Study of Nursing and Nursing Education reported
that "one of the enduring disappointments of the Commission" is that the

efforts to establish a national clearinghouse for nursing research to be placed in the American Nurses' Foundation and supported by public funds "have been singularly unsuccessful."[9]

There are, however, several other projects that include specific strategies for the dissemination of nursing research. In 1981, Project Hope established the International Nursing Interchange (INI) which included a goal of "collection and dissemination of information on nursing practice, education and research to professionals and students through an INI data bank."[10]

Sigma Theta Tau International Honor Society of Nursing is sponsoring an internationally based storage and retrieval system for nursing researchers through the electronic library located in the Center for Nursing Scholarship. The purpose of the electronic library is to provide research dissemination by telephone to nurses who do not have easy access to library resources.

A related issue on research dissemination concerns the process of disseminating research to nurses practicing in clinical areas. Should these nurses be expected to read original research reports rather than reviews of research that summarize research findings? Do such summaries of original research discourage the professional responsibility that each nurse should have to read original research, or do they actually promote an understanding of research and facilitate transfer of research-based results? Should it be the responsibility of the original investigator to write research reports in two formats—one for the scientific community and one for the much larger group of nurses who lack the academic preparation to read and understand original research reports?[11] Although current opinion regarding the answers to these questions varies within nursing's scientific community, all agree that research findings must be disseminated to clinicians so that the current gap between the generation of research findings and their use in practice can be narrowed.

A second issue in the clinical utilization of scientific nursing knowledge is related to the varied contexts in which nurse clinicians and nurse scientists work and their different goals. Nurse clinicians provide individualized patient and family care, focusing on individual differences. Nurse scientists attempt to minimize the impact of individual differences in order to generalize results to larger groups to produce a science of nursing.[12]

A third issue in research utilization is related to the actual utilization of the findings in practice: Who is expected to assume responsibility for carrying out the activities necessary to transfer research-based knowledge into research-based nursing practice? Specifically, should individual practicing staff nurses be expected to make usable changes in their practice on the basis of knowledge gained through research, or is this an organizational responsibility?

Several surveys have shown that staff nurses were relatively unaware of research findings and that they used very little research in their practice. Ketefian's 1975 investigation of the impact of nursing research on nursing practice was designed to determine the extent to which a series of research findings on the mode of temperature determination were being used by nursing practitioners. Her conclusions demonstrated the major gap between knowledge and practice: "A clear picture emerged: The practitioner either was totally unaware of the research literature relative to her practice, or, if she was aware of it, was unable to relate to it or utilize it."[13]

Kirchhoff's 1982 report of a national survey of critical care nurses' coronary precautions revealed that the awareness of published studies had not significantly changed practice.[14]

The majority of practicing nurses have been prepared at the AA or diploma level. It is at the baccalaureate level, however, that nurses are exposed to formal nursing research content designed to prepare them to critically evaluate research studies, which is the initial step in the utilization process. In addition, there are many baccalaureate-prepared nurses who graduated before the relatively recent introduction of research into nursing curriculums. Thus, "the percentage of staff nurses who have been exposed to a nursing research course could be no greater than 10%."[15] In addition, research courses at the baccalaureate level may not include content material related to the actual process of utilizing the results of nursing research in practice.

It is obvious that the individual practicing nurse is expected to use valid research findings to provide scientifically sound patient care. However, it may not be feasible to expect that each practicing nurse will be able to identify, translate, and use relevant research findings in practice:

> The setting for nursing practice plays a large role in whether or not research is perceived as important to practice. For staff members to value research, the importance of research in improving the quality of nursing care would have to be reinforced by administration; members of the staff would have time off to attend nursing conferences, and a small library with current journals would be made available for perusal in spare moments. When few resources are available and when nurses have no voice in policy for the delivery of care, creativity and testing of ideas are rarely visible. There is no incentive for "bucking the system"; and certainly there are few rewards.[16]

At this stage in the progress of utilization of research-based knowledge in practice settings, it would seem that appropriate and effective utilization can be best accomplished through a collaborative process involving the efforts of clinicians, administrators, researchers, and educators:

> Clinicians often begin the process by identifying problem areas, and they are the ultimate users of research-based knowledge. Administrators must facilitate various types of research activities in a number of ways, ranging from providing open encouragement of staff interest to

securing the necessary support and resources. Researchers should include implications for nursing practice in their reports, and make con-
crete and practical suggestions for formatting their findings for use in
the clinical setting. Educators should assist nurses through the systematic review of research, both to help extract research-based knowledge that has validity and relevance for practice and to translate the
criteria for evaluating research findings into terms that clinicians can
use.[17]

MAJOR UTILIZATION PROJECTS

In an attempt to bridge the gap between the conduct of research and its utiliza-
tion in clinical practice, three large-scale utilization projects have received
grant support from the Division of Nursing at the federal level: (1) the Regional
Program for Nursing Research and Development Project carried out by staff
members of the Western Interstate Commission for Higher Education
(WICHE); (2) the Nursing Child Assessment Satellite Training Projects
(NCAST); and (3) the Conduct and Utilization of Research in Nursing (CURN)
Project conducted under the auspices of the Michigan Nurses' Association.

Regional Program for Nursing Research and Development (WICHE) Project

With the goal of increasing the quantity, quality, and use of nursing research
in the western United States, this regional project, headquartered in Boulder,
Colorado, was funded in 1971 by the Division of Nursing. The primary thrust
of the program was "to support collaborative research endeavors among
nurses from different settings and by both prepared and potential nurse researchers." An additional grant, funded in 1974, enabled the project staff to
begin "the first large-scale structured approach to using valid clinical nursing
research findings in the patient care setting."[18]

Three types of research groups were developed during the project: non-
targeted groups, targeted groups, and utilization groups. Each group represented a different approach to nursing research:

> The goal of non-targeted research is the generation of research
> hypotheses from care settings by nurses caring for patients. In con-
> trast to the single investigator–single institution approach that char-
> acterized nursing research in the 1960s, the non-targeted, regional ap-
> proach brings groups of nurses with different skills and backgrounds
> together. . . . The long-term goal of targeted research is to develop
> valid and reliable instruments, composed of indicators known to be

related to change in health status or level for the purpose of assessing quality of nursing care.[19]

The goal of the utilization groups was to help nurses to "locate, evaluate, choose and make plans for using research findings to change the care they provide to patients. . . . [20] Nurses from the western region met in a series of workshops to develop plans for basing changes in nursing care in their own settings on research findings. Dracup and Breu's article "Using Nursing Research Findings to Meet the Needs of Grieving Spouses" (1978) is a report of their own experiences with a utilization project in a coronary care setting developed at one of the regional workshops. In 1978, Krueger et al. provided the following recommendation regarding this large-scale research utilization project: "On the basis of the experience gained in this project, it is apparent that it was ahead of its proper time. When and if nursing research is identified, evaluated, and collated systematically, this project should be repeated on local levels in such a way that it is available to all nurses."[21]

Nursing Child Assessment Satellite Training (NCAST) Projects

Three projects were carried out between 1976 and 1985 with the purpose of translating and disseminating research findings to increase the practicing nurse's awareness of new research and the value of using research in practice. The first project (1976–1978) tested the use of a communications satellite for rapid dissemination of new research results that focused on new assessment techniques in child health. The second NCAST project (1978–1983) provided learners with videotaped parent–child interactions with which to practice assessments. The objective of the third NCAST Project (1983–1985) was to teach public health nurses to use a nursing protocol for the follow-up care of preterm infants and their families.[22]

Conduct and Utilization of Research in Nursing (CURN) Project

This five-year research development project was funded by the Division of Nursing on the federal level from 1975 to 1980. The Michigan Nurses' Association conducted the project with the assistance of faculty and graduate students at the University of Michigan School of Nursing, the Institute for Social Research, and the Michigan State University School of Nursing. The purpose of the project was to improve the practice of nursing through two types of activities: (1) the utilization of existing research findings in the daily practice of registered nurses, and (2) the design and conduct of research that was directly relevant and could be readily transferred to nursing practice.[23]

Thirty-four departments of nursing in hospitals throughout Michigan assisted the CURN Project staff. The research utilization process developed and used by the project's staff consisted of a systematic series of activities that included (1) the identification and synthesis of multiple research studies in a common conceptual area (research base), (2) the transformation of the knowledge derived from a research base into a solution or clinical protocol, (3) the transformation of the clinical protocol into specific nursing actions (innovations) that are administered to patients, and (4) a clinical evaluation of the new practice to ascertain whether it produced the predicted result.[24]

Ten research-based practice protocols were developed by CURN Project personnel:

1. Preventing Decubitus Ulcers
2. Structured Preoperative Teaching[25]
3. Clean Intermittent Catheterization
4. Intravenous Cannula Change
5. Reducing Diarrhea in Tube-Fed Patients
6. Closed Urinary Drainage Systems
7. Distress Reduction Through Sensory Preparation
8. Preoperative Sensory Preparation to Promote Recovery
9. Mutual Goal Setting in Patient Care
10. Pain: Deliberative Nursing Interventions

Each protocol has been published as a separate book (see CURN Project, *Using Research to Improve Nursing Practice,* in the Bibliography and Suggested Readings at the end of this chapter). An additional book (Horsley et al., 1981) provides a guide for implementation of the protocols. Each protocol in the series contains (1) information regarding the need for the change (innovation); (2) a description of the innovation; (3) a summary of the research base provided by the conceptually related research studies that met specific criteria developed by CURN Project personnel; (4) a description of research-based principles (empirical generalizations) guiding the implementation of the innovation; and (5) a description of the implementation and the systematic evaluation of its effects. Each protocol contains a summary of the benefits to be anticipated from successful use of the innovation, as well as additional pertinent materials.

In an effort to determine the extent of use of the CURN models in the practice setting, Brett used research journals and the CURN publications to identify fourteen nursing research findings that meet the CURN project criteria for clinical use.[26] She then surveyed nurses practicing in small, medium, and large hospitals to determine the extent of their awareness of, persuasion about, and use of these research findings. All of the 216 respondents were employed full time and were responsible for the direct care of patients. Eighty-six percent were staff nurses and 14 percent were head nurses. Brett concluded: "The majority of nurses were aware of the average innovation, were persuaded about it, and use the average innovation at least sometimes."[27]

In 1987, Goode and her colleagues described how they used the CURN protocols to utilize research-based knowledge in their own hospital.[28] The already active audit committee was charged by the nursing administrator with reviewing, discussing, and evaluating findings from current research and making recommendations regarding using the research findings in their own hospital. The authors provide three examples of completed research utilization projects. The first project they selected was temperature taking because not only did they want to start with an aspect of patient care to which all of their nurses could relate, but also there was concern about the basis for low temperature readings by the procedure currently in use. As a result of a review and evaluation of the research literature related to temperature taking, the committee found substantial support for making changes in the hospital policies and the procedures for temperature taking. They learned from this project that "Just because that is the way we've always done it is not reason enough to explain our practice."[29]

Subsequent utilization protocols were developed for preoperative teaching about coughing, deep breathing, and exercise and for a standardized teaching program on breast feeding. The authors concluded: "We are in our fifth year of work and the number of utilization projects is increasing. We hope this article encourages nurses to begin research utilization projects. There is nothing more rewarding than instituting a protocol based upon research that improves patient outcomes."[30]

This group of nurses has produced two videotapes based on their utilization experience: *Using Research in Clinical Nursing Practice* (1987) and *Research Utilization: A Process of Organizational Change* (1989).

The CURN protocols provide a model for developing research-based innovation protocols for nursing practice and represent a significant step in transferring research-based scientific knowledge into clinical nursing practice. In addition, "In retrieving, reviewing, and organizing studies into areas of conceptually related research, the [CURN] project staff has developed a system that could well be the backbone of a complete clearinghouse for nursing research into client care."[31]

In summary, research utilization, the final step in the research process, is concerned with using research to improve nursing practice. Efforts toward systematic utilization of the results of research within organizational settings are in the early stages, but several models exist that could serve as guides.

The following Application Activities are designed to help you evaluate your understanding of principles and procedures related to this material.

APPLICATION ACTIVITIES

   I. Dissemination of research findings
       1. Discuss the major benefits and obstacles that you see in the recommendation to identify, evaluate, collate, and publish the findings of nursing research studies.

    2. Who should assume the responsibility for implementing this recommendation? Why?

II. Utilization of research findings in practice

    1. Select two of the CURN protocols that interest you enough to investigate them and explain how the research-based principle in each protocol is really an empirical generalization derived from the research base for each of the protocols.

    2. Select a clinical setting and investigate the extent of knowledge and/or use of the CURN protocols in this setting.

III. Critical evaluation and utilization of research reports

    1. Use the "Guidelines for Evaluating a Research Report" provided in Appendix I to formulate your conclusions regarding the feasibility of utilizing the findings of the study for each of the four studies you have chosen to critique.

    2. Formulate your recommendations regarding the process you would use to utilize the results of one study to initiate change in a practice setting.

REFERENCES

1. Horsley, J. A., J. Crane, M. Crabtree, and D. Wood. 1981. *Using Research to Improve Nursing Practice: A Guide.* New York: Grune and Stratton, pp. 1–2.
2. Horsley, J. 1985. "Using Research in Practice: The Current Context." *Western Journal of Nursing Research,* 7: 135.
3. Halpert, H. 1966. "Communications as a Basic Tool in Promoting Utilization of Research Findings." *Community Mental Health Journal,* 2(Fall): 231.
4. National Commission for the Study of Nursing and Nursing Education. 1970. *An Abstract for Action.* New York: McGraw-Hill, p. 86.
5. Mercer, R. 1984. "Nursing Research: The Bridge to Excellence in Practice." *Image,* 16(Spring): 47.
6. Burns, N., and S. K. Grove. 1987. *The Practice of Nursing Research: Conduct, Critique and Utilization.* Philadelphia: Saunders, p. 627.
7. Diers, D. 1972. "Application of Research to Nursing Practice." *Image,* 5: 7–11.
8. Krueger, J., A. Nelson, and M. O. Wolanin. 1978. *Nursing Research: Development, Collaboration and Utilization.* Germantown, PA: Aspen Systems, p. 337.
9. Lysaught, J. 1981. *Action in Affirmation.* New York: McGraw-Hill, p. 62.
10. "International Nursing Exchange Established." 1981. *Image,* 13(June): 42.
11. Cronenwett, L. R. 1988. "Disseminating Research to Clinicians." *CNR,* 15: 1, 3.
12. Horsley et al. *Using Research to Improve Nursing Practice,* pp. xiii–xiv.
13. Ketefian, S. 1975. "Application of Selected Research Findings in Nursing Practice: A Pilot Study." *Nursing Research,* 24(March–April): 91.
14. Kirchhoff, K. 1982. "A Diffusion Survey of Coronary Precautions." *Nursing Research,* 31(July–August): 196–201.
15. Kirchoff, K. 1983. "Using Research in Practice: Should Staff Nurses Be Expected to Use Research?" *Western Journal of Nursing Research,* 5: 246.
16. Mercer, R. 1984. "Nursing Research: The Bridge to Excellence in Practice." *Image,* 16(Spring): 47.

17. Hefferin, E., J. Horsley, and M. Venturn. 1982. "Promoting Research-Based Nursing: The Nurse Administrator's Role." *Journal of Nursing Administration,* May: 41.

18. Lindeman, C., and J. Kreuger. 1977. "Increasing the Quality, Quantity, and the Use of Nursing Research." *Nursing Outlook,* 25(July): 450.

19. Ibid., pp. 450–452.

20. J. Krueger, A. Nelson, and M. Wolanin. 1978. *Nursing Research: Development, Collaboration and Utilization.* Germantown, PA: Aspen Systems, p. 20.

21. Ibid., p. 337.

22. Crane, J. 1985. "Using Research in Practice: Research Utilization—Nursing Models." *Western Journal of Nursing Research,* 7: 494–497.

23. Krone, K., and M. Loomis. 1982. "Developing Practice-Related Research: A Model That Worked." *Journal of Nursing Administration,* April: 38.

24. Horsley et al., *Using Research to Improve Practice,* p. 2.

25. Four of the studies listed as Suggested Readings for critical evaluation at the end of Chapter 3 make up the research base for this protocol (Felton et al.; Fortin and Kirouac; Johnson et al.; Lindeman and Van Aernam).

26. Brett, J. L. L. 1987. "Use of Nursing Practice Research Findings." *Nursing Research,* 36(November–December): 344–349.

27. Ibid., p. 344.

28. Goode, J. C., et al. 1987. "Use of Research Based Knowledge in Clinical Practice." *Journal of Nursing Administration,* 17(December): 11–18.

29. Ibid., p. 13.

30. Ibid., p. 17.

31. Lysaught, *Action in Affirmation,* p. 64.

BIBLIOGRAPHY AND SELECTED READINGS

Barnard, K. 1980. "Knowledge for Practice: Directions for the Future." *Nursing Research,* 29(July): 208–212.

Bennis, W., K. Beene, R. Chin, and K. Corey. 1977. *The Planning of Change.* New York: Holt, Rinehart and Winston.

Brett, J. L. L. 1987. "Use of Nursing Practice Research Findings." *Nursing Research,* 36(November–December): 344–349.

Burns, N., and S. K. Grove. 1987. *The Practice of Nursing Research: Conduct, Critique and Utilization.* Philadelphia: W. B. Saunders.

Champion, V. L., and A. Leach. 1989. "Variables Related to Research Utilization in Nursing: An Empirical Investigation." *Journal of Advanced Nursing,* 14: 705–710.

Crane, J. 1985. "Using Research in Practice. Research Utilization: Theoretical Perspectives." *Western Journal of Nursing Research,* 7(May): 261–268.

Crane, J. 1985. "Using Research in Practice: Research Utilization—Nursing Models." *Western Journal of Nursing Research,* 7(November): 494–497.

Cronenwett, L. R. 1988. "Disseminating Research to Clinicians." *CRN,* 15: 3, 5.

CURN Project. *Using Research to Improve Nursing Practice.* New York: Grune and Stratton. Series of Clinical Protocols:

Clean Intermittent Catheterization (1982)

Closed Urinary Drainage Systems (1981)

Distress Reduction through Sensory Preparation (1981)

Intravenous Cannula Change (1981)

Mutual Goal Setting in Patient Care (1982)
Pain: Deliberative Nursing Intervention (1982)
Preoperative Sensory Preparation to Promote
    Recovery (1981)
Preventing Decubitus Ulcers (1981)
Reducing Diarrhea in Tube-Fed Patients (1981)
Structured Preoperative Teaching (1981)

Diers, D. 1972. "Application of Research to Nursing Practice." *Image*, 5: 7–11.

Dracup, K. A., and C. S. Breu. 1978. "Using Nursing Research Findings to Meet the Needs of Grieving Spouses." *Nursing Research*, 27(July–August): 212–216.

Duffy, M. E. 1985. "Research Utilization: What's It All About?" *Nursing and Allied Health Care*, 6(November): 474–475.

Fawcett, J. 1982. "Utilization of Nursing Research Findings." *Image*, 14(June): 57–59.

Fawcett, J. 1984. "Another Look at Utilization of Nursing Research." *Image*, 16(Spring): 59–62.

Feldman, H. 1981. "Nursing Research in the 1980s: Issue and Implications." *Advances in Nursing Science*, 3(October): 85–92.

Goode, C. J., M. K. Lovett, J. E. Hayes, and L. A. Butcher. 1987. "Use of Research Based Knowledge in Clinical Practice." *Journal of Nursing Administration*, 17(December): 11–18.

Gould, D. 1986. "Pressure Sore Prevention and Treatment: An Example of Nurses' Failure to Implement Research Findings." *Journal of Advanced Nursing*, 11: 389–394.

Haller, K. B., M. A. Reynolds, and J. A. Horsley. 1979. "Developing Research-Based Innovation Protocols: Process, Criteria and Issues." *Research in Nursing and Health*, 2: 45–51.

Halpert, H. 1966. "Communications as a Basic Tool in Promoting Utilization of Research Findings." *Community Mental Health Journal*, 2(Fall): 231.

Hefferin, E., J. Horsley, and M. Venturn. 1982. "Promoting Research-Based Nursing: The Nurse Administrator's Role." *Journal of Nursing Administration*, May: 34–41.

Hinshaw, A. S., et al. 1987. "Research Challenges for Practice Settings." *Journal of Nursing Administration*, 17(July–August): 20–26.

Horsley, J. A., J. Crane, and J. D. Bingle. 1978. "Research Utilization as an Organizational Process." *Journal of Nursing Administration*, 8(July): 4–6.

Horsley, J. A., J. Crane, M. Crabtree, and D. Wood. 1981. *Using Research to Improve Nursing Practice: A Guide*. New York: Grune and Stratton.

Horsley, J. A. 1985. "Using Research in Practice: The Current Context." *Western Journal of Nursing Research*, 7: 135.

Hunt, M. 1987. "The Process of Translating Research Findings into Nursing Practice." *Journal of Advanced Nursing*, 12: 101–110.

———. 1981. "International Nursing Exchange Established." *Image*, 13(June): 42.

Ketefian, Shaké. 1975. "Application of Selected Research Findings into Nursing Practice: A Pilot Study." *Nursing Research*, 24(March–April): 89–92.

King, D., K. E. Barnard, and R. Hoehn. 1981. "Disseminating the Results of Nursing Research." *Nursing Outlook*, 29(March): 164–169.

Kirchhoff, K. 1982. "A Diffusion Survey of Coronary Precautions." *Nursing Research*, 31(July–August): 196–201.

———. 1983. "Using Research in Practice: Should Staff Nurses Be Expected to Use Research?" *Western Journal of Nursing Research*, 5: 246.

Krone, K., and M. Loomis. 1982. "Developing Practice-Related Research: A Model that Worked." *Journal of Nursing Administration*, April: 38.

Krueger, J. C. 1979. "Research Utilization." *Western Journal of Nursing Research,* 1: 148–152.

――――. 1982. "Using Research in Practice: A Survey of Research Utilization in Community Health Nursing." *Western Journal of Nursing Research,* 4: 244–248.

Krueger, J. C., A. Nelson, and M. Wolanin. 1978. *Nursing Research: Development, Collaboration and Utilization.* Germantown, PA: Aspen Systems.

Lindeman, C., and J. Krueger. 1977. "Increasing the Quality, Quantity, and the Use of Nursing Research." *Nursing Outlook,* 25(July): 450.

――――. 1984. "Dissemination of Nursing Research." *Image,* 16(Spring): 57–58.

Loomis, M. E. 1985. "Knowledge Utilization and Research Utilization in Nursing." *Image,* 17(Spring): 35–39.

Lysaught, J. 1981. *Action in Affirmation.* New York: McGraw-Hill.

Mercer, R. 1984. "Nursing Research: The Bridge to Excellence in Practice." *Image,* 16(Spring): 47–51.

Miller, J. R., and S. R. Messenger. 1978. "Obstacles to Applying Nursing Research Findings." *American Journal of Nursing,* April: 632–634.

National Commission for the Study of Nursing and Nursing Education. 1970. *An Abstract for Action.* New York: McGraw-Hill.

Rettig, F. M. 1981. "Assessing Research for Clinical Use." *AORN Journal,* 33: 873–881.

"Sigma Theta Tau 10 Year Action Plan Strategies." 1982. *Image,* 14(February–March): 3.

Stetler, C. B. 1985. "Research Utilization: Defining the Concept." *Image,* 17(Spring): 40–44.

Ward, M., and S. Moran. 1984. "Resistance to Change: Recognize, Respond, Overcome." *Nursing Management,* 15 (January): 30–33.

Part Three

Data Collection Methods
for the Research Process

THE MATERIAL IN PART III is designed to provide you with the principles and techniques for these three major approaches to data collection: the historical research approach (Chapter 10); the descriptive research approach (Chapter 11); and the experimental research approach (Chapter 12).

10

The Historical Research Approach

Nursing is both a very young profession and a very old one. Even before Greek and Roman soldiers were carried home on their shields—sometimes dead and sometimes wounded—someone has always been charged with the care of the ill or injured.

Before 1859 and the Crimean War, nurses of either sex were often camp followers, prostitutes, and thieves. Florence Nightingale's heroic ministrations to the sick and wounded British soldiers helped to raise nursing to the respectability it enjoys today. However, this respectability did not come about simply as a result of Nightingale's work. Many more subtle battles have been fought against those individuals who have deeply resented the rapid changing of the traditional nursing role.

We do not wish to chronicle Nightingale's life or those of any other heroic characters of nursing. This brief introduction to the founding of modern nursing is intended to set the scene for an examination of the techniques of historical research.

THE NATURE OF HISTORICAL RESEARCH

Historical research deals with what has happened in the past and how those events affect the present. No professional group is more in the forefront of world history than nursing. By its very nature, nursing is always where the action is. Nurses have been active in all areas of the world both in times of conflict and in times of peace, yet nursing history has tended to center around a few semimythologized individuals.

The lives and times of these individuals are important to nursing, but historical research is more than the discovery and adulation of famous individuals. Historical research covers all people and events. Historians piece together the lives of less well known and less controversial individuals to get a picture of the actual lives and times of an era. The historian uses these data to determine the impact of history on the present and occasionally tries to predict the future on the basis of this knowledge.

METHODOLOGY

Essentially, the historian follows the same kind of research format as any other researcher. First, the problem to be investigated must be selected and formulated within the context of existing knowledge and theory. For a historical research study, a hypothesis may be tested. Like any other researcher, the historical researcher must be particularly careful in gathering and interpreting data and in drawing conclusions based on those data. Historical research lends itself to the acceptance of evidence that is hard to verify. The careful researcher must do the utmost to corroborate data and to demonstrate their reliability and validity. Data sources available to the historical researcher fall into two categories, secondary and primary.

SECONDARY DATA SOURCES

Secondary sources are the least trustworthy. They are of two basic types: (1) interpretations by someone else of documented data and (2) hearsay.

Interpretations

The use of interpretations by someone else of documented data is fraught with peril. Historical researchers depend on another person's private frame of reference for information. This means that their interpretations may or may not be totally correct. Just as a television commercial can tell you that almost 50 percent of the people polled preferred one product over another product (leaving out the fact that *more* than 50 percent did not prefer this product), so, too, the historical researcher may choose to emphasize those facts and data that fit his or her hypothesis. This is not good research, but it does exist and can lead to further misinterpretation of data. In fact, the farther a researcher is from the original historical data, the greater the chance of misinterpretation. It is crucial that the historical researcher go back to the original sources whenever possible. The bibliography and footnotes of secondary sources often lead to primary sources, which can then be checked for accuracy of interpretation and used for gathering additional data. No secondary source, no matter how carefully prepared, can provide a total interpretation of all the data. All historians must select and interpret from a variety of sources.

Hearsay

The second, and possibly the most naive, secondary source is hearsay evidence. Hearsay is simply what people think they heard or, even worse, the extension of unproved rumors and gossip. We all know how easy it is to misinterpret and pass along incorrect information. The classic example is the gossip game, in which a group of people sit in a circle and one person starts by whispering a sentence or phrase to the next person. The message is then passed around the circle until it comes back to its original source. It is always interesting to discover how the message has changed along the way. Historical researchers must be extremely careful when dealing with hearsay data. It may be old and valuable or it may totally misrepresent the facts. Every effort must be made to corroborate any piece of hearsay data and to place it into proper historical perspective.

PRIMARY DATA SOURCES

Primary data are of far greater value and importance to the historian than secondary data. Primary data can be found in many forms and in many places.

Oral History

One of the most exciting current historical movements is called *oral history*. With the advent of modern electronic devices, such as the audio- or videotape recorder, it is possible to record the remembrances of older members of the professional community, thus providing records of what took place in past times and in specific places. These older people are invaluable resources and, as they die, their information is lost forever.

Essentially, oral historians transcribe the tapes and reproduce the conversations in writing. These data must be carefully screened, but they do provide an important *primary source*. The oral historian should plan a list of questions for the interviewee to help start the conversation off and to keep it on the subject. The historian should also get permission to reproduce this information. Many things may be said off the record, but they are of no value to the historian. Only evidence for the record can be utilized.

Life History

Life histories or career histories are an extension of the oral history technique. The proposal in Appendix A is designed to elicit a career history of one individual who had a significant impact on the field of nursing.

When researchers gather life or career histories from several individuals who are contemporaries, the researchers can go beyond discussing the lives of the individuals and begin to interpret and discuss the whole cultural milieu in which these individuals worked and lived. For example, if one source says that a certain organization or individual was helpful in developing his or her career, the information is useful only insofar as it relates to that individual. But if a number of individuals name the same organization or individual as influential, the researcher can then draw a broader conclusion.

Published Sources

Published sources are valuable to the historical researcher. There is an increasing trend to store old newspapers, journals, magazines, and other published material on one of the various microform sources. This means that the historical researcher does not have to travel great distances to get to the few remaining copies of the material. Rather, a microform copy can be ordered from the producer and reviewed by using a microform reader, which is readily available in most college and university libraries and in an increasing number of public libraries. The listings available can be found in *Microforms in Print*.

Other published sources available are the original documents themselves. Many items of interest to nurses and nursing can be found in popular literature either in the form of articles about nurses and nursing or as fictional representations of nurses and their role. Early items are indexed in *Poole's Index* and the *Readers' Guide to Periodical Literature*. Neither of these may contain a complete listing, but both will aid in the library search.

Government documents are an excellent source for the historical researcher. Many governments have compiled enormous quantities of official records and documents. In addition to the national government, state and local governments also abound with records. Many source data have been lost over the years as county courthouses and other document repositories have burned accidentally. Yet many other promising avenues of research are open to the researcher who is not afraid of the dust and grime usually found in these seldom-used sources.

Diaries

Diaries can provide an invaluable source of documentation. These are often handed down from generation to generation in a family; the researcher must locate families who still have these documents in their possession and are willing to share their intimate contents. Diary research requires judicious questioning and a substantial amount of careful exploration.

Historical Societies

Often, there will be a local historical group that a researcher can contact. These groups are justifiably proud of the community's history and can provide access to many documents and to individuals with specific knowledge. All of this can be invaluable to an outside researcher.

Official Minutes

Obviously, the availability of minutes and records of meetings is important. It is wise to remember, however, that the minutes of meetings usually reflect an abridged version of what really happened. Acrimonious debate or nonvoted issues often are not shown in minutes. Remember, each legislator has the privilege of editing what he or she has said on the floor of the U.S. House or Senate before such speeches are finally placed in the *Congressional Record*. Thus, the speeches we read are not necessarily verbatim reports of what was actually said.

Audio and Visual Recordings

Current technology has made a great deal of audio and visual source materials available. Records, tape and wire recordings, and film and videotapes all provide invaluable historical insight. Much of this material may be rare and hard to obtain. Locating appropriate sources can be a tedious yet fascinating job.

Eyewitnesses

Eyewitness accounts are always useful. Written eyewitness accounts may be found in newspapers, as oral history, or in diaries. It is crucial that eyewitness accounts receive corroboration from other sources because such accounts may report only a small part of the whole.

Pictorial Sources

Still photographs and other pictorial sources, such as sketches, are extremely valuable items. Certainly Matthew Brady and the other photographers of the American Civil War provided visual portraits of times and places that could only be imagined if we had nothing more than the written documents. Again, even as personal diaries are rich resources, so are family picture albums. They can be used to find out a great deal about the history of a group of people in any locality.

Other Print Sources

Other valid source materials for historical research might be old telephone books and directories, catalogues of local businesses and national concerns, and accounting books and bank records.

Physical Evidence

Do not ignore physical evidence of change throughout the years. For example, there have been many alterations in the various types of equipment used by nurses. Many of the products of technical change that have been added to the repertoire of nursing can be used as source materials for historical research.

COMPUTERS AND HISTORICAL RESEARCH

Like other researchers, historical researchers are turning more and more to the computer for help. In some instances, the computer can be used to locate and reprint historical documents. Some historians have examined numerical data statistically and have drawn conclusions about the conditions of individuals in a given historical period. This use of statistical methodology is called *cliometrics*. Sometimes this method has been used to demonstrate that certain cherished ideas were incorrect. As a consequence, the use of the computer in historical research is somewhat controversial.

VALIDITY AND RELIABILITY

In all cases, the historical researcher must question the reliability and validity of sources by applying both *internal* and *external* criticism to the written document. External criticism deals with the validity of the document: Is it really what it purports to be? Internal criticism deals with the reliability or accuracy of the information. Some of the questions that should be asked include: Is this document consistent with other documents written by this person? Does it have the same style? Does the style match the style of the time? Are the spelling and handwriting consistent with the time? Is what the document saying true? It is very easy to fool a naive researcher with manufactured documents like the so-called Hitler diaries. Caution must be the watchword when dealing with historical material.

In this chapter we discussed the principles and techniques of historical research. Discovering the past through careful documentation can provide many important insights into the present.

APPLICATION ACTIVITY

Reread the historical research proposal in Appendix A. Notice how the researcher carefully delineates her topic and provides careful checks on the validity and reliability of her oral historical data sources to provide accurate data interpretation. Note also how the researcher focuses on primary sources and defends her uses of such sources, while being aware of the potential hazards of historical research. The abstract in Appendix G provides a summary of the results of the completed study.

BIBLIOGRAPHY AND SUGGESTED READINGS

Austen, A. L. 1957. *History of Nursing Sourcebook.* New York: G. P. Putnam's Sons.

Baly, M. 1986. *Florence Nightingale and the Nursing Legacy.* London: Routledge, Chapman and Hall.

Benjamin, J. R. 1975. *A Student's Guide to History.* New York: St. Martin's Press.

Bogue, A. G. 1983. *Clio and the Bitch Goddess: Quantification in American Political History.* Beverly Hills, CA: Sage.

Christy, T. E. 1975. "The Methodology of Historical Research." *Nursing Research,* 24 (May–June): 189–192.

Clark, G. 1969. *Guide for Research Students Working on Historical Subjects,* 2nd ed. London: Cambridge University Press.

Dingwall, R., and C. W. Rafferty. 1988. *An Introduction to the Social History of Nursing.* London: Routledge.

Dock, L. L. 1912. *A History of Nursing.* New York: G. P. Putnam's Sons.

Dock, L. L., and I. Stewart. 1920. *A Short History of Nursing.* New York: G. P. Putnam's Sons.

Fairman, Julie A. 1987. "Sources and References for Research in Nursing History." *Nursing Research,* 36(January–February): 56–59.

Hawkins, J. W. 1987. *The Historical Evolution of Theories and Conceptual Models for Nursing.* Educational Resources Information Center (ERIC) ED 284969.

History of American Nursing Series. New York: Garland Press.

Jones, A. H., Ed. 1987. *Images of Nurses: Perspectives from History, Art and Literature.* Philadelphia: University of Pennsylvania Press.

Kalish, P. A., and B. J. Kalish. 1986. *The Advance of American Nursing,* 2nd ed. Boston: Little, Brown.

Lagermann, E. C., Ed. 1983. *Nursing History: New Perspectives, New Possibilities.* New York: Teachers College, Columbia University.

Moore, J. 1988. *A Zeal for Responsibility.* Athens: University of Georgia.

Rice, M. H., and W. M. Stallings. 1986. *Florence Nightingale, Statistician: Implications for Teachers of Educational Research.* Educational Resources Information Center (ERIC) ED 269452.

Roberts, M. M. 1954. *American Nursing: History and Interpretation.* New York: Macmillan.

Rosenberg, C. 1987. ''Clio and Caring: An Agenda for American Historians and Nursing.'' *Nursing Research,* 36 (January–February): 67–68.

11

The Descriptive Research Approach

This material covers the descriptive research approach and the techniques and tools most frequently used to gather data needed to study present conditions.

THE NATURE OF DESCRIPTIVE RESEARCH

The *descriptive research approach* describes what now exists, but the term is not completely appropriate. Description is also involved in the other two approaches: *Historical research* describes the past, and *experimental research* describes what happens to selected variables in order to predict what will happen as other variables are manipulated by the investigator. *Descriptive research* is used here to refer to research questions based on the present state of affairs and yields both quantitative and qualitative data. Such research may generate new knowledge beyond the study's specific subjects or elements.

DESCRIPTIVE RESEARCH TECHNIQUES

The techniques for gathering data about present conditions are intended to provide information that can be analyzed either quantitatively or qualitatively. The techniques most often used to study present conditions, which can be used to study contrasts (differences), comparisons (likenesses), and relationships, include the following:

1. Electrical and mechanical devices
2. Questionnaires
3. Interviews
4. Rating scales
5. Content analysis
6. Use of available data
7. Unobtrusive measures
8. Nonwritten records
9. Proxemics and kinesics
10. Case studies
11. Psychological and projective tests
12. Sociometrics
13. Delphi technique
14. Observation
15. Phenomenology
16. Ethnography
17. Grounded theory

Each of these techniques will be discussed in greater detail in the following pages.

Electrical and Mechanical Devices to Measure Physiological Responses

By its very nature, nursing research lends itself to the use of highly accurate physiological measurements. There are an increasing number of sophisticated measuring devices available to determine physiological responses. Of course, the classical mechanical devices, such as the sphygmomanometer and the stethoscope, have been developed and refined over many years. In addition, many electronic devices, such as the electrocardiograph, the electroencephalograph, and other instruments, are now available.

As in all research dealing with human subjects, when mechanical or electrical devices are used, researchers have the ethical responsibility to obtain informed consent and to explain the purpose of any device that is used to determine patients' responses. It is extremely frightening to be attached to a mechanical device of some kind without knowing why.

Questionnaires

The term *survey research* is often used to refer to the collection of data about present conditions directly from the study subjects. The most common techniques for survey research are the questionnaire and the interview.

A *questionnaire* is a paper-and-pencil instrument completed by the study subjects themselves. In survey research, the questionnaire is often mailed to the respondents, although it might be administered face to face. An *opinionnaire* is a questionnaire designed to elicit the subjects' opinions. The term *interview* refers to verbal questioning of respondents by the investigator in order to collect data. The interview may be conducted either face to face or by telephone.

Nursing researchers have developed many survey instruments—primarily questionnaires—over the years. The respondents may be nurses, patients, patients' relatives, or doctors, among many alternatives. These survey instruments have been designed to examine attitudes, opinions, feelings, and facts concerning certain areas of nursing. Such instruments can accurately reflect these opinions, feelings, and facts only if they are well developed, well administered, and carefully interpreted.

Longitudinal Studies.   Some investigators with long-term interests use the same measuring instrument repeatedly in order to determine responses on a topic and pinpoint trends and issues. Such studies, known as *longitudinal studies,* are designed to collect data from the same people at regularly stated intervals, ranging from a few days to weeks, months, or even years.

Cross-Sectional Studies.   The vast majority of surveys, however, are one-time *cross-sectional studies.* They study certain aspects of responses of individuals at a certain point in time and are seldom, if ever, conducted again. This is unfortunate because it leads to a proliferation of data-gathering instruments, some of which may not be very good. In addition, the lack of repeated measurement over time prevents the analysis of trends concerning various issues.

Researchers use surveys to gather information from a representative sample of a population. The researcher can specify the location of the population, such as all patients admitted to the emergency room of hospital XYZ, or only those patients admitted to the emergency room between the hours of noon and midnight. Such specificity allows for the use of probability sampling techniques; with good statistical analysis, generalizations can be drawn about the whole population. As discussed in Chapter 6, the researcher who is developing a research proposal must take care to ensure an accurate description of the target population as well as the sample. Whether the population is 24- to 27-year-old postpartum mothers with female infants or any other of the large number of possible combinations, the best research defines specifically who will be surveyed.

With these ideas in mind, we will now describe the steps in designing and carrying out survey research using questionnaires.

Development and Administration.   First, as with any research study, an appropriate research question or problem must be established. The problem statement and the purpose of the study should guide the selection of an appropriate survey research design and the choice of a measuring instrument that meets the criteria of validity, reliability, and usability, as discussed in Chapter 6. The following principles apply to self-developed questionnaires constructed by the investigator for a specific study.

In constructing a questionnaire, care must be exercised so that the items will allow the respondents to provide the information that relates to the study problem and to the purpose of the study. The theoretical or conceptual framework should provide the rationale for the development of the questionnaire.

Questionnaires are constructed to be either open-ended or closed. Open-ended questionnaires allow the respondents a variety of ways to answer questions and permit the researcher to make inferences from the responses to the questions. Closed questionnaires allow for certain structured answers—''yes,'' ''no,'' or a limited selection of choices. Because most survey researchers want to expedite the coding of data and eliminate ambiguity, they usually opt for a closed questionnaire.

The questionnaire must be clear and unambiguous. We tend to assume that people understand what we are talking about, but the naive respondent may not have the same frame of reference as the researcher. The question ''Are the chickens ready to eat?'' is a good example of the ambiguous use of our language. Any question that could have multiple interpretations should also be avoided.

The wording of questions should be concise. Avoid asking a wordy question when a brief one will do. Respondents not familiar with the vocabulary will not give accurate or valid answers. At the same time, respect the respondent's intelligence. This means walking a fine line. The more confusion or mistrust the instrument causes, the less chance there will be that the respondent will return the questionnaire.

Keep the instrument as simple and short as possible. There is something very threatening about an instrument with many pages and a multiplicity of choices. The shorter the instrument (within reason), the more likely it will be completed and returned. Be sure to put relatively simple questions at the beginning of the instrument, allowing the respondent to succeed and be reinforced to continue.

Provide cross-check questions in order to be sure that the respondent is answering consistently. Rewording the same question and asking it again, either positively or negatively, is a good way to provide this insurance, but questions should be sufficiently separated so that the subject will not see through this technique.

Finally, careful development of the instructions for the respondent involves a clear statement of what you want the respondent to do. Validity and reliability must be determined by using any one of the techniques described in Chapter 6. We strongly recommend that a pretest of the questionnaire be conducted in order to correct any problem with the questionnaire before it is administered to the study subjects.

Researchers should probably spend more time formulating their questionnaires than they do analyzing their research data. Well-constructed questionnaires allow for relatively easy interpretation and analysis. Poorly developed questionnaires may cost more in time and effort and prevent the investigator from achieving the purpose of the study.

Mailed questionnaires are answered in much larger numbers if a self-addressed, stamped envelope is included with each questionnaire. Most people are willing to respond but unwilling to subsidize the researcher. If a follow-up letter is sent, it may be wise to send yet another self-addressed, stamped envelope and questionnaire. Granted, this may add to the researcher's expenditures, but all research should be planned to include the total cost of all items.

Cover letters are important and should include the following items:

1. Name of the researcher
2. Address of the researcher
3. Purpose of the study

4. Approximate length of time required to fill out the questionnaire
5. A statement safeguarding the confidentiality of the responses
6. Any other information the researcher feels is important

When using a mailed questionnaire, the investigator should allow a specific amount of time to elapse after the survey instrument has been mailed and should determine an acceptable percentage of responses to be obtained. This is necessary because there are many reasons for nonresponses to any survey, especially if the survey instrument is mailed. Any investigator who expects a 100 percent response will probably never draw any conclusions from the study!

Interviews

There are two basic kinds of interviewing techniques: structured and unstructured. In the *structured interview* the interviewer has a list of prepared questions that the researcher believes will provide a format for the respondent's answers concerning the researcher's project—for example, (1) How friendly do the nurses in ZZZ hospital seem to be? (2) Why do you answer as you do? The interviewer thus guides the respondent to determine what information is elicited and then records the answers.

An *unstructured interview* is more like a conversation. Here the researcher has a general framework of questions to elicit answers concerning the information sought, but uses the respondent's answers to enlarge upon the topic and to ask additional questions. The topics flow from the conversation's progress, and there is no set pattern or ordering of the categories that the researcher is exploring. Unstructured interviews take more time than structured interviews. The researcher must search the record of responses in order to categorize and organize the data elicited.

It is always the responsibility of the researcher to provide adequate training for the interviewers who may be assisting in the collection of the study data. Face-to-face interviewers must be nonthreatening to the respondent. Certain styles of dress and manners may be appropriate in one setting but not in another. Each interviewer must gain rapport and trust with the respondent. Interviewers should be trained to remain neutral when eliciting answers to the survey instrument. Many people will give the answer that they think the interviewer wants to hear rather than what they really believe. Interviewers who encourage such responses, whether overtly or unconsciously, cannot gather valid data.

A pilot or preliminary study is extremely valuable as a part of the training process. Debriefing after a few interviews allows the interviewers to point out flaws not initially discovered in the interview schedules and coding sheets. It also provides for a check on interviewing techniques.

Remember, too, that the interviewer will be doing two separate things during the course of the interview. First, the questions or statements must be given to the respondent and the appropriate response elicited. Second, the interviewer must mark a coded response sheet or record what the respondent says. Obviously, the statements on the response sheet must be organized carefully so that the interviewer can perform these tasks with a minimum of problems. If it is physically difficult to code the responses, the chance of error increases significantly.

It is usually easier to gain interviews if the interviewers have official sanction. When planning to interview members of a community, for example, the researcher might contact local city officials. Frequently they will be willing to provide a letter, badge, or other symbol of official recognition, which gives interviewers easier access to study subjects. It is helpful to remember that in a small community news travels fast. If the interviewing techniques are displeasing, potential respondents may reject the interviewers on the basis of what they have heard from others in the community.

Telephone interviewers should also be selected with care. Respondents visualize the individual on the other end of the line, so the interviewer should have a pleasing telephone voice and should have practiced using the survey instrument a number of times before actually talking to potential respondents.

It is noteworthy that people seem increasingly resistant to responding to telephone surveys. This may be due to a number of factors. First, with the increasing popularity of telephone surveys, individuals find that their time is being demanded more frequently. Second, there have been frequent misrepresentations by telephone solicitors who claim to be conducting a survey but are actually selling a product. Finally, more and more people have come to resent intrusion into their privacy.

Respondents should be given an opportunity to receive the results of the study. After being a respondent in any survey, the individual has an interest in finding out what came about as a result of the study. The offer to provide a summary of the study's results will often entice individuals who might not otherwise participate or respond. Be sure to keep your word; failure to provide the promised information may ruin future research possibilities both for yourself and for others.

Rating Scales

A *rating scale* is a type of data-collecting instrument that allows the respondents to place their feelings or attitudes on a scale. For example:

How would you rate the nursing care in this hospital?

Very good _____ : _____ : _____ : _____ : _____ : _____ Very poor
Please check the appropriate blank.

The number of response options on rating scales may vary considerably. Although five options occur most frequently, and this appears to be the minimum acceptable number, six, seven, or eight options can also be presented. The *Likert Scale* is a rating scale in which each statement usually has five possible responses: strongly agree, agree, uncertain, disagree, strongly disagree. A Likert-type scale may have more or fewer response choices, however.

There is a definite advantage in using even-numbered scales. These are called *forced choice* scales. When given an odd number of choices, subjects may respond to the middle choice and thus appear to be neutral, choosing neither high nor low ratings. If a scale has an even number of options, the subject must respond with a high or low ranking or rating. Given the previous question, the forced choice scale compels the respondent to like or dislike the nursing care.

The nursing care in this hospital is:

Very good _____ : _____ : _____ : _____ : _____ : _____ Very poor

The scale might similarly have been written:

The nursing care in this hospital is very good.
VSA   SA   A   D   SD   VSD

The responses stand for very strongly agree, strongly agree, agree, disagree, strongly disagree, very strongly disagree, respectively. In this instance the respondent would probably be asked to circle the appropriate response.

Sometimes, if the sample size is small, adequate statistical analysis cannot be done. Forced choice scales allow for the collapsing of cells (categories of data), for dichotomization, or for bringing cells together in statistically valid groups. Neutral responses might otherwise have to be discarded or divided, giving an unclear picture of the respondents' feelings or attitudes.

Respondents may be asked to *rank order* their responses from the most important to the least important. This technique can be very effective. If the rank order list is too long, however, the subjects may have trouble keeping the whole list in mind. For example:

Nurses should be capable of participating in research. The following is a list of settings in which nursing research can be carried out. Please rank each in order of importance as a setting for nursing research by placing a ''6'' by the most important, a ''5'' by the second most important, and so on down to number ''1'' (least important).

( ) hospital
( ) community health center
( ) visiting nurses association

( ) hospice
( ) day care center
( ) home health agency

A type of rating scale that has had a great deal of interest and success is called the *semantic differential scale*. This tool consists of a list of bipolar adjectives that may describe a setting, object, profession, or any other variable. For example, if we want to determine how people from different cultural and ethnic backgrounds perceive hospitals, we might construct the following:

Below is a checklist of words that describe a hospital. Please place a check mark in the space that best shows how you feel about hospitals. Be sure to place a check mark on each line.

Hospitals

Good ____ : ____ : ____ : ____ : ____ : ____ : ____ Bad
Busy ____ : ____ : ____ : ____ : ____ : ____ : ____ Quiet
Warm ____ : ____ : ____ : ____ : ____ : ____ : ____ Cold
Clean ____ : ____ : ____ : ____ : ____ : ____ : ____ Dirty

Various analytical techniques can be applied to the items in a semantic differential scale to determine if different subjects perceive the hospital setting in different ways.

Multiple-choice questions have long been a staple of examinations. They may also be used for eliciting research data. For example:

Place a circle around the letter of the response that most accurately reflects your point of view about the following items:

1. People have strong feelings about a national health care program. Which of the following statements best represents your attitude toward national health care?
   a. National health care will cost too much to be practical and should be avoided.
   b. National health care is the only way to provide adequate health care for all people.
   c. National health care should be limited to catastrophic illnesses.
   d. National health care would subvert our free enterprise system.

Note that in this instance respondents may not agree with any of the choices. Care must be exercised in developing this kind of instrument so that experimenter bias does not creep in through the use of slanted questions.

Content Analysis

Up to this point we have been discussing closed or structured measuring instruments: instruments that allow the respondent few or no alternatives in their responses. Frequently, as you probably have experienced, there is a feeling or response of "yes, but . . . " The respondents would like to qualify their answers or provide reasons for them. Open-ended measuring instruments allow respondents to explain why they respond in a particular manner. For example:

> Do you believe that the hospital staff should be differentiated by the color of their uniforms—blue for RNs, green for aides, yellow for LPNs, etc.? Please explain your answer.

This type of instrument lends itself to *content analysis*. The researcher examines the responses to determine the frequently cited reasons, compares adjective use between different groups, or uses one of a large number of potential analytical techniques. As we have already noted, Kalish et al. used content analysis to determine how television portrayed the nursing role.[1]

Obviously, with large samples and many responses, this technique can become tedious. Careful analysis of responses and documents can reveal a great deal that might otherwise be lost if closed or structured measuring instruments were used.

Use of Available Data

The increasing number of nursing studies over the years has created a large pool of *available data*. Studies that give complete reports of the number of respondents and their responses can be reanalyzed using other statistical tools to determine if the original conclusions were accurate. As a result of technological advances, these tools are often more sophisticated than those available to the original researcher. Furthermore, comparisons and contrasts can be made between past and current study responses. For example, a renewed interest in the study of sociobiology has led to a great deal of controversy at the present time. Reanalysis of existing data from sociobiological studies done at the beginning of the century might well be a valid research project at this time. Many such data are open to reinterpretation based on current knowledge and techniques.

Other available data sources include the reports of the large number of specialized statistic-gathering organizations, census tract reports, licensing bureau reports, and the reports of other organizations that gather and report data about people or groups of people. For example, a college placement service might have information about the type and level of employment held by the graduates of the school of nursing. This might lead to conclusions about the success of the school in educating its students and might also point out strengths and weaknesses.

Unobtrusive Measures

Over the years, an increasing number of studies have used *unobtrusive measures*. The researcher decides what needs to be measured and then determines how to measure it without direct intervention. A time-honored way to measure the most popular exhibits in a museum would be to determine the dirtiest display cases at the end of the day; this is done on the assumption that the more people who touch or press their noses against a display case, the dirtier it will be. Over a period of time, certain exhibits would show the most consistent usage.[2]

Similarly, counting the cigarette butts in ashtrays in the waiting room of an emergency facility might provide information if a researcher wanted to determine whether repeated warnings about cigarette smoking and health hazards have had any effect. Anxiety levels could be measured by observing the wear and tear on magazines placed in waiting rooms. Perhaps more stress is exhibited in the office of a dentist than in the waiting room of an emergency facility.

Nonwritten Records

A number of techniques are available to preserve the activities of individuals and groups in an enduring format. In the past, still photographs and pictures were used to analyze the behavior, beliefs, dress, and activities of subjects. With the advent of motion pictures, more details could be captured. Today, these techniques, as well as the technology of video- and audiotapes, can provide long-lasting records for future use and study.

Proxemics and Kinesics

Proxemics studies the use of time and space in communication. Americans, for example, often become uncomfortable when people from other countries or cultures approach and engage them in conversation. The person may be felt to be standing too close, and this makes the American nervous because his or her "body space" is being invaded. The other person is also uncomfortable, and feels that the American is being stand-offish. Both individuals are right. Cultural background defines how far apart individuals should be when communicating. Nurses might design research using videotape technology to study how patients from various cultures interact and react when communicating with nurses from the same and different cultures.

Kinesics is the observation of nonverbal communication. Almost all individuals learn appropriate methods of nonverbal communication, ranging from the smiles and frowns of the very young to the posture with which one carries oneself. Again, videotapes can be used to analyze how individuals react and interact nonverbally regardless of their verbal reactions and interactions.

Case Studies

The use of *case studies* might be considered a particular methodology within the category of descriptive research techniques. Social anthropologists have long been concerned with rather large groups of individuals, especially those sharing a common culture or background. In the case study method, a general population sharing a common background is identified, but the researcher works with a limited number of individuals, ranging from one person to a large sample. (Statistical research carried out on an individual is known as *single-subject research*.) The researcher then carefully observes and documents all the activities, contacts, and other salient actions of the individual(s).

Using the case study method, a nurse might document the activities of several hospital supervisors to determine if differences in leadership styles existed in the obstetrical service as opposed to the intensive care units.

Psychological and Projective Tests

Sometimes a researcher may want to determine more than surface attitudes about something. Perhaps the intent is to understand why a patient feels the way he or she does. Because it is impossible to read a person's mind, inferential instruments must be used. Consistency of responses can indicate a frame of reference, a mind-set, or a set of ideas.

Psychiatry and psychology have developed a number of instruments to determine a patient's feelings. These are called *projective tests* because the patient projects a meaning into materials that are essentially ambiguous or meaningless.

We have all heard of the Rorschach (ink blot) test. An individual is asked to look at a standard series of abstract forms (ink blots) and tell what he or she sees. Because the forms are random in shape, the subject must project or put meaning into them from his or her own beliefs or ideas. By presenting a series of these items, the researcher can draw conclusions about the subject's state of mind.

The Thematic Apperception Test (TAT) is frequently used to determine feelings and ideas. In this test subjects are shown pictures of people in ambiguous situations and asked to describe what is happening. Again, the subject must project his or her own feelings into the situation, allowing the researcher to draw conclusions about the individual.

Projective tests can be very helpful, but the researcher must interpret the responses cautiously. The very nature of the devices can lead to misunderstanding and misinterpretation. Much training is necessary before a researcher puts these devices into use.

As discussed in Chapter 6, we strongly recommend that you go to as many sources as possible to determine if a preexisting measuring instrument is available. Frequently, an appropriate instrument is available, with reliability and validity already established. A few hours of library search with such re-sources as *Mental Measurements Yearbook* or *Tests in Print* may save several weeks of development time.

Sociometrics

Sometimes a researcher wants to determine the social interaction and patterns of leadership roles in a group. This can be determined by the use of sociometric techniques. Essentially, the researcher structures a questionnaire to determine the most desirable or the most favorably perceived individuals in a group. Questions use in sociometrics might include the following:

1. Who is the best nurse on the unit?
2. Which nurses are the most effective? Name three.
3. Which three nurses do you like working with the best?

You may want to develop a sociogram to diagram the responses (Figure 11.1) or you may want to develop a social matrix showing the responses in tabular form (Table 11.1). These techniques can provide some very important information about the group's informal structure, who the informal leaders are, and where the power really lies.

Delphi Technique

One survey technique that has been very popular in the past few years is known as the *Delphi technique*. Named after the famous Oracle of Apollo at Delphi, the process attempts to predict what will be important to the surveyed group in the future.

The Delphi technique consists of identifying a group of experts or persons concerned with a certain area or program. Their concerns about their area or program are elicited and ranked. Once a total list of concerns has been ac-quired, it is given to the experts, who are asked to rank the items on the list in order of importance.

The responses are again tallied by the researcher and sent back to the same panel with totals of responses given. The panel members are then asked to rerank their responses on the basis of the total responses and their peers'

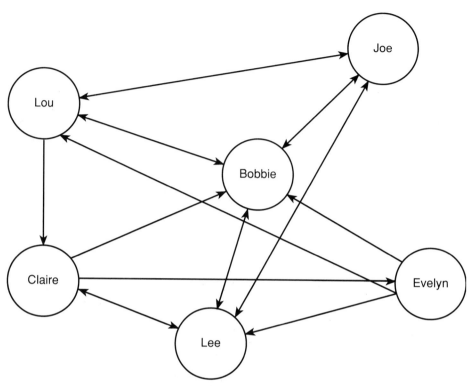

FIGURE 11.1
Sociogram

TABLE 11.1
Social Matrix

	SELECTOR					
Selectee	**Lee**	**Claire**	**Evelyn**	**Lou**	**Joe**	**Bobbie**
Lee	—	X	X		X	X
Claire	X	—		X		
Evelyn		X	—			
Lou			X	—	X	X
Joe	X			X	—	X
Bobbie	X	X	X	X	X	—

evaluations. The researcher can then focus on those items considered the most important by the experts.

For example, we might use the Delphi technique to examine nurses' concerns in a community health agency by sending out the following questions to all, or a sample, of the staff nurses.

> We are attempting to determine the future goals for patient care in a community setting. Please list at least five of your major concerns about nursing service as it is currently practiced in a community setting.

As you can see, each of the respondents then has an opportunity to express concerns and predictions about the future of nursing care in the community.

After the first round of responses is returned, the researcher lists each comment—with similar comments organized into a single topic—and a questionnaire is developed. The same respondents are used in all rounds of questioning so that a letter like the following might be sent to the initial respondents.

> Several weeks ago you were asked to list your major concerns about the patient care in your community. As a result of your responses and those of your peers, we have been able to develop the following list of concerns. We would now like you to rate these concerns on a scale of 1 to 5, with 1 being of little importance and 5 being of great importance.

1. Patient loads are too large for adequate care to be given.

1 2 3 4 5

2. Patients are unable to get additional care from other community agencies.

1 2 3 4 5

After the subjects respond to this questionnaire, the researcher then calculates how each response was evaluated by determining the percentages of the total responses in each category. For instance, the group sampled on the question concerning patient loads might have responded 60 percent 5's, 20 percent 4's and 20 percent 3's. Another survey is then sent to the respondents with a letter that might read like this:

> You and your colleagues have responded to a series of questions concerning nursing care in your community. Each of you was asked to

rank a list of questions as to their importance. Based on your responses, the questions were rated by the percentages in the categories which you see below. Please rate the questions as to their importance again, based on your own beliefs and your knowledge of your peers' responses.

At this point, the subjects may also be supplied with their own previous responses. The subjects then respond and rate the questions as to their relative importance. The researcher reevaluates the scale and determines which items are now considered the most important by the respondents. The researcher then identifies the main areas of concern and makes recommendations.

The Delphi technique has the advantage of identifying the group's major concerns and can be used to make recommendations to alleviate these concerns. It also allows an organization to focus on and take direction toward the future.

Observation

When the researcher is concerned with habits and other attributes that may be difficult to elicit by the use of survey instruments, there are a number of observational techniques that lend themselves to description and analysis of behavior.

The structured checklist is one technique used for observation. What happens and how frequently it happens is recorded to determine the frequency of certain events or activities. For example, a study's purpose might be to determine if laryngectomy patients behave differently as a result of structured preoperative teaching about their surgery, as opposed to a different kind of instruction. The researcher creates a checklist of significant behaviors of the patients being observed in the study. The researcher then determines the frequencies of occurrence and tallies the results. This provides a foundation for interpretations and conclusions about the effect of structured preoperative teaching on the postoperative behavior of laryngectomy patients.

Observation research often requires that several observers be used. This means that there is a potential for differences of observations among the observers. Consequently, the researcher must be extremely careful to train observers by providing common experiences so that observer reliability can be established. Given the example of the laryngectomy patient study, observers could be shown films or videotapes of patients performing a range of behaviors. The observers would then mark the designated activities on their observation checklist, and their perceptions could be checked by the researcher. After a number of training sessions, interobserver reliability could be determined by correlational techniques.

QUALITATIVE STRATEGIES FOR DESCRIPTIVE RESEARCH

As mentioned in previous chapters, beginning researchers should be aware that qualitative research studies are significantly more time-consuming to conduct and analyze than quantitative research studies. Although qualitative research strategies appear deceptively simple on the surface, they require the researcher to spend enough time with the study subjects to obtain and analyze the data. The time required for collecting data can be very long, and data analysis can become very complex because of the many possible ways that the data can be analyzed and reduced to comprehensible information. The qualitative researcher must identify a researchable problem and design the study in the same fashion as the quantitative researcher, although testing hypotheses is neither required nor possible in many instances.

Phenomenology

Phenomenological research is based on the philosophy of phenomenology, which was espoused by Edmund Husserl. Husserl's contention was that "meaning" is a personal experience that can be shared or communicated with others in an objective fashion and can be reduced to an underlying structure that can be understood by all individuals.

The phenomenological researcher develops a research question that can be analyzed by the researcher based on the "feelings" of the research subjects concerning the phenomena being investigated. This can be done by asking the subjects to write their thoughts, feelings, and perceptions concerning the phenomena, as was done by Parse, Coyne, and Smith when they asked their subjects to describe, in writing, a time when they felt healthy.[3] The researchers then reviewed the subjects' writings for common themes, which they reduced to common "meanings."

The researcher may also be directly involved in the experience(s) being examined. In this case, the researcher observes and records the verbal and nonverbal actions of the subjects as well as their reaction(s) to the situation. Data may be collected through notes or other appropriate data-gathering techniques. Because any portion of the information may lead to the determination of "meanings," the researcher must be objective in recording the data.

Partial data analysis may take place during the data collection phase. Since the researcher's goal is to reduce the myriad of observed phenomena to common elements, it may be possible to discover emergent themes very early on while collecting data. It must be noted, however, that the emergent themes or patterns may not contain substantive information and must be carefully scrutinized in light of the total data collected.

Researchers may use a judge panel of experts to determine whether the categories of meaning are valid.[4] Conversely, the researcher may opt to make the decisions concerning the categories of meaning and to establish their relative levels of importance.

Ethnography

Ethnographic research, often referred to as participant observation, may be used when the researcher must catalogue all activities, or as many as possible, that are taking place in a social situation and then determine which activities are significant and which are trivial. This, essentially, is the technique used by social anthropologists or ethnographers. The social anthropological researcher often becomes a participant as well as an observer and attempts to elicit data by using both structured and unstructured interviews and observations.

For example, there are many ways to examine beliefs about diseases and how to effect cures of these diseases. There are also many groups of people in developed as well as underdeveloped countries who practice various kinds of folk medicine to achieve cures. Disease etiology and classification are important to a nurse who is attempting to communicate with a patient. How the illness experience is perceived and described by a subculture is also a critical area for research. For example, the student who wrote the proposal in Appendix D proposed to describe what living in the congregate setting is like from the perspective of the homeless person with AIDS.

Other studies for which participant observation could be used include disease classification among Spanish-speaking migrant workers, the root medicine still practiced in many areas of the rural South, the continuation of various healing activities of American Indian groups, the introduction of herbal cures by different refugee groups, and the use of health foods and herbs in the population at large.

There are four levels of participant observation. The first level is that of a complete observer. If a researcher is working with a group of individuals whose language is not adequately understood or if discourse must be conducted through an interpreter, the researcher will be primarily an observer.

At the second level of participant observation, the researcher may become a partial participant. This could take place where the observer has a degree of fluency in the language and a great deal of knowledge concerning the group being studied. For example, a researcher working in a hospital setting might well fulfill this role. It is clear that the researcher is not a nurse, doctor, or member of the support staff of the hospital. This does not mean the researcher might not help in certain activities. Rather, it simply means that the researcher is nonjudgmental. Thus, the researcher can look for a variety of patterns of behaviors, social interactions, rituals, and other activities that are considered routine by the participants.

The third level of participant observation is that of an observer as participant. In this instance, a member of the group plays a dual role: first as a participating member of the group, with all of the rights and duties required of such a member, and second as an announced observer, where the group members are aware that they are being observed. As an example, a critical care nurse could describe the varieties of activities and interactions that occur between the various staff members in the critical care unit of a hospital. Some of the inter-actions would clearly be related to social and role expectations, rather than those interactions required to care for patients. Here the line between partici-pant and observer is very narrow. Individuals within the group would know they were being observed, yet the observer would be able to perform the role of participant competently.

Finally, there is the role of full participant. The researcher conceals any intent to do research, and the subjects are not necessarily aware of the researcher's purpose. There are strong questions of ethics involved in this type of research. Given the nature of informed consent by subjects in a research setting, total concealment of the research activity may be impossible.

It is the responsibility of the participant observer to make frequent and valid notes. Time considerations force many observers to develop a kind of shorthand for jotting down observations made on the spot. Later, they write down a full description of the event or events. Common sense dictates that such observations be recorded in full as soon as possible so that the researcher does not forget what those scribbles really meant.

The researcher who uses participant observation is limited as to the num-ber of individuals with whom contacts can be made. The first contacts may be with marginal individuals who need social contacts and/or approval and whose information may be unreliable. Therefore, the researcher must be very careful that the data gathered are accurate and valid. A study of witchcraft be-liefs might be extremely hard to document, for example, because of respondents' fear that they might be accused of witchcraft, or that they would become victims of witchcraft if they tell of known witches. Rapport and trust are crucial if the researcher is to obtain any kind of valid information.

Ethnographic researchers employ a technique called *key informant inter-viewing*. Key informants are those individuals whose positions or roles in a so-ciety or institution place them in a position to "know" what is really taking place. The participant observer must identify such individuals and gain their trust in order to have opportunities to interview them. Because key informants may be extremely busy individuals, care must be exercised not to waste their time and to take advantage of time that is unscheduled or at least free enough that the key informant does not feel that the investigator is too intrusive.

Grounded Theory

Grounded theory strategies were first reported by Glaser and Strauss when they examined the politics of pain management in a hospital environment.[5] Because there was little available existing data and no previously developed theory of pain management, the researchers had to collect data with no recourse to established ideas. This led to the strategy of the "constant comparative" method in which all the data being collected are compared to all the data previously collected in order to determine their importance and position in the hierarchy of data analysis. All kinds of data are collected. Written records and any other available data, such as verbal and nonverbal communications, are examined for their potential usefulness in the development of a usable theoretical framework. This means that the data collection and the data analysis stage of the research process occur simultaneously. The data are arranged in categories as patterns emerge. In the initial stages, the categories may be too broad or may be incorrect. As more data are collected, an isolated datum may be fitted into the appropriate category with greater ease.

After the researcher has developed categories, a framework is generated and a central hypothesis or theme may be formed concerning a key or core variable. The core variable is used to explain and simplify the complex structure of interactions that has been observed by the investigators(s).

SUMMARY

In summary, the descriptive research approach is present-oriented in that it describes what now exists. In each case, the techniques and instruments must be carefully selected and evaluated to determine their appropriateness for collecting the study data. Careful attention must be paid to the fundamental questions of validity, reliability, and usability, as well as to time and cost constraints.

In order to apply the principals presented, you should complete the Application Activities listed next.

APPLICATION ACTIVITIES

1. Examine your research problem carefully. Does it require an electric or mechanical measurement? If so, describe the device(s) you might use.
2. If you are using a survey instrument, is there an electrical or mechanical device that might be used in conjunction with it to validate respondents' answers?
3. Look in a nursing journal that publishes research studies. Examine and list techniques for gathering data used by the researchers in at least three issues of the same journal. Is any one technique used more frequently than others?
4. Either write a questionnaire with five to ten questions or develop a struc-

tured checklist of five to ten items designed to help you observe the activities of others. Administer your instrument to a population of your choice. Discuss orally or in writing both the positive and the negative results of this experience.

REFERENCES

1. Kalish, P. A., B. J. Kalish, and J. Clinton. 1982. "The World of Nursing on Prime Time Television, 1950 to 1960." *Nursing Research,* 31(November–December): 358–363.
2. Webb, Eugene, et al. 1966. *Unobtrusive Measures: Non-Reactive Research in the Social Sciences.* Chicago: Rand McNally, pp. 45–46.
3. Parse, R. R., A. B. Coyne, and M. J. Smith. 1985. *Nursing Research: Qualitative Methods.* Bowie, MD: Brady Communications.
4. Omery, A. 1983. "Phenomenology: A Method for Nursing Research." *Advances in Nursing Science,* 5: 49–63.
5. Glaser, B., and A. Strauss. 1967. *The Discovery of Grounded Theory: Strategies for Qualitative Research.* Chicago: Aldine.

BIBLIOGRAPHY AND SUGGESTED READINGS

Anastasi, A. 1976. *Psychological Testing,* 4th ed. New York: Macmillan.

Dobbert, M. L. 1982. *Ethnographic Research.* New York: Praeger.

Glaser, B., and A. Strauss. 1967. *The Discovery of Grounded Theory: Strategies for Qualitative Research.* Chicago: Aldine.

Harrison, L. L. 1989. "Interfacing Bioinstruments with Computers for Data Collection." *Research in Nursing and Health,* 12(February): 57–63.

Kalish, P. A., B. J. Kalish, and J. Clinton. 1982. "The World of Nursing on Prime Time Television, 1950 to 1980." *Nursing Research,* 31(November–December): 358–363.

Lindeman, C. A. 1981. *Priorities within the Health Care System: A Delphi Study.* Kansas City: American Nurses' Association.

Linstone, H., and M. Turoo, Eds. 1975. *The Delphi Method: Techniques and Applications.* Reading, MA: Addison-Wesley.

Omery, A. 1983. "Phenomenology: A Method for Nursing Research." *Advances in Nursing Science,* 5: 49–63.

Osgood, C. E., G. J. Suci, and P. H. Tannenbaum. 1957. *The Structure of Inquiry.* Urbana: University of Illinois Press.

Parse, R. R., A. B. Coyne, and M. J. Smith. 1985. *Nursing Research: Qualitative Methods.* Bowie, MA: Brady Communications.

Poyatos, F., Ed. 1988. *Cross Cultural Perspectives in Nonverbal Communication.* Toronto: Hogrefe.

Rosengren, K. E., Ed. 1981. *Advances in Content Analysis.* Beverly Hills, CA: Sage.

Rosenthal, R. 1966. *Experimenter Effects in Behavioral Research.* New York: Appleton-Century-Crofts.

Sackman, H. 1975. *Delphi Critique: Expert Opinion, Forecasting, and Group Process.* Lexington, MA: Lexington Books.

Turner, A. P. F., I. Karube, and G. Wilson. 1987. *Biosensors: Fundamentals and Applications.* Oxford: Oxford University Press.

Webb, E., D. T. Campbell, R. D. Schwartz, and L. Sechrest. 1966. *Unobtrusive Measures: Nonreactive Research in the Social Sciences.* Chicago: Rand McNally.

Weiman, J. M., and R. D. Harrison, Eds. 1983. *Nonverbal Interaction.* Beverly Hills, CA: Sage.

Werner, O., and G. M. Schoepfle. 1987. *Systematic Fieldwork.* Beverly Hills, CA: Sage.

Yin, R. K. 1984. *Case Study Research.* Beverly Hills, CA: Sage.

12

The Experimental Research Approach

The material in this chapter is designed to introduce you to some basic principles and methods of the experimental design approach. When researching a nursing problem, we seek solutions that we hope will improve patient care and enhance the quality of life for all people. One of the greatest problems we face in seeking solutions to research problems is that we are dealing with human beings, who may report a wide variety of feelings, attitudes, or even misunderstandings. Obviously, the researcher wants to control as many factors as possible. This leads to the use of an experimental approach and the development of experimental design methodology.

THE NATURE OF EXPERIMENTAL RESEARCH

Experimental design is based on the notion of control. Observed instances of an activity may or may not be the cause of an observed consequence. The experimenter wants to determine if the activity was or was not the cause of the effect observed. For example, parents, teachers, and others admonish children not to get their feet wet because the children will catch cold. Although this may seem to be a reasonable admonition, in fact, we know that colds are caused by viruses that are transmitted from one person to another. Wet feet in and of themselves will not cause a person to catch a cold. They may make the person uncomfortable, disturb physiological balance, and lower resistance to infection; but, alone, foot wetting is not the causal factor in colds. Many commonsense ideas are rooted in the folklore of cause and effect; the careful researcher designs experiments to verify if, indeed, the cause does bring about the observed effect.

As has been mentioned, working with human beings makes experimental research extremely difficult. Controls are difficult to apply, and many techniques used on plants and animals are certainly not open to experimenters who work with human subjects. Reexamine the discussion of the protection of human subjects in Chapter 4 to gain a fuller appreciation of the researcher's responsibilities for the protection of human rights.

In nursing research, the investigator may want to vary certain factors that appear to have causal relationships to something else. In the proposal for the study investigating the effect of stockinette caps on the conservation of body heat in newborns (Appendix E), the researcher planned to control as many factors as possible and, where not possible, to compensate for these potential effects.

It is again worthwhile to mention the idea of statistical significance. A desired level of outcome is established prior to carrying out the research plan. Frequently, the result is not statistically significant, and the researcher goes away feeling that the research was for naught. Nothing could be further from the truth. Research studies that yield no statistical significance, if carefully planned and executed, are just as valid as studies that yield statistically significant differences. Beginning researchers sometimes have the idea that their research is not acceptable if no statistically significant difference is found. Most researchers want to reject the null hypothesis. They believe the experimental approach they are using is better than some other approach, and they often have a vested interest in the success of their experiments. They find it terribly disappointing to discover that their great ideas did not work out as expected.

In reviewing the literature, we quickly discover that research journals tend to report studies with highly significant results. This attitude has developed over the years and is potentially damaging to the research process. Editors of some journals will report only those reports that are highly significant but will not report equally valid studies that show no statistically significant differences.

Organizations that give grant funds often like to have significant results. A researcher whose experiments show no significant difference may be less likely to be funded a second time than a researcher whose experiments show such differences. Unfortunately, this has led to a number of false reports by unethical researchers.

We must remember that the field of statistics developed outside of the area of human subject research. Experimental rigor can be applied far more effectively by experimenters who work with biological or physical specimens, and who can more easily control the variables to analyze their experimental results, than by those who work with human subjects.

Finally, even a slight improvement in a condition may be significant to the individuals with that condition, even though the treatment may not be statistically significant as far as the controlled experiment is concerned.

Up to now we have referred frequently to the word *control*, which can be defined as a manipulation or alteration of the experimental conditions in order to limit sources of error. As described in Chapter 6, the purpose of experimental research is to determine if condition X (the cause) will result in response Y (the effect). Condition X is termed the *independent variable*, and response Y is the *dependent variable*.

The nature of control is to restrict the effects of *extraneous variables* that could have an impact on the variables under investigation and could affect the outcome of the research.

Careful controls are also used to avoid side effects that could occur during the course of a potentially harmful experiment. Many useful drugs may be highly toxic or have unpleasant side effects if doses are too large. For example, reports of experiments with rats and mice by the Food and Drug Administration caused a great furor by identifying artificial sweeteners, such as cyclamates and saccharin, as potential carcinogens. These experiments were conducted in such a manner that the quantities of potentially harmful substances to be ingested by the experimental animals were carefully controlled. By varying the quantity levels of the substances, the experimenters could determine differential responses to the substances. Also, the Surgeon General's reports are able to state with higher and higher degrees of certainty that the more one smokes, the greater one's odds of having various medical problems.

Probably the most important control the experimenter uses is that of random assignments of subjects to groups (also called *randomization*). Every subject should have an equal chance of being assigned to any group as the investigator assigns subjects to a control group or an experimental group on a random basis. The purpose of random assignment is to avoid any systematic bias in the groups being studied.

QUASI-EXPERIMENTAL RESEARCH DESIGNS

Sometimes the researcher is not able to design a true experimental study because of constraints imposed in subject selection and/or the setting of the study. In such cases, the researcher may use a quasi-experimental design, in which the investigator is still able to manipulate the independent variable (the experimental condition) and exercise some control over the experiment. However, random assignment of subjects to control or experimental groups is not feasible. For example, the student who wrote the proposal in Appendix F investigating variations in blood loss and placental trapping associated with oxytocin administration used a quasi-experimental design. She was still able to manipulate the independent variable for her study (oxytocin administration time) but was unable to randomly assign the study subjects to the treatment groups. This is in contrast to the true experimental design of the study in Appendix E, in which the researcher plans to randomly assign the study subjects (newborns) to either the experimental or the control group.

EXPERIMENTAL RESEARCH DESIGNS

There are a number of ways to design true experimental research. Each design is characterized by manipulation of the independent variable by the investigator, and by some form of control and randomization. The designs range from simple to extremely complex.

One-Group Pretest–Posttest Design

The simplest type of experimental design is the *one-group pretest–posttest design*. Although this design leaves many things to chance, it is often the only available way to determine the effectiveness of a treatment. Essentially, this design measures what has happened to the experimental group based on the way it was prior to the beginning of the experiment (pretest state), and the differences achieved at the end of the experiment (posttest state).

For example, such a design might be used to study a group of patients who suffer mild angina pain. The experimenter could measure cholesterol level in the patients' blood and then ask the patients to restrict their intake of cholesterol through changes in their diets. After a given period of time, the experimenter would determine whether or not the mild angina pain had been reduced and if the blood cholesterol levels had dropped. If blood cholesterol levels had dropped and angina pain has been reduced, the experimenter might then conclude that lowering cholesterol levels in the blood reduces angina pain. Note that there is a minimal amount of control placed on other variables that might affect the evidence in the study subjects. Changes in stress patterns, weight, exercise patterns, or any one of many other factors might have contributed to the change.

The following table shows the characteristics of the one-group pretest–posttest design:

Number of Groups Used	Pretest?	Treatment?	Posttest?	Strength of Design
1	Yes	Yes	Yes	Weak

Pretest–Posttest Control Group

A second and more sophisticated technique of experimentation is the use of a *control group* to determine if the treatment appears to make a difference. Utilizing the previous cholesterol example, a number of subjects with mild angina pain would be randomly assigned to two groups: an *experimental group* and a *control group*. The experimental group subjects would then alter their diets, while the control group subjects would change nothing. At the end of the experiment, the researcher would determine whether there was a significant difference in the cholesterol levels of both groups. If this difference was significant, and there was a significant difference in the reported incidences of mild angina pain between the experimental and the control group, the experimenter could then conclude that the reduction of blood cholesterol did have an effect on the occurrence of angina.

Note that there was no attempt to match or otherwise compare the members of either group. The only common element of control the control group shares with the experimental group is mild angina pain. Note also the term *mild*. Pain perception varies greatly from individual to individual, and response to pain varies between cultures as well as between the sexes within a culture. In the previous example, not all of these factors were taken into consideration, only the common diagnosis of mild angina pain.

The following table shows the characteristics of the pretest–posttest control group design: X refers to the experimental group; C refers to the control group.

Number of Groups Used	Pretest?	Treatment?	Posttest?	Strength of Design
2	X Yes C Yes	X Yes C No	X Yes C Yes	Weak

Matching Samples

Far more valuable in terms of rigor would be a research design that attempts to match or to pair the control and the experimental group. In the cholesterol study, the experimenter might use simple matching procedures such as height, weight, sex, age, and smoking or nonsmoking, or such sophisticated measurements as psychological stress tests, projective techniques, or any one of literally dozens of methods in order to control for extraneous variables.

A major problem with this type of experimental design is that, unless the subject pool is infinitely large, the experimenter reduces the available sample with each matching or pairing situation. Males can be matched only with other males. Age further reduces the sample size. Eventually, it is entirely possible to reduce the sample down to two very well matched individuals. The problem then becomes one of a large enough sample size to be generalizable to the target population.

The following table shows the characteristics of the matching sample design: X refers to the experimental group; C refers to the control group.

Number of Groups Used	Pretest?	Treatment?	Posttest?	Strength of Design
2	X Yes C Yes	X Yes C No	X Yes C Yes	Weak

Solomon Four-Group Design

A frequently used and highly valid experimental procedure is the *Solomon four-group design*. An experimenter using this methodology randomly divides the sample into four separate groups. Effectively, there are two experimental groups and two control groups.

The first experimental group receives the same procedures as in the pretest–posttest design. Subjects are randomly selected, pretested, given the appropriate treatment, and then given the posttest.

The first of the control groups is given the pretest, no treatment, and then the posttest. Up to this point, the Solomon design is precisely the same as the pretest–posttest control group design. However, group 3 is also defined as an experimental group. In our cholesterol example, it would consist of subjects diagnosed as having mild angina. They would not be given the pretest; that is, their cholesterol level would not be measured at all. However, they would receive the treatment; that is, their intake of cholesterol would be reduced and they would be given the appropriate blood tests at the end of the experimental period.

Subjects in the fourth group in the Solomon design would have nothing done until the posttest. They would not be pretested for cholesterol levels at the experiment's beginning and they would not receive any treatment. Only at the end of the experiment would their blood cholesterol level be measured (posttested) and then compared to the incidence of anginal pain in the other groups.

Because two of the groups (groups 1 and 3) have received the experimental treatment, any differences noted by the experimenter can be more confidently ascribed to the treatment if both experimental groups show similar results at the end of the treatment and there is a significant difference between the experimental and the control groups. Similarly, a lack of significant difference between the four groups enables the investigator to accept the null hypothesis.

The following table shows the characteristics of the Solomon four-group design: X refers to the experimental group; C refers to the control group.

Number of Groups Used	Pretest?	Treatment?	Posttest?	Strength of Design
4	X1 Yes	X1 Yes	X1 Yes	Strong
	C1 Yes	C1 No	C1 Yes	
	X2 No	X2 Yes	X2 Yes	
	C2 No	C2 No	C2 Yes	

Two-Group Random Sample

The experimenter may choose to use only the last two groups of the Solomon design. That is, one group is given the treatment and then posttested with no pretesting, and the control group is given only the posttest. The theory behind this methodology is that the experimenter, adhering rigorously to the random assignment of subjects to the groups, can say that the two groups were essentially the same because random assignment should avoid any systematic bias in the two groups.

This type of design simplifies the experimenter's task and eliminates the effect of a pretest on the subjects. In effect, it maintains the subjects' naiveté. It is also noteworthy that there are some things that cannot be pretested or accurately predicted. Patients who are already suffering from mild angina pain may or may not be suffering from elevated cholesterol levels. The angina pain already exists. If treatment or lack of treatment (cholesterol in the diet) is a factor, there should be a difference between the two groups at the end of the treatment.

The following table shows the characteristics of the two-group random sample design: X refers to the experimental group; C refers to the control group.

Number of Groups Used	Pretest?	Treatment?	Posttest?	Strength of Design
2	X No	Yes	Yes	Strong
	C No	No	Yes	

Nonrandomized Control Group Design

Occasionally, circumstances may preclude random assignment of subjects to groups at the beginning of an experiment. For example, the experimenter may wish to compare a sample of individuals from a local Veteran's Administration hospital with a sample of individuals from a privately funded hospital who are also complaining of angina pain. One of the hospitals may insist on a standardized routine of treatment for angina patients, whereas the other hospital may be available for the experimental treatment.

In this case, the subjects in both samples are given the pretest and one group is given the experimental treatment, but the researcher is not able to control various interaction effects at the beginning of the experiment. In this instance, where it is not possible to develop controls by assigning subjects randomly to control and experimental groups, alternative methods of statistical analysis are required. The method commonly used is the analysis of covariance. As noted in Chapter 7, this statistical technique allows the experimenter to control for varying potential interaction effects after the experiment has been performed.

The following table shows the characteristics of the nonrandomized control group design: X refers to the experimental group; C refers to the control group.

Number of Groups Used	Pretest?	Treatment?	Posttest?	Strength of Design
2	X Yes C Yes	X Yes C No	X Yes C Yes	Control through analysis of covariance can be strong

Counterbalanced Design

A more effective design, or at least one that attempts to remove some of the previously described problems, is the *counterbalanced design*. This design can be used when more than one treatment method is attempted. Each set of subjects is given the treatment at the same point in time during the course of the experiment. This means that sets of subjects become both experimental and control groups for themselves and for another group. Because of the nonrandom nature of group assignments, the experimenter cannot control differences. However, the testing does allow for greater flexibility in the interpretation of results; differences are noted both between groups and within groups. Utilizing the statistical test of analysis of variance, the experimenter may be able to determine that the effects were caused by the treatment.

For example, a group of psychiatric patients might be subjected to a computer program designed to interact with individuals and give the illusion of eliciting feelings. (Such a program exists and may be found on many college campuses as either "Doctor" or "Eliza.") After such interaction, the subjects would then be given a subjective test and their responses scored. At an alternative time, standard psychotherapeutic techniques would be used and the same projective tests would be given. After a number of alternating treatments, types of responses to the projective tests could be measured, and the differences, if any, between the two treatments could be recorded.

A number of variations to this design should be noted. Two or more variables could be introduced, such as another type of treatment in addition to computer and psychotherapy. Perhaps a questionnaire could be utilized with a format such as "I feel _____." Here the subject chooses from a list of adjectives provided and is then asked to tell why he or she feels this way. Or a question such as "How do you feel about _____?" could be asked. Responses to projective techniques could again be used to determine differences between the treatments.

The following table shows the characteristics of the counterbalanced design. (X refers to the experimental group; C refers to the control group.)

Number of Groups Used	Pretest?	Treatment?	Posttest?	Strength of Design
Varies (X's and C's reverse roles in study)	X Yes C Yes	Treatment A X Yes C No	X Yes C Yes	Strong
	X Yes C Yes	Treatment B X No C Yes	X Yes C Yes	

Time Series Design

Most experimental studies fall into two categories: one-shot studies and those that continue over a longer period of time, known as longitudinal studies. As an experimenter you may want to measure the effects of a treatment over a long period of time. You would thus continue to administer the treatment and would measure the effects a number of times during the course of the experiment.

In our cholesterol example, instead of testing patients with mild angina pain only once (at the end of the diet restriction), the design would call for a multiple testing at stated intervals. Chemical or behavioral changes in a human being can be very subtle and difficult to measure. Responses can vary daily, and some intervening but unrecognized variables may lead to incorrect conclusions. Testing over a long period of time helps to reduce such pitfalls and improves the experiment. With a time series experiment, however, variables occurring during and after treatment may go unnoticed by the experimenter and can lead to a false or improper conclusion.

The following table shows the characteristics of the time series design: X refers to the experimental group; C refers to the control group.

Number of Groups Used	Pretest?	Treatment?	Posttest?	Strength of Design
1	Yes	Yes over time	Yes over time	Strong

Control Group Time Series Design

In order to diminish the problems inherent in a time series design, experimenters can use a *control group time series design*. This design requires that a control group be tested simultaneously with the experimental group without being given the treatment. In our cholesterol example, two groups of randomly selected angina patients would receive a sequential series of blood tests over a period of time. The experimenter would then determine if blood cholesterol had diminished significantly between the experimental treatment group and the control group, as well as the frequency and intensity of angina pain. This technique, obviously, provides far greater control than a single time series design and is preferable to the single time series design.

The following table shows the characteristics of the control group time series design: X refers to the experimental group; C refers to the control group.

Number of Groups Used	Pretest?	Treatment?	Posttest?	Strength of Design
2	X Yes	X Yes over time	X Yes over time	Strong
	C Yes	C No over time	C Yes over time	

Factorial Designs

In experimental designs like those we have been discussing, the experimenter identifies one independent variable and one dependent variable. Through the use of various forms of control, the effect of the independent variable on the dependent variable is then measured. However, there may be a time when we find that there are two or more variables that occurred simultaneously and, through interaction, may cause the dependent variable to appear in the way that it did.

Using our cholesterol example, suppose the subjects were overweight when placed on the low-cholesterol diet. In some cases weight might be maintained because, although saturated fat intake is reduced, there is a plethora of nonsaturated fats that could be substituted for the saturated fats.

The experimenter, however, might want to reduce both the weight and the intake of saturated fats of the subjects simultaneously. At the end of the experiment, it might be found that angina pain had been reduced in both intensity and frequency. It would then become very difficult to ascribe the causal effects to either of the two independent variables. Experimenters can more easily control experiments in which one and only one independent variable is introduced, as in the case of a cholesterol intake reduction alone or a weight-loss diet alone. Often the interaction of two or more variables produces more significant results than a single variable does. The experimenter must then use what is called a *factorial design*. In this type of design, subjects are divided into all possible combinations to determine the effect of the independent variables alone and the effect of the interaction of the independent variables.

Such factorial designs can grow to enormous complexity very quickly, but such is the work of researchers. Human beings are enormously complex; even the simplest, most tightly designed and tightly controlled experiment has results that are probably influenced by interaction effects. Factorial designs attempt to get at these interactive effects and determine their impact on the experiment.

The following table shows the characteristics of the factorial design: X refers to the experimental group; C refers to the control group.

Number of Groups Used	Pretest?	Treatment?	Posttest?	Strength of Design
Varies	X Yes C Varies	X Yes C Varies	X Yes C Yes	Strong but can be very complex

Table 12.1 summarizes the experimental designs using the diagrammatic explanation of each design.

Ex Post Facto Designs—Correlations

In *ex post facto research*, changes in the independent variable have already occurred prior to the research. Ex post facto designs are really correlational designs that allow the researcher to infer relationships among variables, rather than draw cause-and-effect conclusions. This can lead to spurious (incorrect) conclusions. Researchers who conclude that a high positive or high negative correlation is necessarily a cause-and-effect relationship have failed to see the whole picture. There is a tendency to oversimplify in drawing conclusions. It has been said that there are two solutions to every problem: one short, simple, and wrong and the other extremely complicated. Indeed, there has been a problem regarding the reports of several regulatory agencies of the federal government, such as the Food and Drug Administration and the Surgeon General's office, both of which have reported a great deal of correlational research. Because of the potential ambiguity in interpretation, industries such as the tobacco industry and the artificial sweetener industry have often attempted—and sometimes succeeded—in responding to these reports with other correlational studies of their own showing lower relationships or no causality at all. This has led to much confusion on the consumer's part because the question of whom to believe looms large when dealing with such complex market issues.

In summary, true experimental research design is characterized by manipulation of the independent variable by the investigator, who exercises some form of control over the experimental situation, including random assignment of subjects to groups (randomization).

TABLE 12.1
Comparison of Experimental Designs

Design	Number of Groups Used	Pretest?	Treatment?	Posttest?	Strength of Design
One-group pretest/ posttest	1	Yes	Yes	Yes	Weak
Pretest/posttest control group	2	X[a] Yes C[b] Yes	X Yes C No	X Yes C Yes	Weak
Matching samples	2	X Yes C Yes	X Yes C No	X Yes C Yes	Weak
Solomon four-group design	4	X1 Yes C1 Yes X2 No C2 No	X1 Yes C1 No X2 Yes C2 No	X1 Yes C1 Yes X2 Yes C2 Yes	Strong
Two-group random sample	2	X No C No	X Yes C No	X Yes C Yes	Strong
Nonrandomized control group	2	X Yes C Yes	X Yes C No	X Yes C Yes	Control through analysis of co-variance can be strong
Counter-balanced	Varies (X's and C's reverse roles in study)	Treatment A: X Yes C Yes Treatment B: X Yes C Yes	Treatment A: X Yes C No Treatment B: X No C Yes	Treatment A: X Yes C Yes Treatment B: X Yes C Yes	Strong
Time series	1	Yes	Yes over time	Yes over time	Strong
Control group time series	2	X Yes C Yes	X Yes over time C No over time	X Yes over time C Yes over time	Strong
Factorial	Varies	X Yes C Varies	X Yes C Varies	X Yes C Yes	Strong but can be very complex

[a] X refers to experimental group(s).
[b] C refers to control group(s).

CONSIDERATIONS IN EXPERIMENTAL RESEARCH DESIGN

In all true experimental studies, the researcher must keep several concerns as high-priority items when designing research.

Generalizability

The researcher should design the experiment so that its findings will be generalizable to the larger target population when sampling techniques are used. Sometimes research studies do not allow for generalization because of sample size, method of subject selection, or various other reasons. In addition, experiments carried out in artificial or restricted laboratory situations often preclude generalizability. Quasi-experimental designs are less generalizable than true experimental designs.

Subject Sensitization

Subjects can become sensitized or knowledgeable about the procedures used. This is especially true where a psychological rather than a physiological response is measured. By its very nature, a pretest gives information about what it is the experimenter wants to discover. Even if questions are masked, subjects will know something about the research. Even physiological measurements can be affected. With our increased knowledge of biofeedback, we can see that subjects may be able to control, voluntarily or involuntarily, many of their physiological responses.

Replicability

Can the research be repeated in another setting with other subjects? If a study can be replicated, and other researchers get similar results, a great deal more confidence can be placed in the conclusions drawn by the original researchers. One of the criteria for developing a scientific research base for utilization in nursing practice is sufficient replication of the studies to ensure the validity of the results of the studies.

Historical Factors

Historical factors may also come into play. If an experiment is carried out over a period of time, events extraneous to the experiment, such as maturation or increased knowledge on the part of the subjects, may cause changes. These events become intervening variables and must be accounted for.

Fatigue

Both the subjects and the researchers can become fatigued, bored, or inattentive during the course of a research study. This means treatment, or response measurement, may not be consistent during the course of an experiment. There comes a time when both subjects and researchers have the feeling of "let's get this thing over with and get out of here." This natural fatigue must be guarded against in order to ensure correct and consistent measurement.

Attrition

In research conducted over a period of time, there may be attrition or loss of subjects. Subjects move, become ill, withdraw because they are tired of the research, or are lost to the experiment for any number of other reasons. This means that an experimenter who starts with too small a sample or samples at the beginning of the experiment may obtain insufficient data for valid analysis.

Hawthorne Effect

Over the years there have been many studies of the Hawthorne effect. The Hawthorne studies were a series of classical studies conducted in the late 1920s and early 1930s at the Hawthorne Plant of the Western Electric Company in Chicago. The *Hawthorne effect* is the term used to describe the psychological reactions to the presence of the investigator or to special treatment during the study, which tends to alter the responses of the subjects. Subjects may change their behavior in an effort to please the experimenter. Again, we caution that experimenters can unconsciously bias subjects merely by their tone of voice or facial expression.

Experimenter Bias

Sometimes experimenter expectations interfere with the gathering of accurate results. Many experimenters have a vested interest in their experiments, and failure to reject the null hypothesis may be a terrible blow to one's ego. A true researcher remains objective and attempts to control as many variables as possible.

Blind Studies

Methods called *blind studies* have been developed to ensure that experimenter bias and the Hawthorne effect are reduced or eliminated. *Single blind* studies may be carried out in one of two ways. In one method of single blind studies, the subjects know whether they are in the experimental group or the control group, but the experimenter does not know which group each subject is in. In the other single blind method, the experimenter knows which group the subjects are in, but the subjects do not know which group they are in. The preferred method of blind studies is the *double blind* study, where only an outside, neutral party has assigned subjects to the experimental and control groups, and neither subjects nor experimenter knows which subjects are in which group.

SUMMARY

In summary, we have discussed the nature of experimental research and a number of the most commonly used experimental research designs, including the one-group pretest–posttest design; the pretest–posttest control group design; the matching sample design; the Solomon four-group design; the two-group random sample design; the nonrandomized control group design; the counterbalanced design; the time series design; the control group time series design; factorial designs; and ex post facto designs. We have also discussed the nature of quasi-experimental research as well as some considerations in experimental research design. Beginning researchers should be aware that there are other less common designs that may be found in the literature.

In order to apply the principles presented, complete the Application Activities that follow.

APPLICATION ACTIVITIES

1. Reread the experimental research proposal in Appendix E. Note how the researcher selected the subjects for inclusion in her study. Which research design did she plan to use?
2. The student who wrote the research proposal in Appendix E was able to implement her proposal. Read the abstract of the study in Appendix G and explain her rationale for using the *t*-test to analyze the data.
3. Read the quasi-experimental research proposal in Appendix F. Note how the researcher planned to select the study subjects. Why is this study a quasi-experiment rather than a true experiment?
4. Locate two published true experimental research reports, and determine what type of experimental design was used in each.
5. Locate two quasi-experimental research reports. Explain why the study designs are quasi-experimental rather than true experimental.

BIBLIOGRAPHY AND SUGGESTED READINGS

Campbell, D. T., and J. Stanley. 1963. *Experimental and Quasi-Experimental Designs for Research*. Chicago: Rand McNally.

Forcese, D. P., and S. Richer. 1973. *Social Research Methods*. Englewood Cliffs, NJ: Prentice-Hall.

Kerlinger, F. H. 1973. *Foundations of Behavioral Research*, 2nd ed. New York: Holt, Rinehart and Winston.

Kidder, L. H., C. M. Judd, and E. R. Smith. 1986. *Research Methods in Social Relations*, 5th ed. New York: Holt, Rinehart and Winston.

Leedy, P. D. 1974. *Practical Research: Planning and Design*. New York: Macmillan.

Polit, D., and B. Hungler. 1987. *Nursing Research: Principles and Methods,* 3rd ed. Philadelphia: J. B. Lippincott.
Solomon, R. C. 1949. ''An Extension of Control Group Design.'' *Psychological Bulletin,* 46: 137–150.
Wiseman, J. P., and M. S. Aron. 1970. *Field Projects for Sociology Students.* Cambridge, MA: Schenkman.

Appendices

Appendix A

Example of a Historical Research Proposal

ERNESTINE WIEDENBACH:
A HISTORICAL NURSING REVIEW
Her Life and Career Contributions

by
SUSAN NICKEL

Reprinted by permission.

STATEMENT OF THE PROBLEM	METHODOLOGY
LITERATURE REVIEW	PLAN FOR DATA ANALYSIS
CONCEPTUAL FRAMEWORK	LIMITATIONS OF THE STUDY
STATEMENT OF THE PURPOSE	REFERENCES
OF THE STUDY	BIBLIOGRAPHY

History makes the deeds of men (and women) live after them. Its function is to transmit knowledge of the past. It is a nation's memory, perpetuating its deeds, its traditions, and even its mistakes, also its aspirations and ideals. It makes the past a part of us, shapes our deeds in many ways, and links past and present with the future, making all one.[1]

STATEMENT OF THE PROBLEM

Historical research deals with what has happened and how those happenings affect the present. More than a mere biography of a few leaders, historical research uses dates to determine the impact of events of the past on the present and occasionally tries to predict the future, based on this knowledge.[2]

Historical research has long been a respected method of inquiry. A major contribution of historical inquiry is in the development of a broader, more complete perspective to enhance our understanding of the present and our approach to the future. Historical research is not merely a collection of incidents or facts; it is a study of the relationships of facts and incidents, of themes or currents of social and professional issues that have influenced the present and the future.[3]

Other professions, such as medicine, law, and education, have placed great importance on their histories and have used their knowledge of the past to guide and inspire their profession in its forward movement. The interest in historical nursing continues to lag. Some of the reasons for the dearth in nursing history include heavy teaching and administrative loads, salaries too meager to permit travel to archive sites, lack of local source material, and uncertainty of an outlet for publication.[4] Notter cited the lack of emphasis on nursing history taught in schools of nursing and the fact that nurses are too action-oriented as other possible causes.

> Research into present day problems without adequate search into the past to examine the course of events which produced the present problems, or bring to light past investigations of the same or similar problems by nurses or others, results in research which only scratches the surface and may even duplicate previous work.[5]

The role of historical research as a guide to the future becomes very clear as the lessons of the past are revealed. Provisions must be made so that nurses of the future may look back and draw both inspiration and direction from the nursing leaders of the past who have overcome obstacles. Ernestine Wiedenbach, B.A., M.A., R.N., P.H.N., C.N.M., has been a leader in the nursing profession since her graduation from the Johns Hopkins Hospital School of Nursing in 1925. Her five-decade career in nursing and nurse-midwifery has spanned a gamut of roles from practitioner to educator, administrator to author, patient advocate to mentor, and philosopher to theorist.

Today, Miss Wiedenbach lives in retirement in Miami, Florida. She is receptive and cooperative toward historical research on her life and career contributions. The value of her oral history of nursing and nurse-midwifery's past, present, and future as she perceives it is immeasurable.

LITERATURE REVIEW

Ernestine Wiedenbach's career has evolved continually through some difficult years for both nursing and our nation. She worked as a public health nurse during the Depression and with the American Nurses' Association/National League for Nurses throughout World War II. When it was not widely accepted, she became a certified nurse-midwife. What prompted this woman from an upper-middle-class background to assume these various roles?

Role theory represents a collection of concepts and a variety of hypothetical formulations that predict how actors will perform in a given role, or under what circumstances certain types of behavior can be expected.[6] The body of scientific knowledge has grown markedly in recent years. Concomitantly, the field of health care has experienced a proliferation of roles. The exponential increase in technology in an extremely short time span and the demands made by consumers seeking ready access to care have caused health professionals to continually redefine and realign their roles. Nursing, like other professions, offers a career ladder for the aspiring. For career development, each upward step features different professional responsibilities, opportunities, and associations.[7] The shortage of primary care physicians created a situation in which clinical nurse specialists and nurse practitioners were hired to perform many clinical activities that were formerly the responsibility of physicians.[8] Brault, in a 1976 California study, found that nurses with higher levels of nursing responsibility were found to produce more favorable patient outcomes.[9] Clark and Affonso state:

> The number of roles which a person enacts also influences role performance ability. Someone with a repertoire of a variety of well practiced, realistic social roles is better able to meet new and critical situations and to deal effectively with others. However, a multiple of role demands may pose serious difficulties to a person's ability to fulfill role obligations unless the allocation of time and resources is handled in a satisfactory manner.[10]

Miss Wiedenbach has expressed her own concept of role theory: ''Role may be conceptualized as a characterization of an individual of designated, distinctive qualities and competencies which (s)he typically manifests both in what (s)he does and in the way in which (s)he does it.''[11] She sees change in role as a behavioral response to the realities within the situation. Five realities noted in Miss Wiedenbach's role theory are: (1) the agent or propelling force, (2) the recipient or consumer, (3) the goal, (4) the means to the goal, and (5) the framework or environment. Role is expressed in any program of deliberate action, tempered by insight and the stock of resources.[12] To summarize, was Miss Wiedenbach's career development a product of the pressures of the health care settings and environment in which she worked, or was it a deliberately planned series of actions?

CONCEPTUAL FRAMEWORK

The previously discussed role theory by Miss Wiedenbach will be used when analyzing data collected as it pertains to her career development. Also utilized as a background will be her central purpose:

to motivate the individual and/or facilitate her efforts to overcome the obstacles which currently or anticipatorily interfere with her ability to respond capably to the demands made of her by the realities in her immediate situation.[13]

Also as a framework will be the three fundamental concepts of her philosophy: (1) reverence for the gift of life; (2) respect for the dignity, worth, autonomy, and individuality of each human being; (3) resoluteness to act dynamically in relation to one's belief.[14]

STATEMENT OF THE PURPOSE OF THE STUDY

The purpose of this study is to contribute to the understanding of the history of nursing and nurse-midwifery by focusing on the life and career evolution of Ernestine Wiedenbach. The principal methodology will be oral history, recorded on video- and audiotapes. Interviews between the investigator and the research subject will be conducted in Miami, Florida.

A goal of the historiographer will be to establish the truth, publish the research findings, and establish a foundation for future historical research.

METHODOLOGY

The first step of this research study will be to gather background data, including a review of: (1) Miss Wiedenbach's writings; (2) the history of nursing in the United States, 1900 to 1970; (3) the birth and development of nurse-midwifery in the United States; and (4) a background history of the United States, 1900 to 1970.

Both primary and secondary source material will be used; however, the principal focus will be the valuable primary source of oral history as recorded from interviews with Ernestine Wiedenbach via audio and video tapings. Oral history is recognized as one of the most exciting current historical movements. The tapings of the remembrances of older members of a professional community provide records of what took place in the past periods of time and in specific places.[15]

The profile of Miss Wiedenbach will focus on: personal data, personality characteristics, education, career evolution, philosophy, contributions, social relationships, reflections on nursing and nurse-midwifery, and predictions for the profession's future. Other primary sources used to substantiate the oral history will be published primary sources, personal writings, diaries, and professional societies' minutes and histories.

Secondary sources involve materials from some other authors. Although secondary sources are less reliable and trustworthy, they will be used as background material for corroboration. Particularly, information obtained from the Ernestine Wiedenbach Reading Room Archives at Yale University may provide interesting secondary sources. Review of these data may necessitate a trip to Yale by the researcher.

The historical research design will be used and all data will be subject to intensive internal and external criticism. External criticism establishes the validity of documents by examining the authenticity of the original material. The purpose of external criticism is to establish that original documents are what they purport to be. Examination of the handwriting, age of the paper, signature, and source are all part of the external criticism to prevent fraud.

Internal criticism establishes reliability of the data. An important part of internal criticism is a broad knowledge of the period in which the data originated. In this study, it would be important to bear in mind that even primary sources are not completely reliable and should be corroborated by two independent primary sources to be established as fact. Material will be categorized as a possibility when supported by only one primary source and a probability when supported by sufficient secondary source backing.

Thus, all information for this historical research must pass the criteria of internal and external criticism for reliability and validity.

PLAN FOR DATA ANALYSIS

The narrative format will be used with synthesis of significant propositions. ''The historian has no obligation to be clever or dull, but she had better be interesting.''[16]

LIMITATIONS OF THE STUDY

Personal bias, projection of meaning, and incorrect interpretation of facts can pose a real problem to the historiographer. Objectivity must be maintained. Also considered as limitations will be the limited research experience of the investigator and time constraints.

REFERENCES

1. Hockett, H. C. 1955. *Critical Method in Historical Research and Writing*. New York: Macmillan, p. 8.
2. Dempsey, P. A., and A. D. Dempsey. 1981. *The Research Process in Nursing*. New York: Van Nostrand, p. 117.

3. Notter L. E. 1972. ''The Case for Historical Research in Nursing.'' *Nursing Research,* 21(November–December): 11.
4. Newton, M. E. 1965. ''The Case for Historical Research.'' *Nursing Research,* 14(Winter): 24.
5. Ibid., p. 23.
6. Hardy, M. E., and M. E. Conway. 1978. *Role Theory: Perspective for Health Professionals.* New York: Appleton-Century-Crofts, p. 24.
7. Ibid., p. 234.
8. Ibid., p. 179.
9. Ibid., p. 174.
10. Clark, A. L., and D. D. Affonso. 1976. *Childbearing: A Nursing Perspective.* Philadelphia: F. A. Davis, p. 50.
11. Wiedenbach, E. 1968. ''The Nurse's Role in Family Planning.'' *Nursing Clinics of North America,* 3(June): 356.
12. Ibid., p. 357.
13. Ibid., p. 358.
14. Ibid., p. 359.
15. Dempsey and Dempsey, *The Research Process,* p. 9.
16. Newton, ''Historical Research,'' p. 23.

BIBLIOGRAPHY

Baker, W. G. 1979. ''Changes in Life Goals as Related to Success in a Nursing Leadership Role.'' *Nursing Research,* 28 (July–August): 234–236.

Christy, T. E. 1975. ''The Methodology of Historical Research: A Brief Introduction.'' *Nursing Research,* 24(May–June): 189–192.

Clark, A. L. and Affonso, D. D. 1976. *Childbearing: A Nursing Perspective.* Philadelphia: F. A. Davis.

Dempsey, P. A., and A. D. Dempsey. 1981. *The Research Process in Nursing.* New York: Van Nostrand.

Hardy, M. E., and M. E. Conway. 1978. *Role Theory: Perspectives for Health Professionals.* New York: Appleton-Century-Crofts.

Hockett, H. C. 1955. *Critical Method in Historical Research and Writing.* New York: Macmillan.

Newton, M. E. 1965. ''The Case for Historical Research.'' *Nursing Research,* 14(Winter): 20–26.

Notter, L. E. 1972. ''The Case for Historical Research in Nursing.'' *Nursing Research,* 21(November–December): 11–12.

Varney, H. 1980. *Nurse-Midwifery.* Boston: Blackwell Scientific.

Wiedenbach, E. 1968. ''The Nurse's Role in Family Planning.'' *Nursing Clinics of North America,* 3(June): 355–365.

Appendix B

Example of a Descriptive Research Proposal

PATIENTS' USE OF AN EMERGENCY CARE FACILITY DURING THE NIGHT HOURS: A DESCRIPTIVE STUDY

by
JANET FIERRO

Reprinted by permission.

INTRODUCTION
    Statement of the Problem
    Literature Review
    Conceptual Framework
    Purpose of the Study
    Definition of Terms
PLAN FOR DATA COLLECTION
PLAN FOR DATA ANALYSIS
LIMITATIONS OF THE STUDY
APPENDIX: GUIDELINES FOR DATA COLLECTION
REFERENCES
BIBLIOGRAPHY

INTRODUCTION

Statement of the Problem

Patients presenting to an emergency room in the night hours with medical problems has been an area of interest and concern. Frequently, the client has been suffering for more than a few hours with the complaint, but has selected the nighttime to seek help. In many parts of the United States, the hospital emergency department stands alone as the one continuously available point of access for patients seeking medical care. The facility is the institutional focal point for treating a myriad of problems, from simple to severe. Since World War II, there has been an increase of more than 600 percent in the number of emergency visits in some hospitals. The national average has increased 10 percent each year.[1]

Health care facilities utilize a skeletal staff in the after hours to perform the routine duties usually handled in the daytime hours. What are the motivating factors that bring patients to the hospital late at night for problems that they have had all day or, in some cases, more than a day? In order to maintain excellence of care, in addition to accessibility to that care, we must study the reasons our clients come out in the middle of the night for help when we have been waiting for them all day!

Basic human needs obviously must be met regardless of the time of day. Dorothea Orem, in her theory of self-care, has postulated that when man has a problem with meeting the requirements necessary for maintenance of present states of health or well-being, he will require intervention to alleviate the deficit.[2] The theory is not specific as to the time of day these deficits must be met; therefore, a more in-depth investigation into the health needs during the night hours has sparked an interest.

Literature Review

Although there is fairly substantial literature on the use of emergency medical facilities, little has been written about the characteristics of the patient who presents during the night hours. A review of the literature did not uncover any articles that described the specific rationale for clients presenting for treatment after hours. But a study by Ross Laboratories from 1957 to 1967 cited the increase of emergency room visits as 175 percent during that period, with up to 60 percent estimated to be of a nonemergency nature.[3] The extensive use of emergency room facilities as a source of primary medical care, whether in the day or night hours, remains a persistent health care delivery problem in the United States. Approximately 33 percent of all visits to physicians are made to a hospital emergency department.[4] Hospital emergency rooms are being utilized regularly for the provision of nonurgent care for concerns usually brought to primary-care physicians.[5]

A Chicago study attributed the increased use of emergency departments to: (1) population factors such as a 2 percent population growth rate per year, an increase in incidence of chronic disease, higher accident rates, and a mobile population; (2) hospital factors reflecting the patient's faith in costly equipment only available in hospitals, public confidence in hospitals, and the view of the hospital as the only place where care is available twenty-four hours a day; (3) external factors including health insurance plan benefits for emergency department care, in contrast to other types of ambulatory care for which no benefits are available; and (4) legal issues.[6]

Brook and Stevenson, in a study of the effectiveness of nonemergency care delivered in an emergency room setting at Baltimore City Hospital, found that only 68 percent of patients referred for follow-up X-ray studies for gastrointestinal complaints actually completed the X-rays, while only 50 percent of these patients were seen in a clinic for any further follow-up of their complaints.[7] A similar study done at Johns Hopkins Hospital revealed almost identical results.[8]

An article from the psychiatric literature reveals documentation that insomnia, persistent or sporadic, often accompanies health deficits.[9] People's constitutions are at the lowest ebb in the middle of the night, with the feelings of defeat and despair overwhelming, according to McCartney.[10] These individuals frequently turn to the emergency department in the middle of the night for help, citing apprehension and helpless feelings as the driving force.

Findings in the field of social psychology were thought to be pertinent, since the low socioeconomic status group accounts for a majority of the patient populations in the emergency department. Persons of this low status give greater priority to meeting immediate needs than to the achievement of long-range goals.[11] The main factor generally distinguishing the poor from the economically more advantaged has been their feelings of helplessness and psychological inability to cope with any further deficits in their already impoverished environment. This concept of social well-being (or lack of it) carries over into their response to health matters, again pointing to the use of the emergency department, as cited by Herzog.[12]

The attitudes of patients are extremely complex, especially in areas that affect choice and usage of health care facilities. Originally, economic reasons were thought to cause some people not to use a service. Now, it is generally accepted that social-psychological reasons are equally or more important.[13] Appropriate utilization of health care service is predicated on a proper attitude toward the service by the patient. An untested assumption in the medical field is that patients who use emergency departments have little interest in developing a patient–physician relationship and use the emergency department in lieu of a private physician. McNamara feels that the attitude and philosophy of the patient using an emergency department may be more ''contemporary,'' as opposed to the ''traditional'' attitude that encompasses a close patient–physician relationship and use of the emergency facility for major traumas only.[14] A study was undertaken to measure the ''contemporary'' or ''traditional'' attitude toward health care of a population using the emergency room.[15] The study assumed that emergent patients use the emergency room by necessity while the nonemergent patient uses the facility for convenience. The corresponding attitude difference should have correlated with the usage pattern—the emergent patient would have a traditional attitude and the nonemergent patient the contemporary attitude. Unfortunately, the results of the study were unable to completely confirm the assumption and indicated that there is no difference regardless of the urgency of the patient's condition. The conflict between attitude and action raises the question: Are patients using the emergency room because they have no other point of entry into the health care system?

The impact of social networks on health behavior and health services utilization has been under investigation for a decade.[16] Berkanovic et al. suggest that under the threat of illness, individuals begin to seek information and support from their network of social contacts.[17] "Strong tie" networks, where there is consultation with few persons, lead to delay behaviors, since group opinion tends to be uniform and tends to support the individual to stay well. "Weak tie" networks, with their diverse contacts, may provide confusing and disparate information, which causes individuals to seek professional advice sooner than they would if their network were of the strong tie variety. Additionally, Horowitz postulated that the type and structure of the network may have less influence on utilization behavior than the type of advice the network members give—that is, whether they advocate seeking medical care quickly in the face of concern or symptoms or espouse delay and non-use of medical care.[18]

A significant relationship between life stress and medical illness was empirically documented by Anderson and Pleticha in 1974.[19] Patients who recently had undergone some stressful life situation presented at their emergency unit and were admitted for medical problems. The investigators randomly sampled 52 emergency room patients treated over a one-week period and interviewed them using the Holmes and Rahe 1967 Social Readjustment Rating Scale to determine life stress (change) units. The results of the investigation confirm the relationship between stressful life events and presentation for medical care. Although the investigators were unable to document any relationship between specific life events and specific illnesses, they validated a relationship between the degree to which an individual was adapting to stressful life events and his perception of the severity of his medical problem. The impact of stress and patients' health deviation self-care is extremely valid and appropriate for a study into patients' use of the emergency department at any time of day or night![20]

In summarizing the literature specifically on patients' use of the emergency units, the reader will note a definite increase over the past decade in the utilization of emergency facilities. Unfortunately, patients seek care for non-acute problems, often draining emergency room personnel from the acute cases. This subject requires further investigation but certainly warrants some documentation in any study on emergency room patients and utilization.

Economics is perhaps the greatest reason people seek care at the emergency room, whether it be because of availability and accessibility or due to the fact that most third-party payments are reimbursed through emergency rooms

and not private doctors. Accessibility over twenty-four hours is the prime reason people use the emergency services, but the literature review fails to reveal
other reasons that patients present after hours.

The motivating factors that bring people to seek health care can be related
to their own support or lack of support systems. The more contemporary attitude about receiving health care from the emergency room physician for non-
acute problems was addressed in relation to the traditional attitude of emergency room for acute cases only, but a direct correlation could not be made
even with such valuable information.

The impact of stress on individuals' lives was reviewed in regard to seeking attention for medical problems. An underlying life stress assessment
would be warranted for any patient who presents to the emergency room regardless of his presenting problem or time of day. As health professionals our
responsibility should be to deliver the appropriate care first and then to educate the consumer.

Conceptual Framework

The goal of the health care services is the health and well-being of individuals,
families, and communities.[21] Orem believes the focus of nursing is to help the
individual achieve health results through therapeutic self-care.[22] She defines
self-care as the practice of activities that the individual personally initiates and
performs on his own behalf in maintaining life, health, and well-being. Essentially, self-care is a person's continuous contribution to his or her own health.

Self-care is founded upon the following premises:

1. Self-care is based on voluntary action that humans are capable of undertaking.
2. Self-care is based on deliberate and thoughtful judgment that leads to the
   appropriate action.
3. Self-care is a requirement of every person and is a universal requisite for
   meeting basic human needs.
4. Adults have the right and the responsibility to care for themselves in
   order to maintain health, life, and well-being.
5. Self-care is behavior that evolves through the combination of social and
   cognitive experiences and is learned through one's interpersonal relationships, communication, and culture.
6. Self-care contributes to the self-esteem and self-image of a person and is
   directly affected by self-concept.[23]

Orem perceives nursing's special concern as the individual's need for self-
care action and the provision and management of it on a continuous basis in
order to sustain life and health, recover from disease or injury, and cope with

their effects.[24] In addition, Orem views nursing as a vehicle for providing assistance to persons who are completely or partially unable to perform their own daily health-related care because of their health situation.

Patients seeking care for problems at any time of the day or night are obviously not able to meet their own self-care needs. These deficits compromise the individual's therapeutic responses, threatening his maintenance of life processes, promotion of normal growth and development, and prevention or control of disease and disability. The nurse in the emergency room must assess clients' limitations in self-care and intervene at the appropriate level. Orem suggests three basic designs of nursing assistance from which the nurse can select a system or combination of systems that will most effectively aid in achieving the desired results for the patient: (1) wholly compensatory, (2) partly compensatory, and (3) supportive-educative.

The patient who needs supportive-educative guidance for self-care requires precious time that is not usually afforded during night hours in an emergency room. Totally incapacitated patients are the primary target for intervention with a minimal amount of manpower. If patients can receive a supportive-educative background prior to discharge from the hospital or even over the telephone once in the home setting, their need to present to the emergency department might be reduced.

The investigator feels strongly that with the proper education, the community can practice self-care and therefore require intervention only when medically necessary. The time to seek attention for nonacute problems is during the day, when staffing of all facilities allows the highest level of care possible.

Purpose of the Study

The purpose of the study is to (1) collect specific data on each medical patient presenting to the emergency department utilizing a basic health assessment tool; (2) classify these patients into one of Orem's three nursing systems; (3) determine, if possible, any motivating factors for these patients presenting during the night hours.

Definition of Terms

Health deviation self-care: Those demands or requirements that arise owing to illness, injury, or life cycle events.[25]
Medical patients: Any patient not asking specifically to see the psychiatrist.
Nursing system: The approaches that the nurse uses to assist patients with deficits in self-care due to a condition of health:
    Wholly compensatory: Patient has no active role in the performance of his care. The nurse acts for and does for the patient.
    Partly compensatory: Both the patient and the nurse perform care measures

requiring manipulative tasks. Distribution of responsibility for performance of care varies with patient's actual physical or medical limitation.

Supportive-educative: Patient is able to perform or can and should learn to
perform required measures of self-care.[26]

Nonacute emergency: Presenting condition does not require the resources of an
emergency department; referral for routine care may or may not be
needed; delay of twenty-four hours would make no appreciable difference
in patients' clinical condition.

Self-care: The practice of activities that individuals personally initiate and perform on their own behalf for maintenance, restoration, or promotion of
health.[27]

Self-care deficit: An inability to engage in self-care, which occurs when the patient is unable to meet the therapeutic self-care demand placed upon
him.[28]

Therapeutic self-care demand: A complex set of objectively established requirements for actions that assist a person with maintenance of present states
of health or well-being or with movement toward estimated desirable
states.[29]

Universal self-care: Basic human needs that are constantly present and must be
met in order to maintain a healthy state. They are air, food, and water;
elimination; solitude and social interaction; activity and rest; protection
from hazards; normalcy.[30]

Veteran: Any man 20 years of age or older who received an honorable discharge
from the Army, Navy, Air Force, or Marines for service to the United
States of America.

PLAN FOR DATA COLLECTION

The researcher will use a descriptive approach to study a selected group of
medical patients presenting to the emergency department at a Veterans' Administration Medical Center. The investigator plans to observe and describe
the sample by means of an interview to gain an assessment of their self-care
deficit and then to later classify the patient into one of Orem's nursing systems.

The target population will be any veteran presenting to the emergency facility for medical problems between the hours of midnight and 6:00 A.M. A
prearranged time will be selected for the researcher to obtain a convenience
sample of at least 30 patients and not more than 50 patients. Only those patients requesting medical treatment will be used in the study; patients requesting to see the psychiatrist will be excluded from the study. If the patient is
unable to communicate and information can be elicited from a significant

other, the patient will still be selected. Due to the nature of the facility, the demographic data on the veteran will be collected by the admission clerk prior to the interview.

Pertinent data on the patient's health will be collected by the investigator, utilizing the standard assessment tool already in existence at the facility. This tool is a single sheet of paper with the top portion for the nursing personnel to write, in SOAP format, a brief assessment. There is an area for vital signs, date and time of day patient presents for treatment, and patient's age and sex. The physician completes the chart by writing his findings, orders, and disposition. This chart becomes part of the patient's permanent record at the facility.

For the purpose of the study and to protect the human rights of the veteran, the author will incorporate the health history, elicited from the patient or the significant other, into a design suitable for selecting one of Orem's nursing systems. The Guidelines for Data Collection (appendix) indicate what the investigator hopes to gain from the assessment interview. Only the information listed in the guidelines will be considered pertinent for the study. The interview will take only a few minutes, as is normal procedure for the facility.

The interviewer (investigator) will ask each client the following information:

1. Main complaint in patient's own words.
2. Brief description of presenting problems. The client will be asked to describe his condition, duration of symptoms, what client has attempted to do for relief of symptoms, and if there are motivating factors for seeking help at this time.
3. Support systems. Patient will be asked if he lives with family or alone and how he manages with present health status.
4. Past history. Patient will be asked to describe past health problems.

Following the interview, the client will be seen by the physician, or, if the client is in acute distress, he will be seen immediately by the physician. The investigator can obtain the interview after the physician has seen the patient or can get it from the family. All patients (or their families) will have an interview by the nurse (investigator).

The initial interview is essential because it is the segment of the nursing process that provides an accurate description of the reasons a patient requires nursing care and determines the kind of nursing required. Once the information has been gathered from the patient and the doctor has made his diagnosis, the investigator will categorize all the pertinent data to help classify the patient.

After the patient has been interviewed by the nurse, examined and evaluated by the doctor, and a diagnosis established, the investigator will incorporate all the information utilizing the Guidelines for Data Collection. To facilitate the lengthy process of categorizing all the information from the assessment and attempting to incorporate it into Orem's design, the investigator will make a nursing diagnosis for each patient. The information will be submitted to a panel of three nurses from a graduate school of nursing who have a background in adult health and Orem's theory of self-care. The panel will decide into which of Orem's nursing systems the patient should be placed (wholly compensatory, partly compensatory, or supportive-educative). By having the panel of experts make the final decision, the investigator hopes to eliminate bias and avoid a judgmental opinion.

PLAN FOR DATA ANALYSIS

Descriptive statistics will be utilized to describe and synthesize the data collected from the sample. Since the purpose of the study is to classify the patients into one of Orem's nursing systems, that will be the primary target. The investigator hopes to gain enough information about each member of the sample to also classify the self-care deficits, determining which were the most frequently seen (see Table B.1).

At the present time, the investigator does not feel qualified to make an attempt at any further discussion of methods of analyzing the data. The majority of the material collected from the client may be so complex that only written description will clarify it. For clarity, the investigator would like to utilize tables and graphs that will display the information neatly and concisely for any reader.

LIMITATIONS OF THE STUDY

The facility being utilized for the study is not equipped to handle pediatric cases and only rarely treats women; therefore, the sample will be adult men. Since most primary-care facilities treat all types of patients, the study might be slightly one-sided in relation to the parameters of demographic data.

TABLE B.1
Percentage from Sample Classified According to Orem's Nursing System

Orem's System	*Percentage*
Wholly compensatory	
Partly compensatory	
Supportive-educative	

A large percentage of night admissions in the emergency room are psychiatric patients. If these patients had been included in the sample, the researcher would have to have included a psychiatric interview tool and would not have felt comfortable dealing with this. The facility has a psychiatric nursing team on all shifts to handle patients requiring mental hygiene.

A better cross-section of the population could be viewed if more time were allowed for selection of the sample. There are definitely trends in the veteran population, with peak admission times being during the winter season when there is an influx of tourists. By limiting the sample selection time, there is also a limit on the cross-section of the population.

APPENDIX: GUIDELINES FOR DATA COLLECTION

  I. Demographic data
      A. Age
      B. Sex
      C. Marital status (determine support system)
 II. Subjective data (what patient perceives of his health)
      A. Signs and symptoms
      B. Duration of problems
      C. What client has done to relieve problems
      D. Medications client is taking
      E. What client hopes to achieve by his visit
III. Objective data (what investigator sees)
      A. Brief description of client's physical self
      B. Interpretation of lab values, EKG, and any treatments accomplished
 IV. Assessment: Universal self-care requisites
      A. Investigator will list any problem seen with universal self-care requisites and devise a nursing diagnosis
  V. Selection of nursing agency (system)
      A. Panel to decide whether client belongs in wholly compensatory, partly compensatory, or supportive-educative system.

REFERENCES

1. Jenkins, A. 1978. "Emergency Department Organization and Management." *American College of Emergency Physicians*, 23(4): 2–6.
2. Orem, D. 1971. *Nursing: Concepts of Practice*. New York: McGraw-Hill.
3. Ross Laboratories. 1967. *Currents in Hospital Administration*. Columbus, OH: Ross Laboratories, p. 1.
4. National Center for Health Statistics. 1977. *Health United States 1976–1977*. DHEW Publication No. (HRA) 77. Washington, DC: U.S. Government Printing Office.

5. Jacobs, A., J. Gavett, and R. Wersinger. 1971. "Emergency Department Utilization in an Urban Community." *JAMA*, 216: 307.
6. Gibson, G. 1970. *Emergency Medical Services in the Chicago Area.* Center for Health Administration Studies. Chicago: University of Chicago.
7. Brook, R., and R. Stevenson. 1948. "Effectiveness of Patient Care in an Emergency Room." *New England Journal of Medicine,* 238: 204.
8. Brook, R. H., M. H. Berg, and P. A. Schecter. 1973. "Effectiveness of Non-Emergency Care via the Emergency Room." *Annals of Internal Medicine,* 78: 333.
9. McCartney, F. 1978. "A Deep but Dazzling Darkness." *Journal of Psychiatric Nursing and Mental Health Services,* 10: 38–39.
10. Ibid.
11. Herzog, E. 1963. "Some Assumptions about the Poor." *Social Service Review,* 37 (12): 397.
12. Ibid.
13. McNamara, J. R. 1979. *Behavioral Approaches to Medicine: Application and Analysis.* New York: Plenum Press.
14. Ibid.
15. Ibid.
16. Berkanovic, E., C. Telesky, and S. Reeder. 1981. "Structural and Social Psychological Factors in the Decision to Seek Medical Care for Symptoms." *Medical Care,* 19(7): 693–709.
17. Ibid.
18. Horowitz, A. 1978. "Family, Kin and Friend Networks in Psychiatric Help-Seeking." *Social Science Medicine,* 12: 297.
19. Anderson, M., and J. Pleticha. 1974. "Emergency Unit Patients' Perception of Stressful Life Events." *Nursing Research,* 23(5): 378–383.
20. Orem, *Nursing: Concepts of Practice.*
21. Ibid.
22. Ibid.
23. Joseph, L. 1980. "Self-Care and the Nursing Process." *Nursing Clinics of North America,* 15(1): 131–143.
24. Orem, *Nursing: Concepts of Practice.*
25. Ibid.
26. Ibid.
27. Ibid.
28. Ibid.
29. Ibid.
30. Ibid.

BIBLIOGRAPHY

Anderson, M., and J. Pleticha. 1974. "Emergency Unit Patients' Perception of Stressful Life Events." *Nursing Research,* 23(5): 378–383.
Berkanovic, E., C. Telesky, and S. Reeder. 1981. "Structural and Social Psychological Factors in the Decision to Seek Medical Care for Symptoms." *Medical Care,* 19(7): 693–709.
Brook, R., and R. Stevenson. 1948. "Effectiveness of Patient Care in an Emergency Room." *New England Journal of Medicine,* 238: 204.
Brook, R. H., M. H. Berg, and P. A. Schecter. 1973. "Effectiveness of Non-Emergency Care via the Emergency Room." *Annals of Internal Medicine,* 78: 333.

Gibson, G. 1970. *Emergency Medical Services in the Chicago Area.* Chicago: Center for Health Administration Studies, University of Chicago.

Herzog, E. 1963. "Some Assumptions About the Poor." *Social Service Review,* 37(12): 389–402.

Horowitz, A. 1978. "Family, Kin and Friend Networks in Psychiatric Help-Seeking." *Social Science Medicine,* 12: 297.

Jacobs, A., J. Gavett, and R. Wersinger. 1971. "Emergency Department Utilization in an Urban Community." *JAMA,* 216: 307.

Jenkins, A. 1978. "Emergency Department Organization and Management." *American College of Emergency Physicians,* 23(4): 2–6.

Joseph, L. 1980. "Self-Care and the Nursing Process." *Nursing Clinics of North America,* 15(1): 131–143.

MacStravic, R. 1978. *Determining Health Needs.* Ann Arbor: Health Administration Press, School of Public Health, University of Michigan.

McCartney, F. 1978. "A Deep but Dazzling Darkness." *Journal of Psychiatric Nursing and Mental Health Services,* 10: 38–39.

McNamara, J. R. 1979. *Behavioral Approaches to Medicine: Application and Analysis.* New York: Plenum Press.

National Center for Health Statistics. 1977. *Health United States 1976–1977.* DHEW Publication No. (HRA) 77. Washington, DC: U.S. Government Printing Office.

Orem, D. E. 1971. *Nursing: Concepts of Practice.* New York: McGraw-Hill.

Ross Laboratories. 1967. *Currents in Hospital Administration.* Columbus, OH: Ross Laboratories.

Appendix C

Example of a Research Report

PATIENTS' USE OF AN EMERGENCY CARE FACILITY DURING THE NIGHT HOURS: A DESCRIPTIVE STUDY

by
JANET FIERRO

Reprinted by permission.

INTRODUCTION

Statement of the Problem

Patients presenting to an emergency room in the night hours with medical problems has been an area of interest and concern. Frequently, the client has been suffering for more than a few hours with the complaint, but has selected the nighttime to seek help. In many parts of the United States, the hospital emergency department stands alone as the one continuously available point of access for patients seeking medical care. The facility is the institutional focal point for treating a myriad of problems, from simple to severe. Since World War II, there has been an increase of more than 600 percent in the number of emergency visits in some hospitals. The national average has increased 10 percent each year.[1]

Health care facilities utilize a skeletal staff in the after hours to perform the routine duties usually handled in the day hours. What are the motivating factors that bring patients to the hospital late at night for problems that they have had all day or, in some cases, more than a day? In order to maintain excellence of care, in addition to accessibility to that care, we must study the reasons our clients come out in the middle of the night for help when we have been waiting for them all day!

Basic human needs obviously must be met regardless of the time of day. Dorothea Orem, in her theory of self-care, has postulated that when man has a problem with meeting the requirements necessary for maintenance of present states of health or well-being, he will require intervention to alleviate the deficit.[2] The theory is not specific as to the time of day these deficits must be met; therefore, a more in-depth investigation into the health needs during the night hours has sparked an interest.

Literature Review

Although there is fairly substantial literature on the use of emergency medical facilities, little has been written about the characteristics of the patient who presents during the night hours. A review of the literature did not uncover any articles that described the specific rationale for clients presenting for treatment after hours. But a study by Ross Laboratories from 1957 to 1967 cited the increase of emergency room visits as 175 percent during that period, with up to 60 percent estimated to be of a nonemergency nature.[3] The extensive use of emergency room facilities as a source of primary medical care, whether in the day or night hours, remains a persistent health care delivery problem in the United States. Approximately 33 percent of all visits to physicians are made to a hospital emergency department.[4] Hospital emergency rooms are being utilized regularly for the provision of nonurgent care for concerns usually brought to primary-care physicians.[5]

A Chicago study attributed the increased use of emergency departments to: (1) population factors such as a 2 percent population growth rate per year, an increase in incidence of chronic disease, higher accident rates, and a mobile population; (2) hospital factors reflecting the patient's faith in costly equipment only available in hospitals, public confidence in hospitals, and the view of the hospital as the only place where care is available twenty-four hours a day; (3) external factors including health insurance plan benefits for emergency department care, in contrast to other types of ambulatory care for which no benefits are available; and (4) legal issues.[6]

Brook and Stevenson, in the study of the effectiveness of nonemergency care delivered in an emergency room setting at Baltimore City Hospital, found that only 68 percent of patients referred for follow-up X-ray studies for gastrointestinal complaints actually completed the X-rays, while only 50 percent of these patients were seen in a clinic for any further follow-up of their complaints.[7] A similar study done at Johns Hopkins Hospital revealed almost identical results.[8]

An article from the psychiatric literature reveals documentation that insomnia, persistent or sporadic, often accompanies health deficits.[9] People's constitutions are at the lowest ebb in the middle of the night, with the feelings of defeat and despair overwhelming, according to McCartney.[10] These individuals frequently turn to the emergency department in the middle of the night for help, citing apprehension and helpless feelings as the driving force.

Findings in the field of social psychology were thought to be pertinent, since the low socio-economic status group accounts for a majority of the patient populations in the emergency department. Persons of this low status give greater priority to meeting immediate needs than to the achievement of long-range goals.[11] The main factor generally distinguishing the poor from the economically more advantaged has been their feelings of helplessness and psychological inability to cope with any further deficits in their already impoverished environment. This concept of social well-being (or lack of it) carries over into their response to health matters, again pointing to the use of the emergency department, as cited by Herzog.[12]

The attitudes of patients are extremely complex, especially in areas that affect choice and usage of health care facilities. Originally, economic reasons were thought to cause some people not to use a service. Now, it is generally accepted that social-psychological reasons are equally or more important.[13] Appropriate utilization of health care services is predicated on a proper attitude toward the service by the patient. An untested assumption in the medical field is that patients who use emergency departments have little interest in developing a patient–physician relationship and use the emergency department in lieu of a private physician. McNamara feels that the attitudes and philosophy of the patient using an emergency department may be more "contemporary," as opposed to the "traditional" attitude that encompasses a close patient–physician relationship and use of the emergency facility for major traumas only.[14] A study was undertaken to measure the "contemporary" or "traditional" attitude toward health care of a population using the emergency room.[15] The study assumed that emergent patients use the emergency room by necessity, while the non-emergent patient uses the facility for convenience. The corresponding attitude difference should have correlated with the usage pattern—the emergent patient would have a traditional attitude and the non-emergent patient the contemporary attitude. Unfortunately, the results of the study were unable to completely confirm the assumption and indicated that there is no difference regardless of the urgency of the patient's condition. The conflict between attitude and action raises the question: Are patients using the emergency room because they have no other point of entry into the health care system?

The impact of social networks on health behavior and health services utilization has been under investigation for a decade.[16] Berkanovic et al. suggest that under the threat of illness, individuals begin to seek information and support from their network of social contacts.[17] "Strong tie" networks, where there is consultation with few persons, lead to delay behaviors, since group opinion tends to be uniform and tends to support the individual to stay well. "Weak tie" networks, with their diverse contacts, may provide confusing and disparate information, which causes individuals to seek professional advice sooner than they would if their network were of the strong tie variety. Additionally, Horowitz postulated that the type and structure of the network may have less influence on utilization behavior than the type of advice the network members give—that is, whether they advocate seeking medical care quickly in the face of concern or symptoms or espouse delay and non-use of medical care.[18]

A significant relationship between life stress and medical illness was empirically documented by Anderson and Pleticha in 1974.[19] Patients who recently had undergone some stressful life situation presented at their emergency unit and were admitted for medical problems. The investigators randomly sampled 52 emergency room patients treated over a one-week period and interviewed them using the Holmes and Rahe 1967 Social Readjustment Rating Scale to determine life stress (change) units. The results of the investigation confirm the relationship between stressful life events and presentation for medical care. Although the investigators were unable to document any relationship between specific life events and specific illnesses, they validated a relationship between the degree to which an individual was adapting to stressful life events and his perception of the severity of his medical problem. The impact of stress and patients' health deviation self-care is extremely valid and appropriate for a study into patients' use of the emergency department at any time of day or night.[20]

In summarizing the literature specifically on patients' use of the emergency units, the reader will note a definite increase over the past decade in the utilization of emergency facilities. Unfortunately, patients seek care for non-acute problems, often draining emergency room personnel from the acute cases. This subject requires further investigation but certainly warrants some documentation in any study on emergency room patients and utilization.

Economics is perhaps the greatest reason people seek care at the emergency room, whether it be because of availability and accessibility or due to the fact that most third-party payments are reimbursed through emergency rooms and not private doctors. Accessibility over twenty-four hours is the prime reason people use the emergency services, but the literature review fails to reveal other reasons that patients present after hours.

The motivating factors that bring people to seek health care can be related to their own support or lack of support systems. The more contemporary attitude about receiving health care from the emergency room physician for non-acute problems was addressed in relation to the traditional attitude of emergency room for acute cases only, but a direct correlation could not be made even with such valuable information.

The impact of stress on individuals' lives was reviewed in regard to seeking attention for medical problems. An underlying life stress assessment would be warranted for any patient who presents to the emergency room regardless of his presenting problem or time of day. As health professionals our responsibility should be to deliver the appropriate care first and then to educate the consumer.

Conceptual Framework

The goal of the health care services is the health and well-being of individuals, families, and communities.[21] Orem believes the focus of nursing is to help the individual achieve health results through therapeutic self-care.[22] She defines self-care as the practice of activities that the individual personally initiates and performs on his own behalf in maintaining life, health, and well-being. Essentially, self-care is a person's continuous contribution to his or her own health.

Self-care is founded upon the following premises:

1. Self-care is based on voluntary action that humans are capable of undertaking.
2. Self-care is based on deliberate and thoughtful judgment that leads to the appropriate action.
3. Self-care is a requirement of every person and is a universal requisite for meeting basic human needs.
4. Adults have the right and the responsibility to care for themselves in order to maintain health, life, and well-being.
5. Self-care is behavior that evolves through the combination of social and

cognitive experiences and is learned through one's interpersonal relationships, communication, and culture.
6.   Self-care contributes to the self-esteem and self-image of a person and is directly affected by self-concept.[23]

Orem perceives nursing's special concern as the individual's need for self-care action and the provision and management of it on a continuous basis in order to sustain life and health, recover from disease or injury, and cope with their effects.[24] In addition, Orem views nursing as a vehicle for providing assistance to persons who are completely or partially unable to perform their own daily health-related care because of their health situation.

Patients seeking care for problems at any time of the day or night are obviously not able to meet their own self-care needs. These deficits compromise the individual's therapeutic responses threatening his maintenance of life processes, promotion of normal growth and development, and prevention or control of disease and disability. The nurse in the emergency room must assess clients' limitations in self-care and intervene at the appropriate level. Orem suggests three basic designs of nursing assistance from which the nurse can select a system or combination of systems that will most effectively aid in achieving the desired results for the patient: (1) wholly compensatory, (2) partly compensatory, and (3) supportive-educative.

The patient who needs supportive-educative guidance for self-care requires precious time that is not usually afforded during night hours in an emergency room. Totally incapacitated patients are the primary target for intervention with a minimal amount of manpower. If patients can receive a supportive-educative background prior to discharge from the hospital or even over the telephone once in the home setting, their need to present to the emergency department might be reduced.

The investigator feels strongly that with the proper education, the community can practice self-care and therefore require intervention only when medically necessary. The time to seek attention for nonacute problems is during the day, when staffing of all facilities allows the highest level of care possible.

Purpose of the Study

The purpose of the study was to (1) collect specific data on each medical patient presenting to the emergency department utilizing a basic health assessment tool; (2) classify these patients into one of Orem's three nursing systems; (3) determine, if possible, any motivating factors for these patients presenting during the night hours.

Definition of Terms

Health deviation self-care: Those demands or requirements that arise owing to illness, injury, or life cycle events.[25]

Medical patients: Any patient not asking specifically to see the psychiatrist.

Nursing system: The approaches that the nurse uses to assist patients with deficits in self-care due to a condition of health:

  Wholly compensatory: Patient has no active role in the performance of his care. The nurse acts for and does for the patient.

  Partly compensatory: Both the patient and the nurse perform care measures requiring manipulative tasks. Distribution of responsibility for performance of care varies with patient's actual physical or medical limitation.

  Supportive-educative: Patient is able to perform or can and should learn to perform required measures of self-care.[26]

Nonacute emergency: Presenting condition does not require the resources of an emergency department; referral for routine care may or may not be needed; delay of twenty-four hours would make no appreciable difference in patient's clinical condition.

Self-care: The practice of activities that individuals personally initiate and perform on their own behalf for maintenance, restoration, or promotion of health.[27]

Self-care deficit: An inability to engage in self-care, which occurs when the patient is unable to meet the therapeutic self-care demand place upon him.[28]

Therapeutic self-care demand: A complex set of objectively established requirements for actions that assist a person with maintenance of present states of health or well-being or with movement toward estimated desirable states.

Universal self-care: Basic human needs that are constantly present and must be met in order to maintain a healthy state. They are air, food, and water; elimination; solitude and social interaction; activity and rest; protection from hazards; normalcy.[30]

Veteran: Any man 20 years of age or older who received an honorable discharge from the Army, Navy, Air Force, or Marines for service to the United States of America.

METHODOLOGY

Research Design

A descriptive approach was utilized to study a selected group of medical patients presenting to the emergency department at a Veterans' Administration Medical Center. The investigator planned to observe and describe the sample by means of an interview to gain an assessment of their self-care deficit and then to later classify each patient into one of Orem's nursing systems.

Study Subjects

The target population was any veteran presenting to the emergency facility for medical problems between the hours of midnight and 6:00 A.M. A prearranged time was selected for the researcher to obtain a convenience sample of at least 30 patients and not more than 50 patients. Only those patients requesting medical treatment were used in the study; patients requesting to see the psychiatrist were excluded from the study. If the patient was unable to communicate and information could be elicited from a significant other, the patient was still selected. Due to the nature of the facility, the demographic data on the veterans were collected by the admission clerk prior to the interview.

Data Collection

Pertinent data on the patient's health were collected by the investigator, utilizing the standard assessment tool already in existence at the facility. This tool was a single sheet of paper with the top portion for the nursing personnel to write, in SOAP format, a brief assessment. There was an area for vital signs, date and time of day patient presented for treatment, and patient's age and sex. The physician completed the chart by writing his findings, orders, and disposition. This chart became part of the patient's permanent record at the facility.

For the purpose of the study and to protect the human rights of the veteran, the author incorporated the health history, elicited from the patient or the significant other, into a design suitable for later selecting one of Orem's nursing systems. Table C.1 illustrates what the author hoped to gain from the assessment interview. Only the information listed in the table was considered pertinent for the study. The interview took only a few minutes, as is normal procedure for the facility.

The interviewer (investigator) asked each client the following information:

1. Main complaint in patient's own words.
2. Brief description of presenting problems. The client was asked to describe

TABLE C.1
Percentage from Sample Classified According to Orem's Nursing System

Orem's System	Percentage
Wholly compensatory	20.2%
Partly compensatory	36.8%
Supportive-educative	43.0%

his condition, duration of symptoms, what client had attempted to do for relief of symptoms, and if there were motivating factors for seeking help at this time.

3. Support systems. Client was asked if he lived with family or alone and how he managed with present health status.
4. Past history. Patient was asked to describe past health problems.

Following the interview, the client was seen by the physician, or, if the client was in acute distress, he was seen immediately by the physician. The interview could be obtained after the physician had seen the patient or from the family. All patients (or their families) had an interview by the nurse (investigator).

The initial interview was essential because it was the segment of the nursing process that provided an accurate description of the reasons a patient required nursing care and determined the kind of nursing required. Once the information had been gathered from the patient and the doctor had made his diagnosis, the investigator categorized all the pertinent data to help classify the patient.

After the patient had been interviewed by the nurse, examined and evaluated by the doctor, and a diagnosis established, the investigator incorporated all the information utilizing Table C.1. To facilitate the lengthy process of categorizing all the information from the assessment and attempting to incorporate it into Orem's design, the investigator made a nursing diagnosis for each patient. The information was submitted to a panel of three nurses from a graduate school of nursing who have a background in adult health and Orem's theory of self-care. The panel decided into which of Orem's nursing systems the patient should be placed. By having the panel of experts make the final decision, the investigator eliminated bias and avoided a judgmental opinion.

FINDINGS

The sample consisted of 38 male patients who presented to the emergency department of a VA medical facility during a one-month period between the hours of midnight and 6:00 A.M. A predesigned health assessment tool was utilized for each member of the sample.

After all the necessary information was gathered from the sample, the investigator turned the data over to a panel of experts on the nursing theorist, Dorothea Orem. The three members from the panel of experts were asked to select one of Orem's nursing systems after reading the data collected on each client. Three different-colored pens were provided to distinguish each panelist. Table C.1 demonstrates the percentage of the sample that the panel felt belonged in each of Orem's classifications. The figures were calculated by adding the total number of selections for each of the three categories and determining what percentage of the whole sample those figures represented. The ages of the sample ranged from 20 to 89 years of age. The majority of the patients from the sample fell in the age group of 60 to 69. Table C.2 illustrates the age range of the sample.

A cross-section of the chief complaint of the patient will make it easier for the reader to have a better understanding of the types of clients seen at the facility. The largest single motivating factor for patients presenting to the emergency room was pain. When asked how long they had had the pain, nearly 75 percent responded that the pain had been there for more than twelve hours. The same percentage of subjects felt that the inability to sleep or cope with the pain was the primary reason for coming to the facility during the night hours. Only four members of the sample stated that it was a more convenient time for them to pursue their problem. Table C.3 illustrates the type of presenting problem and the number of subjects in each category.

From the sample of 38, only 10 patients, or 26.3 percent of the sample, were admitted to the facility. The remainder were treated and released. This figure of 26.3 percent justified the 20.2 percent of the sample in Orem's wholly compensatory nursing system. Since the nursing system is for patients who are totally dependent on care, one would hope that they were all admitted.

DISCUSSION

Interpretation of the Findings

The main focus of this investigation was to study the types of patients presenting to an emergency care facility during the night hours. By utilizing a basic health assessment tool, it was hoped to find some motivating factors for clients presenting during the nighttime. Since the literature was not helpful in elicit-

TABLE C.2
Sample by Age Group

Age Range	Frequency
20–29	5
30–39	5
40–49	6
50–59	8
60–69	11
70–79	2
80–89	1

TABLE C.3
Chief Complaint According to Sample

Complaint	Frequency
Abdominal pain	6
Chest pain	4
ENT problem	2
Inebriation	4
Limb or back pain	12
Respiratory dysfunction	6
Skin rash	2
Urinary/bowel dysfunction	2

ing motivating factors for bringing clients to the facility, the author had hoped to find this out by a select sample. Patients apparently are embarrassed to tell a nurse that they were afraid of what was wrong with them. Pain is definitely magnified in the dark, night hours and certainly does prevent people from resting. However, pain that has been going on for weeks needs more evaluation than can be offered during the night hours with only one physician on duty. The study was not designed well enough to gain deeper insight into a patient's perception of what an emergency room is for.

Limitations of the Study

The study was limited by the small sample ($N = 38$). A larger sample would have allowed the researcher to view a more complete cross-section of the population. The study was further limited by using a one-month time frame for gathering the sample.

The nurses on the panel of experts were not all proficient in emergency nursing, and one panelist had no concept of primary care. Had all the members of the panel experienced night duty in an emergency facility, this limitation could have been avoided.

Recommendations for Further Study

The investigator would recommend that a similar study be done allowing the patient to have an opportunity to share his real reason for seeking health care during the night hours. An anonymous mail-in questionnaire with a list of factors/reasons to be checked off by the previously treated patient might accomplish this goal.

Implications for Nursing

With as much as 43 percent of the sample placed in Orem's supportive-educative system, one can clearly see that these were nonurgent cases. A recommendation for a "hotline," available for patients to call in during the night hours, might add a touch of reassurance and advice to the frightened individual. The investigator feels strongly that this hotline could be handled by nursing personnel and would have an impact on the amount of clients presenting unnecessarily.

Availability and accessibility to health care are essential for every human being; this point needs no clarification. But if the facility operates more efficiently during certain hours, our patients should plan on being there during that time. Nursing has a job to do in order to improve quality of care. Orem has taught nurses that our clients must practice "self-care." Now it is our responsibility to instruct them on how to achieve that care.

SUMMARY

The purpose of this descriptive study was to use Orem's theory of self-care to classify medical patients presenting to an emergency care facility between midnight and 6:00 A.M. at a Veterans' Administration Medical Center. Data on the health of 38 subjects were collected using the facility's standard assessment tool. The investigator interviewed each subject using an interview schedule designed to incorporate responses within one of Orem's nursing systems. The largest percentage of subjects (43 percent) were categorized as supportive-educative, 36 percent as partly compensatory, and 20.2 percent as wholly compensatory. The largest single motivating factor for subjects presenting to the emergency facility was pain. Nearly 75 percent stated that the pain had been present for more than twelve hours, and the inability to sleep and to cope with pain was the primary reason for coming to the facility during the night hours. It was recommended that a nursing hotline be made available for patients to call in during the night hours for advice and reassurance. This could impact on the number of nonurgent clients presenting during the night hours.

APPENDIX: GUIDELINES FOR DATA COLLECTION

    I. Demographic data
        A. Age
        B. Sex
        C. Marital status (determine support system)
    II. Subjective data (what patient perceives of his health)
        A. Signs and symptoms
        B. Duration of problems
        C. What client has done to relieve problems

  D. Medications taking
  E. What client hopes to achieve by his visit
III. Objective data (what investigator sees)
  A. Brief description of client's physical self
  B. Interpretation of lab values, EKG, and any treatments accomplished
IV. Assessment: Universal self-care requisites
  A. Author will list any problem seen with universal self-care requisites and devise a nursing diagnosis.
V. Selection of nursing agency (system)
  A. Panel to decide whether client belongs in wholly compensatory, partly compensatory, or supportive-educative system.

ADDENDUM BY THE INVESTIGATOR

At the time this paper was at the typist for final corrections, the Social Service Department at the Veterans' Administration was already utilizing the study. They had hoped to justify having a social worker on duty during the evening and night hours. A review of the data collected on the sample indicated that approximately 20 percent of the patients would have benefited from a social worker before being discharged from the facility!

Our facility is now utilizing a social worker during the evening hours and on weekends. The results of this study had a significant impact on initiating further studies by the Social Service Department at the facility. Nurses who take the time to carry out a research study are further benefiting their patients and the institution.

REFERENCES

1. Jenkins, A. 1978. "Emergency Department Organization and Management." *American College of Emergency Physicians*, 23(4): 2–6.
2. Orem, D. 1971. *Nursing: Concepts of Practice*. New York: McGraw-Hill.
3. Ross Laboratories. 1967. *Currents in Hospital Administration*. Columbus, OH: Ross Laboratories, p. 1.
4. National Center for Health Statistics. 1977. *Health United States 1976–1977*. DHEW Publication No. (HRA) 77. Washington, DC: U.S. Government Printing Office.
5. Jacobs, A., J. Gavett, and R. Wersinger. 1971. "Emergency Department Utilization in an Urban Community." *JAMA*, 216: 307.
6. Gibson, G. 1970. *Emergency Medical Services in the Chicago Area*. Chicago: Center for Health Administration Studies, University of Chicago.
7. Brook, R., and R. Stevenson. 1948. "Effectiveness of Patient Care in an Emergency Room." *New England Journal of Medicine*. 238: 204.
8. Brook, R. H., M. H. Berg, and P. A. Schecter. 1973. "Effectiveness of Non-Emergency Care via the Emergency Room." *Annals of Internal Medicine*, 78: 333.

9. McCartney, F. 1978. "A Deep but Dazzling Darkness." *Journal of Psychiatric Nursing and Mental Health Services,* 10: 38–39.
10. Ibid.
11. Herzog, E. 1963. "Some Assumptions about the Poor." *Social Service Review,* 37(12): 297.
12. Ibid.
13. McNamara, J. R. 1979. *Behavioral Approaches to Medicine: Application and Analysis.* New York: Plenum Press.
14. Ibid.
15. Ibid.
16. Berkanovic, E., C. Telesky, and S. Reeder. 1981. "Structural and Social Psychological Factors in the Decision to Seek Medical Care for Symptoms." *Medical Care,* 19(7): 693–709.
17. Ibid.
18. Horowitz, A. 1978. "Family, Kin and Friend Networks in Psychiatric Help-Seeking." *Social Science Medicine,* 12: 297.
19. Anderson M., and J. Pleticha. 1974. "Emergency Unit Patients' Perception of Stressful Life Events." *Nursing Research,* 23(5): 378–383.
20. Orem, *Nursing: Concepts of Practice.*
21. Ibid.
22. Ibid.
23. Joseph, L. 1980. "Self-Care and the Nursing Process." *Nursing Clinics of North America,* 15(1): 131–143.
24. Orem, *Nursing: Concepts of Practice.*
25. Ibid.
26. Ibid.
27. Ibid.
28. Ibid.
29. Ibid.
30. Ibid.

BIBLIOGRAPHY

Anderson, M., and J. Pleticha. 1974. "Emergency Unit Patients' Perception of Stressful Life Events." *Nursing Research,* 23(5): 378–383.

Berkanovic, E., C. Telesky, and S. Reeder. 1981. "Structural and Social Psychological Factors in the Decision to Seek Medical Care for Symptoms." *Medical Care,* 19(7): 693–709.

Brook, R., and R. Stevenson. 1948. "Effectiveness of Patient Care in an Emergency Room." *New England Journal of Medicine.* 238: 204.

Brook, R. H., M. H. Berg, and P. A. Schecter. 1973. "Effectiveness of Non-Emergency Care via the Emergency Room." *Annals of Internal Medicine,* 78: 333.

Gibson, G. 1970. *Emergency Medical Services in the Chicago Area.* Chicago: Center for Health Administrative Studies, University of Chicago.

Herzog, E. 1963. "Some Assumptions about the Poor." *Social Service Review,* 37(12): 389–402.

Horowitz, A. 1978. "Family, Kin and Friend Networks in Psychiatric Help-Seeking." *Social Science Medicine,* 12: 297.

Jacobs, A., J. Gavett, and R. Wersinger. 1971. ''Emergency Department Utilization in an Urban Community.'' *JAMA*. 216: 307.

Jenkins, A. 1978. ''Emergency Department Organization and Management.'' *American College of Emergency Physicians*, 23(4): 2–6.

Joseph, L. 1980. ''Self-Care and the Nursing Process.'' *Nursing Clinics of North America*, 15(1): 131–143.

MacStravic, R. 1978. *Determining Health Needs*. Ann Arbor: Health Administration Press, School of Public Health, University of Michigan.

McCartney, F. 1978. ''A Deep but Dazzling Darkness.'' *Journal of Psychiatric Nursing and Mental Health Services*, 10: 38–39.

McNamara, J. R. 1979. *Behavioral Approaches to Medicine: Application and Analysis*. New York: Plenum Press.

National Center for Health Statistics. 1977. *Health United States 1976–1977*. DHEW Publication No. (HRA) 77. Washington, DC: U.S. Government Printing Office.

Orem, D. E. 1971. *Nursing: Concepts of Practice*. New York: McGraw-Hill.

Ross Laboratories. 1967. *Currents in Hospital Administration*. Columbus, OH: Ross Laboratories.

Appendix D

Example of a Qualitative Research Proposal

HOMELESS PERSONS WITH AIDS LIVING IN A CONGREGATE FACILITY: AN ETHNOGRAPHIC STUDY

by
SUZAN E. NORMAN

Reprinted by permission.

INTRODUCTION AND STATEMENT OF THE PROBLEM
LITERATURE REVIEW
PURPOSE OF THE STUDY
PLAN FOR DATA COLLECTION
    Study Design
    Setting
    Sample
    Data Collection Techniques
PLAN FOR DATA ANALYSIS
LIMITATIONS OF THE STUDY
ETHICAL CONSIDERATIONS
NURSING IMPLICATIONS
APPENDIX A: INTERVIEW SCHEDULE
APPENDIX B: INFORMED CONSENT FORM—
   LIVING IN SUNRISE MANOR
BIBLIOGRAPHY

INTRODUCTION AND STATEMENT OF THE PROBLEM

Acquired immunodeficiency syndrome (AIDS) is now the leading cause of death in the United States in men under 45 years of age. It is reported that over 100,000 persons in the United States have been diagnosed as having AIDS. Nearly half of these persons with AIDS (PWAs) have died (Center for Disease Control, 1989).

The author wishes to thank Dr. Lydia DeSantis for her professional guidance and editorial assistance in preparing this proposal.

Most PWAs are not hospitalized until an AIDS-related infection with serious physical or psychological debilitation necessitates admission. As such, most PWAs live at home, alone, with friends or family. The financial burden to PWAs is often unmanageable. It can be devastating to someone who prior to diagnosis had inadequate insurance coverage. For PWAs without insurance or family support, the ramifications of having AIDS are overwhelming and can result in one's becoming homeless.

At present there exist but a few shelters or congregate living facilities in the United States that offer food and shelter for homeless PWAs. Having AIDS is saturated with its own unique set of physical, psychological, and social puzzles. Being homeless is accompanied by a multitude of problems. Being a homeless PWA is a contemporary condition, and the needs of this group have not been clearly identified.

There are over 4 million homeless in the United States. According to a recently published study, the typical homeless person in South Florida has a high school education, a family to support, a drug and/or alcohol problem, and nowhere to turn for help. In Dade, Broward, and Palm Beach counties there are about 17,000 individuals who, despite their "homelessness," do not fit the stereotypical "skid row" street bums. Fifty percent are families headed by single women. Fifty-five percent suffer from untreated psychiatric illnesses. Approximately 30 percent have untreated drug and alcohol addictions. It is estimated that 11 percent of the homeless in Miami alone have AIDS (Dewar, 1989).

Despite the apparent interest and the abundance of published information on and about PWAs and homelessness, the literature has focused on the person either caring for PWAs or on those persons living with PWAs. Literature describing what it is like to be a homeless PWA from the PWA's perspective is lacking, but is a necessary first step in addressing the needs and planning appropriate interventions for this growing population.

LITERATURE REVIEW

The literature considers HIV-infected [human immunodeficiency virus infected] individuals from a multiplicity of ethnic cultures and subcultures within these ethnic groups. Even though issues pertaining to specific cultural groups are mentioned, the predominant discussion and source of knowledge is not from an emic perspective (that of the participant). For example, what it is like to live in the United States as a black American male intravenous drug user may change dramatically once this male becomes infected with HIV or is labeled as having AIDS. The cultural rules and expected behaviors may be significantly transformed. How this individual perceives his world may also be modified.

In an investigation by Kelly et al. (1987), physicians' attitudes toward

AIDS patients were explored. Kelly concluded that one of the strongest attitudes was that PWAs are responsible for their illness. In an ethnographic study, Denker (1986) examined the perspectives of health care workers toward pediatric AIDS patients in a large metropolitan city hospital. Seven major themes or domains emerged from this study. These included (1) care, (2) knowledge regarding AIDS, (3) geography within the patient care unit, (4) infection control, (5) fears and doubts, (6) growth and development, and (7) beliefs, feelings, and emotional responses. Denker concluded that most of the fears concerning caring for the pediatric AIDS patients were based on "unknowns"—fears rooted in the uncertainties of viral spread. Education and on-the-job experience with pediatric AIDS patients were the most important factors in decreasing health care workers' unfounded fears.

Freidson (1974) noted that individuals with sexually transmitted diseases were often held in lower respect by medical professionals. The attitude of health care workers has reinforced the stigma of AIDS, with the result that high-risk groups (regardless of their seropositivity status) are even further feared by society. If an illness is discredited by the medical (professional) community, there appears to be more likelihood of stigmatization of the affected persons.

Almost all aspects of AIDS can be considered a social phenomenon. The characterization of high-risk individuals as being primarily the homosexual and drug addict groups made AIDS a stigmatized disease almost immediately. The uncertainties of AIDS are endless, and being labeled as an HIV-infected individual or a PWA may be an obstacle to social interaction, employment, and insurance qualification. As such, the positive characteristics of an individual may be ignored.

Not since the plagues of the sixteenth century and the views of syphilis during the seventeenth century has a disease earned so much social consequence. The social response to AIDS has been such that even highly educated health care professionals interpret the disease as a punishment for social and sexual deviance (Kelly et al., 1987).

In twentieth-century America, AIDS has clearly been related to certain types of antisocial behavior. Fear generated by the uncertainties of AIDS is a common emotional response of all groups (Cassens, 1985). As recently as 1986, children with AIDS made headlines and were banned from attending public school. Headlines such as "Gay plague, lethal scourge, and mysterious epidemic" (McCombie, 1986, p. 457) have fashioned AIDS into a highly stigmatized disease. Persons infected with HIV, as well as suspected (by the public) of infection, have been openly shunned and alienated. The media have often referred to the blameless innocent victims (children and hemophiliacs) being infected by the guilty (homosexuals and intravenous drug abusers).

In Goffman's (1963) classic work, *stigma* was defined as an attribute, an undesired differentness, that discredits or disqualifies the individual from full social acceptance. This ''differentness'' was not in itself cause for social disqualification, but rested upon an interactional process through which this differentness was given social significance and meaning. It was the public's reaction, therefore, that measured the inner strength of a social norm (Shoham and Rahav, 1970).

Some diseases are clearly more biophysically discrete or recognizable. Venereal diseases have been associated with clandestine or immoral sexual activities. Freidson (1974) states that in certain cases, such as venereal disease, there is a moralistic judgment of blame and the indisposed is held responsible for the diseased state. The concept of stigma as some type of repercussion of norm violation is almost universal. The interpretation of such marks or signs is culturally defined, and the position of the one doing the stigmatizing is influential.

Research reports and articles in the medical, nursing, and behavioral sciences are saturated with articles about AIDS, its etiology and pathogenesis; its impact on sexual behaviors and practices, drug addiction, health care delivery, employment, and discrimination issues (Kelly et al., 1987). These reports, however, have only minimally addressed the perspectives and attitudes of PWAs.

PURPOSE OF THE STUDY

The purpose of this study is to describe what it is like to be a homeless PWA living in a congregate facility.

PLAN FOR DATA COLLECTION

Study Design

A naturalistic inquiry using ethnographic methodology will be the approach used to conduct this investigation. Ethnography is a method by which a culture or subculture can be described. The final product of the ethnographic method is a written report based on the description and analysis of the culture of concern.

Ethnography has been defined in the nursing literature as the systematic process of observing, detailing, describing, documenting, and analyzing the lifeways or particular patterns of a culture (or subculture) (Leininger, 1985). Ethnographic methodology is an ideal way to identify behaviors and generate knowledge that will establish the groundwork for further research. Homeless PWAs living in a congregate facility can be considered a subculture whose lifeways are as yet unidentified. The ethnographic approach provides the most appropriate means for describing what living in the congregate setting is like from the perspective of PWAs.

Setting

A church-affiliated congregate living facility opened in 1988 in South Florida. It accepts PWAs who have nowhere else to go and who otherwise would probably be forced to live on the streets. All persons living in this setting have a diagnosis of AIDS or have had an AIDS-related infection or complication. This congregate residence has been selected as the field setting for the researcher's ethnographic study. For anonymity, this residence will be given the fictional name "Sunrise Manor."

Sample

The sample for this study will be drawn from those PWAs living full time at Sunrise Manor. The sampling approach will be a purposive sample of convenience. Residents' charts, containing medical, family, and social histories, will be available for the investigator's review. To avoid preconceived views toward residents and the risk of biasing sample selection, the investigator will not review the charts until after the participants have been selected.

Four to six residents (male and female) will be interviewed in a series of in-depth interviews. It is also anticipated that the staff will be observed as they interact with the residents and will be spoken with informally. It is contemplated that the investigator will spend 15 to 30 hours a week in the field setting.

Data Collection Techniques

Data will be obtained primarily by observation and participant observation. Participant observation will combine straight observation and both unstructured and structured interviews. An interview schedule will be developed before each formal interview. After analysis of each interview, new questions will be generated and, if possible, follow-up interviews will be scheduled. Questions will be of the grand-tour and mini-tour variety (as discussed in Spradley, 1979). An example of the initial interview schedule is attached (Appendix A).

A tape recorder will be used whenever possible during formal and informal interviews. Once transcribed, the tapes will be kept for review in order to listen to the residents' articulation and exclamation and in order to facilitate a further appreciation of their moods. At the completion of this study, the tapes will be erased.

Because the investigator anticipates the use of photography as adding an important dimension to the data base and as facilitating content analysis, a camera will be used (when permitted and appropriate) to capture germane scenes. Photographs allow the researcher to witness an event, situation, or condition through the camera and simultaneously to become a participant observer. This is accomplished by using the camera as an instrument or tool of social inquiry and education. All photographs, including negatives, will be destroyed upon completion of the study. In addition to photographs, hand-drawn sketches, and maps and floor plans of the living quarters and private and public areas of Sunrise Manor will be interpreted throughout the data presentation process to better orient the reader to the setting.

PLAN FOR DATA ANALYSIS

According to Lincoln and Guba (1985), within the ethnographic paradigm, data analysis is not a matter of reduction but of induction. Inductive analysis begins with the data analysis, rather than from established theories or hypotheses. The investigator will use the transcriptions of the interviews and field notes as the source of data analysis. Words and word combinations will be selected so that the researcher can identify the significant area for analysis. Recurrent combinations will generate conceptualizations, understandings, and trends from the perspective of PWAs living in Sunrise Manor.

LIMITATIONS OF THE STUDY

Since the sample will be drawn from a group of homeless PWAs living in a specific setting, the conclusions cannot be generalized to all PWAs living in congregate facilities, or to all homeless.

ETHICAL CONSIDERATIONS

The protocol for this research study, initial interview schedule, and informed consents will be submitted to the appropriate institutional review boards responsible for the protection of human subjects involved in research. Three different consent forms will be written; one will be for resident participation in the ethnographic study; two will be for permission to be photographed (resident and staff forms). A copy of the resident participation informed consent form can be found in Appendix B.

All study participants will be asked to sign informed consents prior to formal interviews and photograph sessions. Confidentiality of the subjects and informants (staff) will be maintained by not identifying them by name. Data will be recorded with special code names, so that there is no link between these codes and the subject's identity. Names of the subjects and informants will be known only to the investigator, who will hold this information in the strictest confidence, coded, and securely stored in a locked file (in the home of the investigator) for a period of not less than three years.

Once agreeing to participate in this study, all participants will be informed that they are free to withdraw from the study at any time. They will also be informed that if the content of the interviews causes emotional discomfort or stress, they are free to terminate the interview at that time and also are at liberty to refuse to answer any question. All participants will be informed that their participation in this study or their wish not to participate will not, in any way, affect their status at Sunrise Manor.

NURSING IMPLICATIONS

Being homeless is accompanied by a multitude of problems. Having AIDS is saturated with its own distinctive set of physical, psychological, and social puzzles. The medical, especially the neurological, problems that are common in AIDS further increase and aggravate the existing gravity of the person's life prior to becoming homeless.

Being a homeless PWA is a "contemporary condition," and it is anticipated that the description derived from this ethnography will present new dilemmas for health care professionals and society. Finding answers to such dilemmas will necessitate that the nurse look beyond the health care setting for practical answers.

As the numbers of AIDS cases multiply, the need for facilities such as Sunrise Manor will undoubtedly increase. AIDS is not a problem that lends itself to simple or immediate solutions, and descriptions of homeless PWAs in other parts of the country are necessary to understand the magnitude and intricacies of the AIDS dilemma. The intent of this study is to establish the first description of what it is like to be a homeless PWA living in a congregate facility from the PWAs' perspective. The findings from this investigation will enhance the knowledge base of the nursing profession with regard to the needs of this population and assist with planning appropriate interventions.

APPENDIX A: INTERVIEW SCHEDULE

1. What is it like for you to live in Sunrise Manor?
2. What was it like for you before you moved in?
3. How are things here compared to where you were before?
4. How do you spend the day?

APPENDIX B: INFORMED CONSENT FORM—
LIVING IN SUNRISE MANOR

1. *Purpose:* You are being asked to participate in a research study in which you will be asked to describe your thoughts and feelings as a person living in Sunrise Manor. The reason for conducting this study is to understand what it is like to live in Sunrise Manor and to determine how the experience can be made more beneficial to the residents.

2. *Procedure:* The study will consist of three to five interviews that the Investigator will conduct over a period of 2–3 months. The interviews will last approximately 60 minutes. You will be asked to respond to questions about what it is like to live in Sunrise Manor and what things were like for you before you moved in. The interviews will be tape recorded and the tape recordings will be erased once the tapes have been typed. At your request, the tape recorder will be turned off at any time during the interview(s). Toward the end of this study, a request may be made to take photographs of resident activities in Sunrise Manor. The photographs will be used to assist in describing the residence and its social activities. The photographs will not be published or displayed in any manner. The photographs will be destroyed at the end of the study. Only persons granting permission to be included in photographs will be.

3. *Risks:* There are no anticipated physical risks involved by participating in this study. If you feel that the content of an interview is causing you feelings of stress or emotional discomfort, please know that you may end the interview.

4. *Benefits:* There is no direct benefit to you for participating in this study. The results of this study may help health care providers gain understanding and make necessary changes to improve your living environment while in Sunrise Manor.

5. *Confidentiality:* Names will not be used in the reporting of any information you tell the Investigator. All information which refers to, or can be identified with you, will remain confidential to the extent permitted by law. The results of this study will be reported as group results.

6. *Participation is voluntary:* Your participation in this study is voluntary. If you decide to participate and later decide that you do not wish to continue, you may at any time withdraw your consent and stop your participation, without affecting your status at Sunrise Manor. You may refuse to answer any question without affecting your status at Sunrise Manor or your continued participation in this study.

7. *Whom to contact for answers:* If there are any questions at any time regarding this study or your participation in it, you are always free to consult with the Investigator [Suzan Norman: (305) 000–0000].

8. I have read and received a copy of this informed consent form.

_____   _____
SIGNATURE OF INVESTIGATOR, DATE   SIGNATURE OF PARTICIPANT, DATE

SIGNATURE OF WITNESS _____ DATE _____

BIBLIOGRAPHY

Cassens, B. J. 1985. "Social Consequences of AIDS." *Annals of Internal Medicine, 103:* 768–771.

Center for Disease Control (CDC). October 1989. *HIV/AIDS Surveillance Report.*

Denker, A. L. 1986. "An Ethnography of AIDS Care." Unpublished manuscript, University of Miami, School of Nursing.

Dewar, H. 1989. "Homeless Don't Fit Image." *Miami Herald,* April 27, Section B: 1B–2B.

Freidson, E. 1974. *Profession of Medicine: A Study of the Sociology of Applied Knowledge.* New York: Dodd & Mead.

Goffman, E. 1963. *Stigma.* New York: Simon and Schuster.

Kelly, J. A., J. S. St Lawrence, et al. (1987). "Stigmatization of AIDS Patients by Physicians." *American Journal of Public Health, 77(7):* 789–791.

Leininger, M. M. 1985. *Qualitative Research Methods in Nursing.* New York: Grune & Stratton.

Lincoln, Y. S., & E. G. Guba. 1985. *Naturalistic Inquiry.* Beverly Hills, CA: Sage Publications.

McCombie, S. C. 1986. "The Cultural Impact of the 'AIDS' Test: The American Experience." *Social Science Medicine, 23(5):* 455–459.

Shoham, S. G., & G. Rahav. 1970. *The Mark of Cain.* St. Lucia: University of Queensland Press.

Spradley, J. P. 1979. *The Ethnographic Interview.* New York: Holt, Rinehart & Winston.

Appendix E

Example of an Experimental Research Proposal

THE EFFECT OF STOCKINETTE CAPS ON CONSERVATION OF BODY HEAT IN NEWBORN INFANTS

by
SARAH J. KLINGNER

Reprinted by permission.

STATEMENT OF THE PROBLEM

Heat regulation in the newborn involves avoiding increased or decreased temperature. Hypothermia in the newborn can result in detrimental effects, including failure to gain weight, hypoxia, acidosis, pulmonary vasoconstriction, hypoglycemia, kernicterus, and clotting disorders. In order to prevent neonatal compromise caused by hypothermia, it is necessary to implement adjunct therapy for temperature regulation. Therefore, it is useful to investigate clinically the comparative effectiveness of different external methods of temperature regulation.

This study will investigate the effect of one method—the use of stockinette caps—in reducing hypothermia. The study is important to nursing because nurses are the primary caretakers of the newborn, and clinical investigation of nursing procedures for prevention of neonatal hypothermia is clearly related to the nursing role.

REVIEW OF THE LITERATURE

Some background information on the following topics is essential to the study: (1) principles of thermoregulation, (2) consequences of thermal imbalance, and (3) current approaches to decreasing cold stress.

Principles of Thermoregulation

Some decrease in newborn temperature is an inevitable part of birth. Dahm and James (1972) note that an initial cold stimulus may play an important role in the onset of breathing. There is also evidence that peripheral vasoconstriction due to cold stress increases systemic vascular resistance and would thereby reduce right-to-left shunting of blood through the *ductus arteriosus* (Gandy et al., 1964). They concluded that initial cold stress should be kept to a minimum. Adamsons (1966, p. 605) writes that

> Under usual delivery room conditions, deep body temperature of the newborn falls 2 or 3 degrees centigrade. The fall is most rapid in the initial minutes after birth, at which time the rates of fall of deep body and skin temperatures are about 0.1 degrees C per minute and 0.3 degrees C respectively, corresponding to a heat loss of approximately 200 calories per kilogram per minute.

Several factors contribute to this heat loss in the newborn (Lutz and Perlstein, 1971; Stern, 1978; Hey and Katz, 1970). These include:

- Separation from the maternal body and amniotic fluid as a heat source.
- Large surface area in relation to body weight.
- Low ambient (environmental) temperature and humidity.
- Convective losses due to cooler air currents moving over the infant's skin.
- Conductive losses, caused by cooler objects coming in contact with the infant's skin; these could include cold blankets, towels, instruments, and bassinette.
- Radiation losses, occurring when heat transfers to cooler objects not actually in touch with the body; this would include cold windows, walls, or incubator walls.
- Evaporative losses, resulting from the infant's wet skin coming into contact with the dry, air-conditioned climate of the delivery room; or by exhalation of fluid from the infant's lungs.

Adult humans are homeothermic beings; that is, they are able to maintain a stable temperature despite a change in the environment. An infant's ability to maintain his or her temperature is not as well developed as an adult's; it is therefore critical that he or she be kept in a temperature zone which is beneficial. This temperature zone, sometimes termed a neutral thermal environment or neutral zone (Stern, 1968, p. 902),

is a range of environmental temperature at which heat production, usually measured as oxygen consumption, is minimal yet sufficient to maintain the body temperature. As the temperature of the environment falls below this zone, oxygen consumption rises sharply, reflecting the increase in heat production needed to maintain body temperature. In newborns, the range is 32 degrees to 34 degrees centigrade.

Normal term infants respond to a cold environment by two primary mechanisms: reduction of heat loss, and increase of heat production. (*Note:* This study will be limited to term infants because preterm or small-for-gestational-age babies have greater problems with heat regulation.)

Reduction of heat loss occurs primarily through vasoconstriction of the peripheral blood vessels. This action serves to increase the core temperature, while simultaneously decreasing the peripheral circulation. Reduction of heat loss may also be achieved by a change in posture which decreases the exposed skin surface.

Adamsons et al. (1965) reported that infants in a cold environment rarely slept, but instead displayed various degrees of physical activity which increased as temperature decreased. They also noted that shivering was a common occurrence, even in infants less than fifteen minutes of age. However, there is some doubt as to whether newborns shiver as regularly as adults, and whether this is an effective mechanism for heat regulation (Stern, 1968).

An increase in heat production is achieved by an increase in metabolic rate in response to cold. This process is referred to as chemical or nonshivering thermogenesis (Motil and Blackburn, 1973; Williams and Lancaster, 1976; Fardig, 1980). Fardig reports (p. 20) that

> Chemical or non-shivering thermogenesis is a metabolic process mediated by norepinephrine that allows oxygen consumption to be raised without increased muscular activity. Heat thus generated warms the blood circulating through brown fat (adipose tissue) and maintains temperature of the body core. Heat is transferred along an internal gradient from the core to the body surface, modulated by vasoconstriction, and then along an external gradient from the skin to the environment, controlled largely by environmental conditions.

Consequences of Thermal Imbalance

These research findings indicate that even newborn infants are able to regulate decreases in their own body temperature through reduction of heat loss, or increase of heat production. However, thermal imbalance can occur through the failure of internal thermal regulation mechanisms or extremes in external temperature.

Thermal imbalance results in a number of sequential consequences. Therefore, the mechanism of thermal regulation has developed as a genetic response to the negative consequences of thermal imbalance. These include (Williams and Lancaster, 1976, pp. 355–360):

- Increased metabolic consumption of calories during thermogenesis, which may lead to loss of or failure to gain weight.
- Increased oxygen consumption during thermogenesis, which may lead to hypoxia, acidosis, pulmonary vasoconstriction, and other complications.
- Increased glucose consumption, which may lead to hypoglycemia.
- Release of fatty acids into the blood through nonshivering heat production process, which may lead to kernicterus at relatively low levels of indirect bilirubin.
- Clotting disorders.

The newborn responds to chilling by increasing his metabolic rate, which results in the partial diversion of metabolic energy to the production of body heat, rather than the laying down of new tissue (Korones, 1981, p. 81).

A prolonged increase in the metabolic rate of the newborn infant is associated with increases in oxygen consumption, which may lead to a number of consequences, including hypoxia, acidosis, pulmonary vasoconstriction, and other complications. When the newborn responds to chilling by increasing his metabolic rate, this automatically entails increased oxygen consumption (Korones, 1981, p. 91). A hypoxic infant may progress to metabolic and respiratory acidosis, caused by a conversion to anaerobic metabolism and an increase in lactic acid production (Williams and Lancaster, 1976, p. 357). In comparing the recovery rate from acidosis at birth, Gandy et al. found that vigorous infants left exposed to room temperature (25 degrees centigrade) did differ from those in whom body temperature was maintained (by external heat sources) at about 37 degrees centigrade. The similar rate of recovery of pH in the "cool group" was achieved by an increased elimination of carbon dioxide to compensate for persistent metabolic acidosis (Adamsons, 1966, p. 608).

Other respiratory complications, such as vasoconstriction, may result from acidosis. Korones reports (1981, p. 91) that

> Lowered oxygen tension is apparently related to diminished effectiveness of ventilation, which is a consequence of pulmonary vasoconstriction caused by the release of norepinephrine that occurs in response to cold stress.

Because hypothermia results in a fall in blood glucose, the hypothermic infant is also frequently hypoglycemic. Hypoglycemia is a decrease in blood glucose level caused by exertion or the use of calories to raise the baby's temperature. The ability of the newborn to survive is not enhanced by the necessity of using scarce blood glucose for heat maintenance (Stern, 1978, p. 33).

The fall in serum glucose levels is also accompanied by an increased release of fatty acids (Williams and Lancaster, 1976, p. 358). The increase in NEFA in the blood may lead to another problem—the development of hyperbilirubinemia. This is an excess of unconjugated (not linked to albumin) bilirubin in the blood. In this free state, it causes jaundice, which in turn may lead to kernicterus, a form of brain damage (Sinclair, 1966).

Finally, severe hypothermia appears to interfere with certain clotting factors, and therefore increases the risk of bleeding. Some authors have noted an increase in pulmonary and cerebral hemorrhage in cold-stressed babies. However, such bleeding is also associated with asphyxia. Thus the bleeding may result from a combination of factors (Williams and Lancaster, 1976, p. 358).

Current Approaches to Reducing Cold Stress

The failure of a newborn to maintain heat therefore results in a number of negative conditions. To prevent their occurrence, researchers and clinicians have developed a variety of techniques for increasing the conservation of body heat, thereby reducing the morbidity and mortality which can result from cold stress. These include:

- Reducing convective heat losses by covering the infant with blankets, keeping it out of drafts or air conditioning, and raising the ambient (environmental) temperature.
- Reducing conductive losses by using warm blankets or towels, placing the baby in a preheated warming unit.
- Inhibiting radiant heat loss by putting the infant under radiant heat lights; keeping bassinettes away from cold walls or outside windows; transporting infants in double-walled incubators (isolettes).
- Reducing evaporative heat loss by drying the infant well as soon after birth as possible, using dry warm towels, and delaying bathing the infant until its temperature is stabilized.

In this connection, it is important to consider not only the sources of heat loss, but the way in which heat loss occurs. According to Stothers (1981, p. 530),

> The brain of the newborn infant uses a large proportion of the total oxygen consumption and therefore generates much of the total heat he produces. Due to the fairly high cerebral blood flow, it is likely that most of this heat would be transferred to the body, but as the surface area of the head represents 20–28% of the total body surface area, heat losses from the head must represent a substantial proportion of the whole.

The Role of Caps in Preventing Heat Loss

A number of investigators have emphasized the importance of covering the infant's head as a means of reducing heat loss through radiation, conduction, and convection.

In a randomized, controlled trial of 104 newborns, DeSaintonge et al. (1979) studied the effect of caps on heat loss. Fifty-four infants wore woolen caps lined with gamgee, while the second group wore no caps. All infants were dressed in diaper, gown, and blanket, and had temperatures monitored periodically for the first 120 minutes of life. All infants were placed in cribs away from drafts and away from overhead radiant warmers. At the end of the initial 30 minutes, it was found that the rate of decline in rectal temperatures was significantly lower in the group with caps.

The benefit of lined woolen caps was confirmed in a study done by Stothers in 1981. This researcher studied a group of 23 term infants to determine the efficacy of head coverings. One group of 13 infants had temperatures taken (1) naked, (2) with a lined woolen (gamgee) cap, and (3) with a cummerbund of the same fabric around the abdomen. The remaining 10 infants were studied while wearing caps of tubegauze. The extent of heat loss was measured in each group. The total heat loss in the first group was only 75 percent, when wearing caps, of the heat loss when naked. The cummerbund provided no detectable benefit. The ten infants wearing tubegauze caps showed no appreciable difference in temperature when naked, as compared to when wearing tubegauze caps.

The conclusions of Stothers's study were similar to those of Aikens (1977), who concluded that there was no significant difference in the rectal temperatures, in the first hour after birth, in infants with or without tubegauze caps.

In summary, this review of the literature has discussed the principles of thermoregulation, the consequences of thermal imbalance, current approaches to reducing cold stress, and the role of caps in preventing heat loss. First, with respect to thermoregulation, it has concluded that the newborn's ability to maintain temperature is not as well developed as an adult's. It is therefore critical that the newborn be kept in a neutral thermal environment. Second, if this is not done, thermal imbalance may result in a sequence of responses (failure to gain weight, hypoxia, acidosis, pulmonary vasoconstriction, hypoglycemia, kernicterus, and clotting disorders) which are deleterious to health. Third, and consequently, researchers have developed a variety of techniques for conserving body heat. Fourth, some research has focused on the use of caps for this purpose, in that the newborn's high cerebral blood flow and large surface area of the head cause substantial heat loss.

Despite the logic of the hypothesis that the use of caps is an effective method of conserving body heat, research has not conclusively validated this hypothesis. For example, some studies (DeSaintonge et al., 1979; Stothers, 1981) have validated the effectiveness of caps for this purpose; while others (Aikens, 1977) have not. While the reasons for these disparate conclusions are not always clear from the information presented in published research findings, it is evident that these studies used different types of caps, different sampling methods, and different methodologies for measuring the extent of heat loss.

In view of these different approaches to researching the problem, and disparate conclusions reached, further research is needed.

CONCEPTUAL FRAMEWORK

Roy's adaptation model will be used as a basis for interpreting the data collected in this study. According to this model, man is a biopsychosocial being in constant interaction with his changing environment. Man's positive response to this environment is known as the process of adaptation. In general, a positive adaptive response is one that maintains the integrity of the individual, while a negative or maladaptive response does not. The role of nursing is to promote the person's adaptation to achieve integrity.

Integrity is achieved by human behaviors which are geared toward adaptation in four modes. These include physiological needs, self-concept, role function, and interdependence. The physiological needs are further divided into the following categories: exercise and rest; nutrition; elimination; fluid and electrolytes; oxygen; circulation; and the regulation of temperature, the senses, and the endocrine system.

The use of caps as a nursing approach to regulation may serve to promote one adaptive response of man. The adult is able to maintain a body temperature relatively independent of his environment. If the body warms, man is able to lose heat by sweating, increasing skin circulation, and heat radiation. If the body cools, heat production may be increased by increasing chemical or physical responses, such as those described in the previous section.

However, as discussed in the review of the literature, the newborn is not as able to achieve thermoregulation through internal mechanisms. The newborn infant is primarily (if not exclusively) concerned with the physiological mode. Therefore, the comparative utility of alternative external thermoregulation methods must be investigated.

STATEMENT OF PURPOSE

The purpose of this study is to test the following hypothesis: The amount of heat loss in newborns wearing stockinette caps for 30 minutes after birth is significantly less than the amount of heat loss in newborns not wearing stockinette caps for 30 minutes after birth.

DEFINITION OF TERMS

Temperature: Degree of heat of a body, in degrees Fahrenheit, measured under the arm with a Filac electronic thermometer, model number F-1010. (*Note:* The rationale for the use of axillary temperatures is presented in Eoff et al., 1974, pp. 457–460.)

Normal newborn temperature: Between 35.5 and 37.5° C (Lutz and Perlstein, 1971, p. 17). This converts to 96.0 and 99.5 degrees Fahrenheit.

Heat loss: Amount of heat dissipated in a given period of time (in degrees Fahrenheit).

Hypoglycemia: Occurs when whole blood glucose is less than 30 mg/100 ml (serum glucose less than 35 mg/100 ml) during the first three days of life. Because blood sugar levels normally fluctuate widely, two low readings are necessary for a positive determination (Korones, 1981, p. 304).

Severe hypoglycemia: Whole blood glucose is less than or equal to 20 mg/ml (North Shore Medical Center newborn nursery policy).

Newborn: An infant between five minutes and three hours old.

Term: Infants with a gestational age of 37–42 weeks (Korones, 1981, p. 109).

Gestational age: Assessment of maturity on the basis of neurological signs (L. Dubowitz et al., as cited in Korones, 1981, p. 109).

Weight: In pounds and ounces, converted to grams.

Apgar: A scoring system for the clinical evaluation of infants, based on heart rate, respiratory effort, muscle tone, reflex irritability, and color (Korones, 1981, p. 69).

Complications: Those complications or procedures which alter the physiologic status (e.g., meconium staining, general anesthetic, shoulder or face presentations, maternal temperature abnormalities during labor or birth, cesarean sections, infant temperature abnormalities, or multiple births).

Normal: A mother who does not have preexisting medical problems, including diabetes, renal disease, cardiac abnormalities, or hypertension; a newborn infant who is not diagnosed as having any abnormality at birth.

Ambient temperature: The temperature of the delivery suite, measured in degrees Fahrenheit.

Humidity: Relative to the maximum saturation point of the air, measured as a percentage of relative humidity.

Radiant warmer: A unit which contains overhead heating elements which emit infrared rays which are focused downward on the area occupied by the infant.

Stockinette cap: A single-layered cap made of closely knit cotton fabric, typically used medically to protect skin when applying a cast.

Delivery room: The hospital room, designed for that purpose, where the infant is born.

PLAN FOR DATA COLLECTION

Research Approach

This study is a clinical experiment which will provide data for descriptive and inferential statistics.

Study Subjects

A sample of 40 newborns meeting the following criteria will be selected: term birth, equivalent gestational age, weight greater than or equal to six pounds, Apgar scores greater to or equal to 7 at 1 minute and at 5 minutes, without complications, born into ambient temperatures between 66 and 72 degrees, and 60 percent relative humidity.

These newborn infants will be selected by sampling from among the mothers admitted to the labor and delivery area. The mother will have had a normal antepartal and intrapartal course up to the time of sampling. Normal in this case has been previously defined in the "Definition of Terms." Babies of selected mothers who agree to participate in the study will automatically be part of the sample, unless complications occur, such as Apgar scores less than 7 or gestational age less than 37–42 weeks.

Those infants selected for the convenience sample will be placed in one of two groups, the experimental group and the control group, on the basis of the mother's Social Security number. Those mothers without Social Security numbers will be excluded from the sample. Those newborns having mothers with odd Social Security numbers will be placed in the control group; those newborns having mothers with even Social Security numbers will be placed in the experimental group. Thus, 20 newborns will be assigned by the researcher to each group.

Techniques for Data Collection

Data will be collected from newborns in the delivery suite of a 300-bed private hospital in southeast Florida by the researcher, who will be providing infant care.

Data will be collected from groups of newborns selected on the basis of similar physical characteristics, with one group wearing stockinette caps and the other not wearing them.

Data collection techniques will control for the following causes of temperature variation in the newborn, other than the experimental variable (use of stockinette caps):

- Thermometer will be calibrated before each use.
- Radiant warmer will be checked before each use.
- Receiving blankets will be warmed in the radiant warmer used for the newborn.
- Stockinette caps will be warmed in the radiant warmer with the receiving blanket.
- Ambient temperature wall thermometers and humidity gauges for the delivery room will be checked prior to the birth.

All newborns in the sample will have their axillary temperatures measured in the delivery room within the first 5 minutes after birth by the researcher, and recorded on the data collection sheet.

With the Filac electronic thermometer, the temperature appears on a LED (light-emitting diode) screen when the temperature reaches its maximum. All infants will be placed under radiant warmers and dried with warm, dry towels, then wrapped in one warmed cotton receiving blanket.

Apgars will be taken at 1 and 5 minutes after birth, in accordance with normal hospital procedure. Those newborns having abnormally low Apgars will be excluded from the sample.

Those infants in the experimental group will be fitted with stockinette caps within 5 minutes of birth, and after their initial temperatures are recorded. Newborns will remain in the delivery room under the radiant warmer for 30 minutes. Their second temperature will be taken at 30 minutes after birth by the researcher, and recorded on the data collection sheet.

All newborns will then be moved to the newborn nursery, in accordance with normal hospital procedure. At this time they will be weighed and assessed for gestational age. Those newborns not falling within normal ranges will be excluded from the sample.

Data collected will be recorded on the Newborn Data Collection Sheet (Appendix A).

Pilot Study

In order to test the appropriateness of data collection techniques and the utility of the Newborn Data Collection Sheet, a pilot study will be conducted by sampling a total of ten (10) newborns. The study will be carried out as described here. Those subjects selected for the pilot study will be used as subjects of the subsequent study, if revisions of data collection techniques or instrument prove unnecessary.

Human Rights

Prior to the inclusion of any newborn in the sample, its parents will be given a letter informing them of the purpose of the study, reassuring them of anonymity, requesting their voluntary cooperation, and offering to share with them the results of the study. Parents must sign the informed consent letter prior to the inclusion of their infant in the study. A sample letter is presented in Appendix B.

Assumptions

Several assumptions have been made for the purpose of this study:

1. Axillary temperature is as accurate a method of measuring temperature as are rectal or oral methods.
2. Infants of multiparous mothers are no different with respect to temperature than are infants of primiparous mothers.
3. The sex of the infant does not affect its body temperature.
4. Maternal factors such as age, parity, and race do not affect the outcome.

Limitations

This study is applicable only to infants exhibiting the characteristics described in the section on data collection. Since the sample is nonrandom and is relatively small in size, extreme care should be taken before attempting to generalize these findings to the general population.

PLAN FOR DATA ANALYSIS

Data will be analyzed using the student's *t*-test for significant differences between groups. The temperature for all infants in the sample will be measured
twice—first when the infant is born, and second after 30 minutes. The extent of
temperature loss is the difference between these two measurements.

The hypothesis states that the experimental group (i.e., those infants with
stockinette caps) will show a smaller degree of heat loss than the control group
(i.e., infants without them). Thus, since the direction of difference between the
experimental and control groups is predicted, the hypothesis is unidirectional
(i.e., rejected if data analysis shows no significant difference between the degree of heat loss between the two groups, or a significantly greater degree of
heat loss in the group with the stockinette caps). Significance will be measured
at the .05 level of probability.

Table E.1 shows results for the experimental group. An identical table will
be used to present and analyze the data for the control group.

TABLE E.1
Extent of Heat Loss—Experimental Group

Patient No.	Extent of Heat Loss
1	
2	
3	
4	
5	
6	
7	
8	
9	
10	
11	
12	
13	
14	
15	
16	
17	
18	
19	
20	

Total heat loss: _____

Mean heat loss (Total heat loss/20) =

The effect of intervening variables (infant's sex and weight) will be controlled for by using chi-square to determine whether significant differences between the experimental and control groups have inadvertently occurred. The effects of these variables will be considered nonsignificant if there are no significant differences (at the .05 level of probability, for the sample size of 20 in each group) between the two groups. A summary of the demographic data for all subjects will be presented in a demographic data table (Table E.2).

TABLE E.2
Summary Demographic Data Table

Variable	Experimental Group	Control Group
Infant's sex		
Value of chi-square:		
Infant's weight		
Value of chi-square:		

The mean heat loss of the two groups will be compared using a mean heat loss table (Table E.3).

TABLE E.3
Mean Heat Loss

	Mean Heat Loss	t-test Value
Experimental Group (n = 20)		
Control Group (n = 20)		
Significance at .05 level of probability: _____		

SUMMARY

This study will investigate clinically the effectiveness of stockinette caps in reducing hypothermia by externally regulating the temperature of newborns. The subjects will be 40 infants from the newborn nursery of a private hospital, selected according to preset criteria to ensure that they and their mothers are equivalent and normal. Subjects will be randomly placed in an experimental group (stockinette caps) or a control group (no caps); temperatures will be measured at 5 minutes and 30 minutes after birth; the extent of temperature loss will be recorded on a data collection instrument and the significance of differences in mean heat loss between the two groups will be examined using the student's *t*-test (one-tailed).

APPENDIX A: NEWBORN DATA COLLECTION SHEET

Environmental Data:

Delivery Room Temp. _____ Humidity _____

Infant Data:

Infant's hospital number _____

Sex _____ Weight: lb. _____ oz. _____ gm. _____

Gestational age _____

Birth date _____ Time _____

Apgars: 1 min. _____ 5 min. _____

Group: Experimental _____ Control _____

Maternal Data:

Mother's Social Security no. (last digit): _____

Mother's hospital number _____

Complications? Yes _____ No _____

(If yes, identify: _____)

Temperatures:

(1) Initial reading _____ Time _____

Time hat applied (if exp.) _____

(2) Second reading _____ Time _____

Time transferred to nursery _____

(3) Difference in readings (1) and (2) _____

APPENDIX B: INFORMED CONSENT LETTER

Dear Mother-to-be:

I am a nursing student conducting a research study at _____. I am requesting that you and thirty-nine other mothers participate in this study, in order to find out whether the use of stockinette caps is an effective method of reducing heat loss in newborn infants.

The study involves placing caps on some infants and no caps on others. Each infant's temperature will be measured immediately after birth and then again after thirty minutes. By measuring and comparing the temperature loss for infants with and without caps, the study will determine whether these caps should be used routinely to reduce heat loss in newborn infants.

In order for the study to be accurate, you will not know in advance whether or not your baby will receive a cap. However, because such caps are not routinely used at _____ at this time, their use is experimental. Thus, there are no risks or benefits involved in your participation. There is also no additional cost to you for your participation.

Your records and results will not be identified as pertaining to you specifically without your express permission. Your physician will consider your records highly confidential. However, in rare circumstances, the U.S. Department of Health and Human Services (DHHS) may request a copy of your records. If this happens, the DHHS request will be honored. If you decide to participate in this study, you will also be giving consent for the investigator and her assistants to review your medical records as may be necessary for the purpose of this research study.

Although mothers and infants who assist in this study will remain anonymous, I encourage you to call me about the study if you have any questions. I will also be happy to share the results of the study with you when it is completed.

Cordially,

Sara J. Klingner

I consent to having my newborn participate in this study.

Parent's signature: _____ Date: _____

REFERENCES

Adamsons, K. 1966. "The Role of Thermal Factors in Fetal and Neonatal Life." *Pediatric Clinics of North America*, 13(3): 599–613.

Adamsons, K., G. Gandy, and L. James. 1965. "Thermal Factors and Oxygen Consumption of Newborns." *Journal of Pediatrics*, 66(3): 495–508.

Aikens, R. 1977. "Hats and Lamps in the Prevention of Neonatal Hypothermia." *Nursing Mirror Midwives Journal*, 144: 65–66.

Dahm, L., and L. James. 1972. "Newborn Temperature and Calculated Heat Loss in the Delivery Room." *Pediatrics*, 49(4): 504–513.

DeSaintonge, D., D. Cross, M. Hathorn, S. Lewi, and J. Stothers. 1979. "Hats for the Newborn Infant." *British Medical Journal*, 2: 570–571.

Eoff, M., R. Meier, and C. Miller. 1974. "Temperature Measurement in Infants." *Nursing Research* 23(6): 457–460.

Fardig, J. 1980. "A Comparison of Skin-to-Skin Contact and Radiant Heaters in Promoting Neonatal Thermoregulation." *Journal of Nurse-Midwifery*, 25(1): 19–28.

Gandy, G., K. Adamsons, N. Cunningham, W. Silverman, and L. James. 1964. "Thermal Environment and Acid–Base Homeostasis in Human Infants During the First Few Hours of Life." *Journal of Clinical Investigation*, 43:751 (as cited in Adamsons, 1966).

Hey, E., and G. Katz. 1970. "The Optimum Thermal Environment for Naked Babies." *Archives of Disease in Childhood*, 45: 328–333.

Korones, S. 1981. *High-Risk Newborn Infants: The Basis for Intensive Nursing Care*, 3rd ed. St Louis: C. V. Mosby.

Lutz, L., and P. Perlstein. 1971. "Temperature Control in Newborn Babies." *Nursing Clinics of North America*, 6(1): 15–25.

Motil, K., and M. Blackburn. 1973. "Temperature Regulation in the Neonate: A Review of the Pathophysiology of Thermal Dynamics and Methods for Environmental Control." *Clinical Pediatrics*, 12: 635–639.

Sinclair, J. 1966. "Prevention and Treatment of the Respiratory Distress Syndrome." *Pediatric Clinics of North America*, 13(3): 711–730.

Stern, L. 1968. "Adaptation to Extrauterine Life." *International Anesthesiology Clinics*, 6(3): 875–909.

Stern, L. 1978. "Physiology of the Newborn Infant: II. Thermoregulation." *Progress in Pediatric Surgery*, 12: 23–40.

Stothers, J. 1981. "Head Insulation and Heat Loss in the Newborn." *Archives of Disease in Childhood*, 56: 530–534.

Williams, J., and J. Lancaster. 1976 "Thermoregulation of the Newborn." *American Journal of Maternal Child Nursing*, 1:355–360.

BIBLIOGRAPHY

Adamsons, K. 1966. "The Role of Thermal Factors in Fetal and Neonatal Life." *Pediatric Clinics of North America*, 13(3): 599–613.

Adamsons, K., G. Gandy, and L. James. 1965. "Thermal Factors and Oxygen Consumption of Newborns." *Journal of Pediatrics*, 66(3): 495–508.

Adamsons, K., and M. Towel. 1965. Thermal Homeostasis in the Newborn. *Anesthesiology*, 26(4): 531–547.

Aikens, R. 1977. "Hats and Lamps in the Prevention of Neonatal Hypothermia." *Nursing Mirror Midwives Journal*, 144: 65–66.

Crouch, J., and J. McClintic. 1971. *Human Anatomy and Physiology*. New York: Wiley.

Dahm, L., and L. James. 1972. "Newborn Temperature and Calculated Heat Loss in the Delivery Room." *Pediatrics*, 49(4): 504–513.

Davis, V. 1980. "The Structure and Function of Brown Adipose Tissue in the Neonate." *JOGN Nursing*, 9(6): 368–372.

DeSaintonge, D., D. Cross, M. Hathorn, S. Lewi, and J. Stothers. 1979. "Hats for the Newborn Infant." *British Medical Journal*, 2: 570–571.

Eoff, M., R. Meier, and C. Miller. 1974. "Temperature Measurement in Infants." *Nursing Research,* 23(6): 457–460.

Fardig, J. 1980. "A Comparison of Skin-to-Skin Contact and Radiant Heaters in Promoting Neonatal Thermal Regulation." *Journal of Nurse-Midwifery,* 25(1): 19–28.

Fenner, A., and M. List. 1971. "Observation of Body Temperature Regulation in Young Premature and Full-Term Newborns While Being Connected to a Servo Control Temperature Unit." *Biology of the Neonate,* 18: 300–310.

Gandy, G., K. Adamsons, N. Cunmningham, W. Silverman, and L. James. 1964. "Thermal Environment and Acid–Base Homeostasis in Human Infants During the First Few Hours of Life." *Journal of Clinical Investigation,* 43:751 (as cited in Adamsons, 1966).

Glass, L., W. Silverman, and J. Sinclair. 1968. "Effect of the Thermal Environment on Cold Resistance and Growth of Small Infants after the First Week of Life." *Pediatrics,* 41(6): 1033–1046.

Hey, E., and G. Katz. 1970. "The Optimum Thermal Environment for Naked Babies." *Archives of Disease in Childhood,* 45: 328–333.

Klaus, M., A. Fanaroff, and R. Martin. 1979. "The Physical Environment." Chapter 5 in M. Klaus and A. Fanaroff, Eds., *Care of the High-Risk Neonate* (pp. 94–106). Philadelphia: W. B. Saunders.

Korones, S. 1981. *High-Risk Newborn Infants: The Basis for Intensive Nursing Care,* 3rd ed. St Louis: C. V. Mosby.

Lutz, L., and P. Perlstein. 1971. "Temperature Control in Newborn Babies." *Nursing Clinics of North America,* 6(1): 15–25.

Motil, K., and M. Blackburn. 1973. "Temperature Regulation in the Neonate: a Review of the Pathophysiology of Thermal Dynamics and Methods for Environmental Control." *Clinical Pediatrics,* 12: 635–639.

Mount, L. 1966. "Basis of Heat Regulation in Homeotherms." *British Medical Bulletin,* 22(1): 84–87.

Porth, C., and L. Kaylor. 1978. "Temperature Regulation in the Newborn." *American Journal of Nursing,* 78: 1691–1693.

Roy, C. 1976. *Introduction to Nursing: An Adaptation Model.* Englewood Cliffs, NJ: Prentice-Hall.

Scopes, J. 1966. "Metabolic Rate and Temperature Control in the Human Baby." *British Medical Bulletin,* 22(1): 88–91.

Sinclair, J. 1966. "Prevention and Treatment of the Respiratory Distress Syndrome." *Pediatric Clinics of North America,* 13(3): 711–730.

Stern, L. 1968. "Adaptation to Extrauterine Life." *International Anesthesiology Clinics,* 6(3): 875–909.

Stern, L. 1978. "Physiology of the Newborn Infant: II. Thermoregulation." *Progress in Pediatric Surgery,* 12: 33–40.

Stothers, J. 1981. "Head Insulation and Heat Loss in the Newborn." *Archives of Disease in Childhood,* 56: 520–534.

Swafford, L., and James, L. 1972. "Newborn Temperature and Calculated Heat Loss in the Delivery Room." *Pediatrics,* 49(4): 504–513.

Williams, J., and J. Lancaster. 1976 "Thermoregulation of the Newborn." *American Journal of Maternal Child Nursing,* 1:355–360.

Appendix F

Example of a Quasi-Experimental Research Proposal

VARIATIONS IN THIRD-STAGE BLOOD LOSS AND PLACENTAL TRAPPING ASSOCIATED WITH OXYTOCIN ADMINISTRATION

by
MARY K. KIRCHER

Reprinted by permission.

INTRODUCTION
CONCEPTUAL FRAMEWORK
LITERATURE REVIEW
STUDY PURPOSE
RESEARCH DESIGN
SAMPLE AND SETTING
METHOD AND INSTRUMENT
    Data Analysis
    Limitations
ETHICAL CONSIDERATIONS
NURSING IMPLICATIONS
APPENDIX A: DATA SHEET
APPENDIX B: INFORMED CONSENT
REFERENCES

INTRODUCTION

Labor comprises those processes that result in the expulsion of the products of conception by the mother (Varney, 1980, p. 169). For purposes of clinical organization, care providers often divide labor into specific stages with respect to uterine physiology and activity.

While there are many references in the literature regarding the distinctiveness of each labor stage, most sources agree on the following descriptive components:

1. The first stage of labor extends from the time regularly occurring uterine contractions are strong enough and persist long enough to encourage cervical thinning and dilating until the time the cervix has opened sufficiently to allow the fetal head to leave the uterus.
2. The second stage of labor encompasses the moment cervical dilatation is complete until the birth of the baby.
3. The third stage of labor extends from birth to the delivery of the placenta.
4. The fourth and final stage of labor involves the one hour following placental expulsion wherein the uterus attempts to constrict and shrink itself in an effort to control bleeding (Varney, 1980, p. 277).

It is the third stage of labor that serves as the focal point of this study. From a physiological perspective, this interval involves separation and expulsion of the functional placental unit. The actively contracting upper uterus is the motivating force behind release of the placenta from the inner uterine wall. Pritchard and MacDonald (1980) assert that as a result of contraction and retraction, this upper segment becomes progressively thicker, with a resultant decrease in the size of the uterine cavity. The sudden reduction in cavity capacity after fetal delivery is accompanied by a reduction in the size of the placental attachment site. Pritchard and MacDonald go on to explain that as the placenta tries to adapt itself to the diminished area, it buckles as a result of its limited elasticity, and its weakest layer subsequently separates from the uterine wall. After the placenta has separated, the pressure exerted upon it by the converging uterine walls causes it to slide downward into the flaccid lower segment of the uterus and eventually out of the body.

Accompanying placental separation is the physiologic loss of a volume of blood, which escapes the vessels supplying nourishment to the uterine muscle fibers and the placental attachment site until contraction of the muscular uterine wall can effectively interrupt this blood supply. Myles (1981) observes a blood loss averaging 120–240 cc in conjunction with an uncomplicated vaginal delivery, while Pritchard and MacDonald (1980) associate any loss under 500 cc with the norm.

The risk of hemorrhage or excessive blood loss in the third stage of labor lies with ineffective contraction of the muscular myometrial layer of the uterus, often due to retention of small portions of the placental unit or substandard myometrial tone. These instances permit continued blood loss from primarily the highly vascular placental implantation site, and may lead to such complications as dangerously low blood pressure, rapid pulse, shock, and even death. While references vary in their definition of hemorrhage, many agree with

Pritchard and MacDonald's guidelines (1980) of blood loss in excess of 500 cc as evidence of third-stage hemorrhage.

The body's inherent mechanism for stimulation of sufficient contraction in the third stage of labor is thought to be related to oxytocin, a naturally occurring pituitary hormone (Dawood, 1978). While little definitive information exists about the actual release and circulating levels of oxytocin in pregnancy and labor, the discovery of a synthetic analog to oxytocin in the mid-1950s sparked the interest of physicians in augmenting the intrinsic supply of oxytocin with an extrinsic introduction of the derivative to encourage effective myometrial activity and thus protect the woman from excessive blood loss.

The use of oxytocin per se in the third stage of labor incites little controversy. But the variations in administration timing have been argued at length with respect to the possibility of intense contractility interfering with the release of the placenta by the uterus. So while blood loss is thought to be minimized by administration of synthetic oxytocin after the placenta separates from the uterine wall, the concept of enhanced control of blood loss by introduction of oxytocin prior to placental separation is often unacceptable, given the prospect of a placenta trapped within the uterus.

This study will investigate the existence of significant variation in uterine blood loss with the administration of intravenous oxytocin following delivery of the anterior fetal shoulder as opposed to delaying administration until after placental separation. The investigation will likewise explore any significant variation in the incidence of placental trapping with the two methods of oxytocin administration.

CONCEPTUAL FRAMEWORK

Active pharmacologic management of the third stage of labor is common today and is thought to be important as a means to encourage early delivery of the placenta, thereby reducing the risk of postpartum hemorrhage (Sorbe, 1978). The utilization of synthetic oxytocics (Oxytocin, Pitocin, Syntocinon) is perhaps the most frequently employed method of this management.

A tremendous number of studies have been undertaken to ascertain the particulars of blood loss in the placental stage of labor and the maternal morbidity associated with inadequate hemostasis in this interval. Nature has fundamental methods of promoting control of blood loss in the third stage of labor. As early as 1543, the Belgian scientist Vesalius dissected a female cadaver and identified the muscular uterine wall. And late in the following century, Eustachio illustrated the vascular supply to the uterus while noting the enclosure of blood vessels within interlacing layers of muscle cells (Wynn, 1977). It is now accepted that the contraction and retraction of uterine muscle fibers that bring about placental separation also act as "living ligatures" by compressing the blood vessels and effectively controlling blood loss (Myles, 1981).

The augmentation of this natural process is by no means a recent institution. As early as 1668, European obstetric writings mention the use of crude oxytocic extracts by midwives (Hendricks et al., 1962). Often mentioned in Indian lore are medicinal agents used to stimulate "a weary uterus or coax out a stubborn fetus." Englemann (1881), as cited in Speert (1980), commented on the use of barks, leaves, fruits, and tree roots with dramatic oxytocic properties by the Oaxaca Indians of Mexico and the Catawbas of the Carolinas (Speert, 1980, p. 31).

Physicians began to augment the natural hemostatic process following extensive physiologic research by Sir Henry Dale, an English investigator who, in 1906, demonstrated the stimulating action of a posterior pituitary extract (oxytocin) on the uterus of a pregnant cat (Speert, 1980). The first human introduction of this pure pituitary derivative came several years later, when British obstetrician Blair Bell demonstrated "the uterus contracting into a ball with subsequent moderate relaxation and minimal blood loss" following the administration of oxytocin to two women undergoing cesarean section (Dawood, 1978, p. 1).

With the initial discovery of the chemical properties of oxytocin and subsequent creation of its synthetic derivation by du Vigneaud in 1953, the drug gained notoriety. Then, as oxytocic utilization became more widespread, physicians noted a marked decrease in the incidence of hemorrhage and its accompanying complications after delivery, which will be discussed in greater depth in the literature review. This brief history of the introduction of oxytocics into routine obstetric protocol provides a foundation from which to extrapolate the significance of succeeding pharmacologic investigations.

While the administration of oxytocics to control bleeding is not to be disputed here, the widespread delay in oxytocic administration until after placental separation has been a much debated point of practice. Late second-stage use of oxytocics has produced evidence of retained or trapped placentas following a uniform tetanic contraction and/or, likewise, the threat to trapping of an undiagnosed second twin (Mayes and Shearman, 1956; Bonham, 1963). However, it has since been shown that such a tetanic contraction is most often associated with a rapid intravenous infiltration of oxytocin or with the early administration of ergotamine (also an oxytocic), as opposed to the controlled delivery of a titrated oxytocin (Oxorn and Foote, 1981).

It is the purposive action of oxytocin that provides the conceptual framework for this investigation. If the extent of oxytocin administration is to stimulate physiologic uterine contracting as an enhancement to the inherent hemostatic process of the uterus, it would seem logical that the oxytocin should be introduced prior to complete emptying of the uterine contents at the conclusion of the third stage of labor. This practice would hasten placental separation and, thus, diminish prolongation of the third stage, which is associated with the increased risk of postdelivery hemorrhage (Hibbard, 1964). In this age of early discharge from the hospital or birth center following an uncomplicated vaginal delivery, it would seem vital to ensure adequate control of bleeding as rapidly as possible, as the client will be under direct observation for only a limited time postpartum. It can be suggested, then, that the late second-stage administration of oxytocin is a means of promoting early and effective uterine involution and of preventing postpartum hemorrhage.

LITERATURE REVIEW

A review of the literature relating to the contractile system of the uterus is essential to complete understanding of the effect of oxytocin on the myometrium. While it was much earlier demonstrated that the uterus is composed of smooth muscle fibers whose involuntary control rests with the autonomic nervous system, Haughton (1873), as cited in Wynn (1977), postulated about the polar orientation of uterine contractions. Bozler (1938) extended that theory through testing on animals whose uteri closely resembled that of the human. His idea was that myometrial muscle fibers are surrounded by a polarized excitable membrane of their own which, when stimulated, contract in an "all or none" fashion. Alvarez and Caldeyro-Barcia (1950) and Caldeyro-Barcia and Poseiro (1959) have done the most extensive inquiry into the character of uterine activity patterns. They designed a logical description of those components accompanying a uterine contraction wave through monitoring of intra-abdominal and intrauterine pressure changes. These studies demonstrated that, while the uterus undergoes a continuous low-level contractile activity (tonus), the introduction of an external stimulus can alter the degree of myometrial tone through enhancement of membrane excitability.

Csapo and Marshall (1961) were able to support Caldeyro-Barcia's hypotheses and added that the external stimulus responsible for enhanced contractility of the myometrium is calcium ion concentrations. This conclusion led to further investigation by Csapo and Marshall involving measurement of electrical responses of animal myometria to the addition or removal of concentrated calcium solution. Addition of a variety of hormonal derivatives led to including oxytocin in a solution bathing inactive muscle tissue, which resulted in an immediate change in the excitability of the tissue. The researchers concluded that the effect of the oxytocin upon myometrial contractility is one of driving the cell membrane toward excitement by changing the intracellular concentration of calcium.

It is indeed the role of a permeability-altering stimulus which oxytocics assume. Oxytocics are purported to increase the myometrial cell membrane permeability to calcium. Since the inside of the cell is more negatively charged than the positively charged calcium ions, the result is an electrical stimulus for the muscle to contract (Wyeth Laboratories, 1982). Oxytocics produce physiologic, rhythmic uterine contractions through "organizing" primarily the upper-uterine segment fibers to contract at the same time. This produces relatively infrequent contractions of high intensity and relatively complete relaxation between contractions (Caldeyro-Barcia and Heller, 1961).

While little experimentation on the utilization of synthetic oxytocin in the third stage of labor has been documented in the United States, many studies have been conducted abroad, particularly in Europe. Mayes and Shearman (1956) administered 5 units of oxytocin intravenously to a group of 25 patients following delivery of the anterior fetal shoulder, noting blood loss of less than 10 oz (300 cc) in 23 cases and less than 5 oz (150 cc) in 20 of these 23 cases. Placental expulsion was generally quite rapid, with 21 of the third stages completed within two minutes and only one manual extraction.

Fugo and Dieckmann (1958) created a double blind study comparing variation in blood loss and duration of third stage with the utilization of ergotamine and oxytocin given intravenously when the anterior fetal shoulder was visible at the vaginal opening. While these variations were not found to be significant, it is noted that over 80 percent of those receiving oxytocics in the late second stage of labor experienced blood loss of less than 100 cc, and greater than 66 percent of those participating had a third stage of less than three minutes' duration. Mulla (1959) recorded third-stage blood loss in 180 consecutive patients who were given 5 units of oxytocin intravenously at the presentation of the anterior fetal shoulder. Bleeding in 175 of the 180 patients was noted to be less than 50 cc. Luby et al. (1959) studied 50 consecutively delivering women who received 5 units of oxytocin intravenously and 5 units intramuscularly with delivery of the fetal head. They concluded that oxytocin effectively shortens the duration of the third stage of labor by several minutes without significantly increasing the incidence of manual placental removal.

American researchers Hibbard and Andrews (1960) were involved in extensive clinical testing of oxytocin for pharmaceutical firms following du Vigneaud's synthesis of a chemical analog to the naturally occurring hormone. These investigators administered 10 units of oxytocin intramuscularly following delivery of the fetal head to 2,800 patients, while only 41 women received the 10 units of oxytocin intravenously at the same point in labor. It is interesting to note that blood loss with intramuscular administration was "less than 500 cc" in 96 percent of these cases, while all of those receiving the intravenous oxytocin experienced "minimal blood loss, ranging between 50 and 100 cc" (Hibbard and Andrews, 1960, p. 145). Length of the third stage of labor in all 2,841 cases was of 3 to 7 minutes' duration.

In 1962, the incidence of third-stage blood loss exceeding 600 cc was 9.5 percent with the routine administration of oxytocics at the end of the third stage of labor in a West Indies hospital. This prompted researchers Clarke and

Douglas (1962) to investigate alternative methods of preventing hemorrhage. By giving oxytocin at the delivery of the anterior fetal shoulder and ergotamine following placental separation, they discovered that the incidence of blood loss exceeding 600 cc diminished to 5.9 percent and that the length of the third stage decreased from an average of 10.7 to 7.6 minutes.

Hibbard (1964) summarized the results of multiple studies on the effects of oxytocin in the management of normal labor thus: "Oxytocin induces strong rhythmic uterine contractions and encourages separation of the placenta, thereby reducing the incidence of postpartum hemorrhage" (1964, p. 1486).

Hibbard joined with Fleigner (1966) in order to look at the active management of the third stage of labor during the period of 1953–1962 in a Liverpool hospital. The incidence of blood loss exceeding 600 cc during that time span was 5 percent and the number of third stages lasting less than 5 minutes was 61 percent. In addition, the rate of placental retention was listed at 0.5 percent. Following these researchers' institution of the administration of a combination of oxytocin and ergometrine as soon as possible after the emergence of the fetal head, the incidence of blood loss exceeding 600 cc decreased to 1.8 percent. And the number of third stages lasting less than 5 minutes had risen to 87 percent, while the rate of placental retention remained unchanged at 0.5 percent.

A definitive study regarding the pharmacologic management of the third stage of labor was conducted by Swedish researcher Sorbe (1978), who compared the effects of oxytocin and ergotamine on uterine blood loss and placental separation time. An experimental sample of 1,049 women was divided into similar-sized groups, with one subject group receiving oxytocin 10 units intravenously immediately following delivery of the anterior fetal shoulder and the other group receiving ergotamine (2 mg) at the same point in labor. Blood loss in the two oxytocic groups was reduced by one-third with respect to the control group, who did not receive an oxytocic until delivery of the placenta. The mean duration of the third stage of labor did not vary significantly between the two experimental groups. However, partial retention and/or trapping of the placenta was significantly ($p < 0.01$) more frequent among women in the ergotamine group than those in the experimental or control oxytocin groups. Sorbe summarized the results of his study by noting that ergotamine produces an unphysiologic uterine spasm of long duration that affects primarily the lower uterine segment, while oxytocin produces a more physiologic uterine contraction affecting primarily the uterine fundus, which encourages early placental separation. Sorbe went further to assert that

> Oxytocin given intravenously in adequate doses offers distinct advantages over ergotamine in the reduction in the incidence of postpartum hemorrhage without disturbance of the physiological placental sepa-

ration mechanism, and this drug should be given at delivery of the anterior fetal shoulder for greatest efficacy (1978, p. 697).

In summarizing this literature review, it is apparent that oxytocin does indeed supplement the physiologic hemostatic mechanism of the uterus in the third stage of labor. These many studies provide supportive evidence that the drug's purpose is enhanced through administration prior to termination of the third stage of labor without substantial evidence of the increased occurrence of placental trapping.

STUDY PURPOSE

The purpose of this study is to test the following hypotheses:

1. Multiparous women involved in an uncomplicated vaginal delivery who receive a controlled titration of intravenous Pitocin in the late second stage of labor will experience significantly less blood loss than women whose controlled titration of intravenous Pitocin is delayed until the late third stage of labor.
2. Multiparous women involved in an uncomplicated vaginal delivery who receive a controlled titration of intravenous Pitocin in the late second stage of labor will experience no significant increase in the incidence of placental trapping over those women whose controlled titration of intravenous Pitocin is delayed until the late third stage of labor.

For the purposes of this study, the following terms are defined:

Multiparous: A woman who has completed one or more pregnancies to the stage of fetal viability.

Uncomplicated vaginal delivery: Birth has progressed without medical/obstetrical difficulty for mother or infant.

Controlled titration: Infusion rate of the intravenous solution is regulated at a moderate velocity of 125 cc/hour through utilization of infusion pump.

Late second stage: Delivery of the anterior fetal shoulder.

Level of significance: Statistically defined at the .05 level.

Late third stage: Point of placental separation from uterine wall.

Placental trapping: Inability of the placenta to escape the uterine cavity within a 15-minute time span after the birth of the baby, as cited in Bonham (1963), Hibbard and Fleigner (1966), and Sorbe (1978), due to premature constriction of the lower segment of the uterine body.

Pitocin: Brand name of a synthetic oxytocin manufactured by Parke-Davis Pharmaceutical Company.

RESEARCH DESIGN

A quasi-experimental approach will be utilized in this study of the influence of oxytocin administration at different points in labor upon third-stage uterine blood loss and placental trapping.

SAMPLE AND SETTING

Forty-five study subjects will be selected through nonprobability convenience sampling upon admission to the labor unit of a community hospital whose obstetrical service manages 650 to 700 deliveries annually. Subjects will be placed in one of three categories: (1) *group I*, receiving no oxytocin per protocol of their care provider; (2) *group II*, receiving oxytocin after delivery of the anterior fetal shoulder per protocol of their care provider; (3) *group III*, receiving oxytocin following placental separation per protocol of their care provider.

A numerical coding system utilizing the group number and chronological order in the study (i.e., the thirteenth client in the group receiving no oxytocin will be coded 113) will identify each client.

Criteria for subject participation in this investigation include the following client characteristics:

1. Parity of 1 through 3
2. Age of 17 through 35
3. Weeks of gestation 37 through 42
4. Estimated fetal weight greater than 5 lb but less than 10 lb
5. Prepregnancy maternal weight not exceeding 180 lb
6. Pregnancy weight gain not exceeding 35 lb
7. Admission Hgb not less than 10 gm
8. Length of active labor greater than 2 hours but not exceeding 14 hours
9. No anticipated use of general or epidural anesthesia
10. No excessive use of narcotics or tranquilizers in labor (no more than Demerol 100 mg, Nisentil 40 mg., Vistaril 100 mg, and/or Phenergan 50 mg).

Those clients specifically excluded from this investigation include:

1. History of previous postpartum hemorrhage
2. History of previous manual removal of the placenta
3. Previous D&C within one year of establishing this pregnancy (whether diagnostic or following a miscarriage)

4. Presence of polyhydramnios or multiple gestation
5. Accompanying complications of pregnancy (anemia, hypertension, etc.)
6. Prolonged rupture of membranes of greater than 12 hours duration prior to the onset of labor
7. Use of oxytocin at any time prior to the second stage of present labor

METHOD AND INSTRUMENT

According to the protocol of the care provider, those subjects receiving oxytocin will have a 500 cc flask of intravenous fluid with 20 units of the drug piggybacked into the primary intravenous line and the flow rate regulated by infusion pump at 125 cc/hour. Blood loss will be collected in a standard water basin from the time of umbilical cord ligation until the uterine fundus is palpably firm within 10 minutes of placental expulsion. A gauze sponge will be applied to the episiotomy to absorb drainage from this incision site throughout the entire collection procedure to attempt to prevent this blood from being included in the collected volume of uterine blood loss. This collected blood will then be transferred to a measuring cylinder with demarcated volume equivalents for final evaluation. Blood loss will also be assessed through the comparison of percentage change in predelivery and postpartum hematocrit levels.

The data sheet (Appendix A) was developed in accordance with the study criteria to document the data necessary for testing the outlined hypotheses. Reliability of the measurement tool will be established by utilization of the same measuring cylinder for every blood collection situation, as well as the performance of each measurement by the same researcher. In addition, practitioners doing the actual blood loss collection will follow the specific collection technique demonstrated to each individual practitioner by the same researcher. Content validity of the data sheet will be established by submitting the tool to two certified nurse-midwives and one professor of nursing research.

Data Analysis

The data for each of the dependent variables (blood loss, change in hematocrit, and incidence of placental trapping) will be analyzed using an analysis of covariance (ANCOVA) to determine whether or not the variation in experimental means of the three participant groups is significant, as hypothesized in the purpose of this study. The level of significance for rejection of the hypotheses will be at the .05 level (see Table F.1).

TABLE F.1
Analysis of Covariance Significance Tests

Sources of Variation	Degrees of Freedom	Sum of Squares	Mean Squares	F
Blood loss				
Hematocrit changes				
Placental trapping				

Limitations

One primary limitation of this study involves the usefulness of postpartum hematocrit levels as an accurate indicator of third-stage blood loss. These laboratory values represent hematologic status following all labor stages, including blood loss in the immediate postpartum period, which in many cases may far exceed intrapartum blood loss. Of concurrent concern is the amount of time elapsed from delivery to obtaining the postpartum hematocrit level. Uniformly, all involved practitioners obtain this sample on the second postpartum day at 7 A.M. However, a difference of as many as 23 hours may separate one subject from another with respect to time elapsed since delivery. A final limitation involves generalization of study results related to the small sample size and the nonprobability participant selection procedure.

ETHICAL CONSIDERATIONS

Subjects meeting the previously outlined participation criteria will be approached for explanation and securing of consent for involvement in the study (see Appendix B). Confidentiality will be maintained through client identification by the previously identified coding system. The subject will not be exposed to any undue physical harm, since those women who receive no oxytocin would not receive the drug per practitioner protocol even in a nonexperimental situation, and those women receiving oxytocin would have received the drug regardless of the existence of the investigative study.

NURSING IMPLICATIONS

Nursing plays a vital role in the knowledgeable assessment and management of postpartum hemorrhage. The results of this investigation will enhance the present body of obstetrical nursing knowledge, promote more comprehensive nursing care for intrapartum/postpartum women, and provide a basis for further nursing investigations.

APPENDIX A: DATA SHEET

Patient Number _____

Gravida _____ Para _____

Age _____

Weeks of gestation _____

Estimated fetal weight _____ Actual fetal weight _____

Prepregnancy weight _____ Pregnancy weight gain _____

    Admission: Hgb _____ Hct _____
    Postpartum: Hgb _____ Hct _____

Length of labor (hours) _____

Length of third stage (minutes) _____

Placental trapping: Yes _____ No _____

Manual placental removal: Yes _____ No _____

Medications in labor (type and amount) _____

Type of anesthesia: None _____ Local _____ Pudendal _____

    Paracervical _____

Episiotomy: None _____ Midline _____ Mediolateral _____

Laceration: None _____ 1 _____ 2 _____ 3 _____ 4 ____

    Other _____

Pitocin received: None _____ After anterior shoulder _____

    After placenta _____

Measurable blood loss (cc) _____

Complications/additional data: _____

_____

APPENDIX B: INFORMED CONSENT

This form documents your invitation to participate in a study investigating uncomplicated vaginal deliveries in women who have had one or more babies. Some blood loss is considered normal with any birth, and this study will measure the actual amount of bleeding that accompanies delivery.

    Your doctor is aware that this study is being conducted and he agrees to your participation. Your participation will not jeopardize your care in any way; any treatment deemed necessary by your doctor will be provided. This participation is completely voluntary and you are free to withdraw from the study at any time without your decision affecting any of the care you receive at Mercy Medical Center.

Your records and results will not be identified as pertaining to you specifically without your express permission. Your physician will consider your records highly confidential, and code numbers will be used as a method of record identification to ensure that confidentiality. However, in rare circumstances, the United States Department of Health and Human Services (DHHS) may request a copy of your records. If this happens, the DHHS request will be honored. If you decide to participate in this study, you will also be giving consent for the investigator and her assistants to review your medical records as may be necessary for the purposes of this study.

I have had any questions answered and voluntarily give my consent to participate in this study.

SIGNATURE   DATE

WITNESS

REFERENCES

Alvarez, H., and R. Caldeyro-Barcia. 1950. "Contractility of the Human Uterus Recorded by New Methods." *Surgical Obstetrics and Gynecology,* 91(1): 1–13.

Bonham, D. 1963. "Intramuscular Oxytocics and Cord Traction in Third Stage of Labor." *British Medical Journal,* 2: 1620–1623.

Bozler, E. 1938. "Electrical Stimulation and Conduction of Excitation in Smooth Muscle." *American Journal of Physiology,* 122(3): 614–623.

Caldeyro-Barcia, R., and H. Heller. 1961. *Oxytocin: Proceedings of an International Symposium.* New York: Pergamon Press.

Caldeyro-Barcia, R., and J. Poseiro. 1959. "Oxytocin and Contractility of the Pregnant Human Uterus." *Annals of the New York Academy of Science,* 75: 813–830.

―――. 1960. "Physiology of the Uterine Contraction." *Clinical Obstetrics and Gynecology,* 3(2): 386–408.

Clarke, G., and C. Douglas. 1962. "A Comparison of Oxytocic Drugs in the Third Stage of Labor." *Journal of Obstetrics and Gynecology of the British Empire,* 69: 904–909.

Csapo, A., and J. Marshall. 1961. "Hormonal and Ionic Influences on the Membrane Activity of Uterine Smooth Muscle Cells." *Endrocrinology,* 68(June): 1026–1035.

Dawood, M. 1978. "The Role of Oxytocin in Human Labor." *Resident and Staff Physician,* July: 45–52.

Fugo, N., and Dieckmann, W. 1958. "A Comparison of Oxytocic Drugs in the Management of the Placental Stage of Labor." *American Journal of Obstetrics and Gynecology,* 76(6): 141–146.

Hendricks, C., T. Eskes, and K. Saameli. 1962. "Uterine Contractility at Delivery and in the Puerperium." *American Journal of Obstetrics and Gynecology,* 83(7): 890–906.

Hibbard, B. 1964. "The Third Stage of Labour." *British Medical Journal,* 6:1485–1488.

Hibbard, B., and J. Fleigner. 1966. "Active Management of the Third Stage of Labour." *British Medical Journal,* 2: 622–623.

Hibbard, L., and A. Andrews. 1960. "Synthetic Oxytocin." *California Medicine,* 92(February): 143–146.

Luby, R., et al. 1959. "Clinical Experience with Synthetic Oxytocin (Syntocinon): A Study of Fifty Cases in the Third Stage of Labor." *American Journal of Obstetrics and Gynecology,* 77(January): 50–54.

Mayes, B., and R. Shearman. 1956. "Experience with Synthetic Oxytocin: The Effects on the Cardiovascular System and Its Use for the Induction of Labor and Control of the Third Stage." *Journal of Obstetrics and Gynecology of the British Empire,* 63(12): 812–818.

Mulla, N. 1959. "The Oxytocics in Obstetrics." *Journal of the International College of Surgery,* 31(February): 174–180.

Myles M. 1981. *Textbook for Midwives,* 9th ed. London: Churchill Livingstone.

Oxorn, H., and W. Foote. 1981. *Human Labor and Birth,* 3rd ed. New York: Appleton-Century-Crofts.

Pritchard, J., and P. MacDonald. 1980. *Williams Obstetrics,* 16th ed. New York: Appleton-Century-Crofts.

Sorbe, B. 1978. "Active Pharmacologic Management of the Third Stage of Labor: A Comparison of Oxytocin and Ergometrine." *Obstetrics and Gynecology,* 52(6): 694–697.

Speert, H. 1980. *Obstetrics and Gynecology in America: A History.* Baltimore: Waverly Press.

Varney, H. 1980. *Nurse-Midwifery.* Boston: Blackwell Scientific.

Wyeth Laboratories. 1982. Oradell, NJ: Medical Economics Company, Charles Baker, publisher.

Wynn, R. 1977. *Biology of the Uterus.* New York: Plenum Press.

Appendix G

Abstracts of Two Completed Studies

ERNESTINE WIEDENBACH: A HISTORICAL NURSING REVIEW OF HER LIFE AND CAREER CONTRIBUTIONS

by
SUSAN NICKEL

THE EFFECT OF STOCKINETTE CAPS ON CONSERVATION OF BODY HEAT IN NEWBORN INFANTS

by
SARAH J. KLINGNER

Reprinted by permission.

ERNESTINE WIEDENBACH: A HISTORICAL NURSING REVIEW OF HER LIFE AND CAREER CONTRIBUTIONS

One need only mention family-centered maternity care and the name of Ernestine Wiedenbach comes to mind. With "clarity of central purpose," which has become her hallmark, Wiedenbach, over a four-decade nursing career, became an early advocate of prepared childbirth, nurse-midwifery graduate education, and nursing theory. Her numerous books and journal articles on nursing practice, education, and theory represent Wiedenbach's legacy to the profession of nursing.

The purpose of this descriptive historical research was to contribute to the understanding of the history of nursing and nurse-midwifery in the United States by focusing on the life of Ernestine Wiedenbach. The principal primary source was Miss Wiedenbach's oral history as recorded during a series of taped audio and video interviews. The historiographer investigated the nursing archives at Yale University where Miss Wiedenbach founded and directed the nurse-midwifery graduate program from 1956 to 1966. Also utilized were Wiedenbach's personal papers, writings, scrapbook, and interviews with her peers. The historical research design was used, and all data were subjected to intense internal and external criticism.

The findings of this study revealed an innovative practitioner, esteemed educator, and prolific author who responded to Florence Nightingale's challenge to discover and define the laws of nursing. Wiedenbach's prescriptive theory of nursing stands out as an important and early achievement of the nursing profession. This study hopefully will prove to be a source of inspiration and direction to future nurses and also provide a base for further historical research on Ernestine Wiedenbach.

THE EFFECT OF STOCKINETTE CAPS ON CONSERVATION OF BODY HEAT IN NEWBORN INFANTS

This study investigated clinically the effectiveness of stockinette caps in reducing hypothermia in externally regulating the temperature of newborns. The subjects were 20 infants from the newborn delivery room of a private hospital who met the following criteria: term birth, equivalent gestational age, weight greater than or equal to 6 pounds, Apgar scores greater than or equal to 7 at 1 minute and 5 minutes, without complications, born into ambient temperatures between 66° and 72° F, and 60 percent relative humidity. Subjects were randomly placed in an experimental group (stockinette caps) or a control group (no caps). Temperatures were measured 5 minutes and 30 minutes after birth, the extent of temperature loss was recorded on a data collection instrument, and the significance of differences in mean heat loss between the two groups was examined using the student's t-test (one-tailed). Analysis of data did not indicate that the difference in heat loss between the two groups was significant at the .05 level of probability. In view of the contradictory findings in the literature concerning the effectiveness of stockinette caps in reducing neonatal heat loss, further research is necessary.

Appendix H

Guidelines for Writing a Research Proposal

The senior author formulated the following guidelines used by beginning research students over the past several years.

The guidelines are useful in writing proposals for both quantitative and qualitative studies. Components of the guidelines may be modified for qualitative proposals. For example, in grounded theory design there may be no review of the literature prior to collecting the data related to the study problem. There also will be no theoretical framework, since the purpose of the grounded theory approach is to develop theory. A proposal for ethnographic research may require a detailed presentation of the qualifications of the researcher or researchers involved in the study, since they are the primary data collection instruments.

Your instructor may want to use these guidelines to evaluate your proposal. (Assigning points to items based on a 100-point total facilitates assignment of a final [percentage] grade.)

GUIDELINES FOR WRITING A RESEARCH PROPOSAL

Name _____   Date _____

Instructor _____

Title of research proposal _____

Comments

A. Statement of the problem
   1. Introduction presents study's general subject area and narrows the focus to a specific problem area.
   2. Enough background material is presented to acquaint the reader with the problem's importance.

Comments

3. The problem is important enough that it will contribute to general knowledge in the nursing field.
4. The problem is novel and/or the study is timely.
5. It is feasible to conduct research on the problem.

B. Literature review
1. An adequate survey of the literature has been made on the problem.
2. The literature references are pertinent to the problem.
3. The literature citations are well documented.
4. The organization of related evidence is logical.
5. The literature review is summarized.

C. Theoretical or conceptual framework
1. Applicable to the research being done.
2. Useful for clarifying concepts and relationships contained in the research.

D. Statement of the purpose of the study
1. Contains a clear statement of:
   a. what the researcher intends to do (i.e., observe/describe/classify, etc.).
   b. where the data will be collected (study setting).
   c. from whom the data will be collected (study subjects).
2. Statement form is appropriate for the study problem (declarative statement/question/hypothesis).

E. Definition of terms
The terms in the study are defined so there is no question in the reader's mind as to what the researcher means.

F. Plan for data collection
1. The research approach (design)—historical, descriptive, experimental—is described and appropriate for the purpose of the study.

Comments

    2. Study subjects
       a. The target population is described.
       b. The kinds and numbers of subjects are appropriate.
       c. The sampling approach (method) is appropriate.
    3. Techniques for data collection
       a. The data collection instrument is appropriate for the research problem.
       b. The data can be quantified for analysis.
       c. Plans for determining the instrument's reliability are included.
       d. Plans for establishing the instrument's validity are included.
       e. The instrument's limitations are recognized.
       f. Plans for pretesting the instrument are included (as applicable).
    4. Procedure for data collection
       a. Steps in the procedure are stated clearly and concisely.
       b. Data collection procedure is appropriate for the study.
       c. Protection of human rights is assured.
    5. Assumptions underlying the study are stated if significant.
    6. Study's limitations are appropriate.
G. Plan for data analysis
    1. Data analysis is consistent with sample and instrument(s).
    2. Statistical procedures are appropriate for the data.
    3. Rationale for statistical procedure is correctly formulated.
    4. Dummy charts/graphs/tables are included.
H. Additional components
    1. The title of the research proposal is appropriate.
    2. Correct grammar is used.

Comments

3. Correct spelling and punctuation are used.
4. Reference format
   a. Citation (footnote) references are listed in consistent and correct format.
   b. Bibliographic entries are listed in consistent and correct format.

FURTHER NOTES

Now that you have a tentative draft of the major sections of your research proposal, reread the draft to be sure you have a logical development of ideas within each section and throughout the proposal. You may want to exchange your proposal with a classmate and use the evaluation guidelines.

In addition to the criteria listed in the guidelines, in the procedure part of the data collection section you may want to include a timetable for the various steps to be followed in carrying out the research project, as well as an estimate of the expenses associated with the research project. Research proposals written for funding require that a budget of projected expenses be included. Guidelines for funding such proposals are very specific regarding the budget information that must be included.

The title of your proposal should accurately reflect the relationship between the variables being studied and the population of the study. The title can be most easily formulated from the information in the purpose of the study section and should reflect this purpose well enough to communicate it to others. Ask yourself if someone reading the title in an index would know what your study is about. A well-formulated proposal title can usually serve as the title for the final report of the study.

Remember to use the future tense and to refer to yourself as ''the investigator'' or ''the researcher.'' In terms of proposal length, rarely does a final proposal written by a beginning researcher exceed twenty to twenty-five typed, double-spaced pages, including bibliography and appendixes.

Appendix I

Guidelines for Evaluating a Research Report

As an aid in estimating the study's general level of acceptability, our students have found it helpful to tally the *yes* responses and divide them by the total possible responses: *yes/total*. This provides a percentage that can be used to estimate the study's *general* level of acceptability. One major caution: Some components of the guidelines are more critical than others. This general evaluation method must be accompanied by logic and judgment. For example, an inadequate title is not as critical to the study's acceptability as an inadequate interpretation of data. Likewise, if the whole data collection section is unacceptable, the study's findings are not valid.

GUIDELINES FOR EVALUATING A RESEARCH REPORT

Yes   *No*   *N/A*

(N/A = Not Applicable)

A. The problem
 1. The problem is clearly identified.
 2. The problem is researchable (data can be collected and analyzed).
 3. It is feasible to conduct research on the problem.
 4. The problem is significant to nursing.
 5. Background information on the problem is presented.
B. Review of the literature
 1. The review is relevant to the study.
 2. The review is adequate in relation to the problem.
 3. Sources are current.

    4. Documentation of sources is clear and complete.
    5. The relationship of the problem to previous research is clear.
    6. There is a range of opinions and varying points of view about the problem.
    7. The organization of the review is logical.
    8. The review concludes with a brief summary of the literature and its implications for the problem.

C. Theoretical or conceptual framework
    1. It is applicable to the research.
    2. It is clearly developed.
    3. It is useful for clarifying pertinent concepts and relationships.

D. Statement of the purpose of the study
    1. The statement form is appropriate for the study: declarative statement, question, hypothesis(es).
    2. The statement form is clear as to:
        a. what the researcher plans to do.
        b. where the data will be collected.
        c. from whom the data will be collected.
    3. Each hypothesis states an expected relationship or difference between two (2) variables.
    4. There is a clear empirical or theoretical rationale for each hypothesis.

E. Definition of terms
Relevant terms are clearly defined, either directly, operationally, or theoretically.

F. Data collection
    1. Study subjects
        a. The target population is clearly described.
        b. The sample size and major characteristics are appropriate (the sample is representative).
        c. The method for choosing the sample is appropriate.

Yes   No   N/A

   d. The sample size is adequate for the problem being investigated.
2. Data collection instruments
   a. Instruments are appropriate for problem and method.
   b. Rationale for choosing instruments is discussed.
   c. Each instrument is described as to purpose, content, strengths, and weaknesses.
   d. Instrument validity is discussed.
   e. Instrument reliability is discussed.
   f. If the instrument was developed for the study:
      1. rationale for development is discussed.
      2. procedures in development are discussed.
      3. reliability is discussed.
      4. validity is discussed.
3. Procedures
   a. The research approach is appropriate.
   b. Steps in the data collection procedure are described clearly and concisely.
   c. The data collection procedure is appropriate for the study.
   d. Protection of human rights is assured.
   e. The study is replicable from the information provided.
   f. Appropriate limitations of the study are stated.
   g. Significant assumptions are stated.
G. Data analysis
   1. The choice of statistical procedures is appropriate.
   2. Statistical procedures are correctly applied to the data.

    3. Tables, charts, and graphs are clear and well labeled.

    4. Tables, charts, and graphs are pertinent.

    5. Tables, charts, and graphs reflect reported findings.

    6. Tables, charts, and graphs are clearly discussed in the text.

H. Conclusions and recommendations

    1. Results are discussed in relation to the study's purpose.

    2. Results are discussed in relation to the theoretical or conceptual framework.

    3. Interpretations are based on the data.

    4. Generalizations are warranted by the results.

    5. Conclusions are based on the data.

    6. Conclusions are clearly stated.

    7. Recommendations are plausible and relevant.

I. Summary

    1. The summary restates the problem.

    2. The summary restates the methodology.

    3. The summary restates the major findings and conclusions.

    4. The summary is clear and concise.

J. Other considerations

    1. The investigator(s) is qualified.

    2. The title is appropriate, accurately reflecting the problem.

    3. The abstract presents a concise summary of the study.

    4. The article is well organized and flows logically.

    5. Grammar, sentence structure, and punctuation are correct.

    6. References and bibliography are accurate and complete.

Evaluator's conclusions regarding the general level of acceptability of the study:

Evaluator's conclusions regarding the feasibility of using the study findings to implement an innovation in a practice setting (clinical/teaching/administration):

Appendix J

A Statistical Primer

The purpose of this statistical primer is to provide the reader with the basic information needed to compute many of the statistics that were described in Chapter 7. Not all of the statistics described in Chapter 7 are included because of the complexity of the mathematical operations required. If you need more explanation concerning the statistics presented in this statistical primer, please refer to Chapter 7 or to the Glossary. The authors assume that readers have a basic knowledge of algebra and understand how to substitute numerical values for algebraic symbols. Many statistics have a variety of formulas for determining their answers. This means you may find other formulas in other texts.

DESCRIPTIVE STATISTICS

Descriptive statistics do exactly what the term says—they describe the data. In all cases, we do not compare descriptive statistics to determine if the differences found are statistically significant. To do that, we must use inferential statistics.

There are two categories of descriptive statistics. One category describes *central tendency* or how the scores appear to center or be grouped together. Measures of central tendency include the mean, the median, the mode, and the percentile rank. The other category of descriptive statistics describes *dispersion* or *variability*—that is, how far the scores spread on the scale being used. Measures of dispersion include the range, the standard deviation, and the variance.

Measures of Central Tendency

The Mean. The mean is the number found when you divide the sum of the scores by the total number of scores. This can be done with either grouped or ungrouped data. For ungrouped scores, the formula looks like this:

$$\frac{\Sigma_X}{N} = \overline{X}$$

where Σ = the sum
X = the scores
N = number of scores
$\overline{X}$ = the symbol for the mean

Thus, if your scores were:

$$7, 2, 8, 9, 4$$
$$\Sigma X = 30$$
$$N = 5$$
$$\overline{X} = 6$$

For grouped scores, the formula looks like this:

$$\frac{\Sigma Fx}{N} = \overline{X}$$

where Fx = the frequency of the scores.

If your scores were grouped—that is, you do not see each score, only how many scores fall within a group—then you compute the mean in a slightly different fashion. In this example of grouped scores, the interval, called the *class interval*, is 3. The midpoint is the middle of the class interval.

Class Interval	Midpoint of Interval (x)	Frequency (F)	Frequency of Midpoint (Fx)
24–26	25	1	25
21–23	22	2	44
18–20	19	1	19
15–17	16	3	48
12–14	13	4	52
9–11	10	1	10
6–8	7	1	7
3–5	4	1	4
0–2	1	1	1
		Sum $\overline{15}$	$\overline{210}$

N   = 15 (the total number of frequencies)
ΣFx = 210 (multiply each midpoint by its frequency and then add)

$$\overline{X} = \frac{Fx}{N} = \frac{210}{15} = 14$$

The Median.   The median is the number that divides a set of scores in half. Half of the scores are above the median and half of the scores are below the median. To find the median, the scores must be arranged in order from low to high. For example,

$$5, 6, 7$$

Here the median is 6. If there is an even number of scores, such as

$$5, 6, 7, 8$$

then the median falls halfway between the two middle scores. That is, the median in this example is 6.5.

If several scores are the same, such as

$$5, 5, 6, 6, 7, 8, 9$$

and the number of scores is odd, we need only to count to the middle score to find the median. In this case, the median is 6. If several scores are the same, such as

$$5, 6, 6, 6, 6, 7, 8, 9$$

and the number of scores is even, we then find the lower limit of the scores, which in this case is 5.5. Then we treat the series of numbers 6, 6, 6, 6 as if they occupy only one interval. We need only two of the 6's to find the median, so the arithmetic becomes

$$5.5 + \frac{2}{4} = 5.5 + 0.5 = 6$$

The Mode. The mode is the most frequently occurring value. It is found by examining the data and counting. This is true whether the data are grouped or ungrouped.

Percentile Rank. The percentile rank is the point below which a percentage of scores occurs. The median is always the 50th percentile. To find the percentile rank, you may use the following formula:

Percentile = Number of scores less than observed score divided by the number of scores times 100.

To find the percentile rank of the 7 in 6, 7, 8, 9, we count the number of scores below 7. The only score below 7 is 6, so the formula looks like this:

$$\frac{1}{4} (100) = 0.25(100) = 25$$

The score of 7 is at the 25th percentile.

Measures of Variability or Dispersion

The Range. Sometimes, we are only concerned with how far the scores are spread apart. This is called the *range*. To find the range we subtract the lowest score from the highest score. The result is the range. For example if we have the series of scores

$$3, 4, 7, 9, 11$$

The range equals 11 minus 3, or 8.

Standard Deviation. The standard deviation tells us how widely distributed scores are from the mean. If the standard deviation is small, the distribution of scores around the mean is small. If the standard deviation is large, the distribution of scores around the mean is large. To find the standard deviation, we use the following formula:

$$SD = \sqrt{\frac{\Sigma(X - \bar{X})^2}{N}}$$

If we have the following scores (X):

X	$\bar{X}$	$X - \bar{X}$	$(X - \bar{X})^2$
11	7	+4	16
10	7	+3	9
8	7	+1	1
4	7	−3	9
2	7	−5	25
Sum			60

$$SD = \sqrt{\frac{60}{5}} = \sqrt{12}$$

$$SD = 3.46$$

Another way to show this would be to make a diagram:

			$\bar{X}$			
				8	10	11
X = 7			7			
	2	4				
$X - \bar{X}$	−5	−3		+1	+3	+4
$(X - \bar{X})^2$	25	9		1	9	16

$$\Sigma(X - \bar{X})^2 = 60$$

$$SD = \sqrt{\frac{60}{5}} = \sqrt{12}$$

$$SD = 3.46$$

The Variance. The *variance* is another measure of the distances of individual scores from the mean. To compute the variance, you must square the standard deviation:

$$V = SD^2$$

Using the previous example, where the standard deviation was 3.46, the variance would be 3.46 squared, or 12. The variance is more difficult to interpret than the standard deviation but provides additional information, which can be used when we compare groups using analysis of variance techniques.

Z-Scores.   Z-scores or standard scores tell us how far a score is from the mean in units of standard deviation. The formula for Z-scores is:

$$Z = \frac{X - \overline{X}}{SD}$$

$$X = \text{raw score}$$

Suppose two professors were teaching the same course. If each gave a different, but equally valid, test on the same information to their own students and wanted to compare the test scores of selected students, they would have to use the Z-scores of the students to determine which ones had a higher score.

Professor A's Test	*Professor B's Test*
$\overline{X} = 86$	$\overline{X} = 81$
$SD = 5$	$SD = 6$
Professor A's student's score $= 88$	Professor B's student's score $= 88$

If we diagram this information, we find:

Professor A's student's results:

$$\overline{X} \qquad \text{Score} \qquad \overline{X} + SD$$

$$86 \Big| \qquad 88 \Big| \qquad\qquad 91 \Big|$$

$$\underline{\qquad}\Big|\underline{\quad 2 \quad}\Big|\underline{\qquad\qquad}$$

$$SD = 5$$

$$|\underline{\qquad\qquad\qquad\qquad}|$$

$$Z = \frac{2}{5} = 0.4$$

Professor B's student's results

$$\overline{X} \qquad\qquad \overline{X} + SD \qquad\qquad \text{Score}$$

$$81 \Big| \qquad\qquad 87 \Big| \qquad\qquad 88 \Big|$$

$$\underline{\qquad}\Big|\underline{\quad SD = 6 \quad}\Big|\underline{\qquad}$$

$$|\underline{\qquad\qquad\quad 7 \qquad\qquad}|$$

$$Z = \frac{7}{6} = 1.17$$

Mathematically, the problem looks like this: The Z-score for Professor A's student would be:

$$Z = \frac{88 - 86}{5} = 0.4$$

The Z-score for Professor B's student would be:

$$Z = \frac{88 - 81}{6} = 1.17$$

Because of the higher Z-score, Professor B's student deserves a higher grade.

STATISTICAL TESTS

Parametric Statistical Tests

Parametric statistical tests rest on two basic assumptions. The first assumption is that data are distributed in a normal fashion: That is, the data approximate a normal curve in their distribution. The second assumption is that the data are at least at the interval level of measurement.

Before we discuss parametric tests, we need to consider the meaning of rejection or acceptance of the null hypothesis. The investigator sets a region of rejection or an alpha level before beginning the investigation. This may be set as .05 on a two-tailed test, or as minus .05 or plus .05 on a one-tailed test. The investigator sets the alpha level indicated by the purpose of the study. A .05 alpha level is used here as an example. Basically, the investigator is saying that the chance that the differences found between the groups being studied are a result of random events is very small. At the .05 alpha level of significance, the researcher is saying that there are only 5 chances out of 100 that the rejection of the research hypothesis is the result of statistical errors (see Figures J.1, J.2, and J.3).

t-Test.   The *t*-test is used to determine whether the differences between the means of two different sets of scores are statistically significant. There are different formulas depending on whether the samples are related or not. In either case, the formula looks formidable, but it is really not that complex. The test is pooling the standard deviations of the two sets of scores. The formula for the *t*-test for independent samples is:

$$t = \cfrac{\overline{X}_1 - \overline{X}_2}{\sqrt{\cfrac{\Sigma X_1^2 - \cfrac{(\Sigma X_1)^2}{N_1} + \Sigma X_2^2 - \cfrac{(\Sigma X_2)^2}{N_2}}{(N_1 + N_2) - 2}\left(\cfrac{1}{N_1} + \cfrac{1}{N_2}\right)}}$$

where $\overline{X}_1$ = mean of sample 1
$\overline{X}_2$ = mean of sample 2
N_1 = number of subjects in sample 1
N_2 = number of subjects in sample 2
df = degrees of freedom, in this case $N_1 + N_2 - 2$

Suppose we had a number of patients who had been randomly assigned to two different groups and we wanted to determine whether a new type of treatment would be more beneficial than the standard treatment. We could give one group (the experimental group) the new treatment and the other group (the control group) the standard treatment.

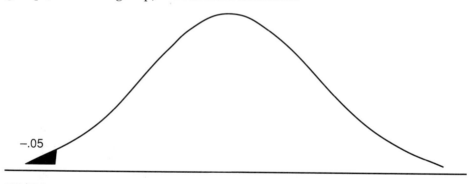

FIGURE J.1
Normal Curve Showing One-Tailed Test with Negative .05 Level of Significance

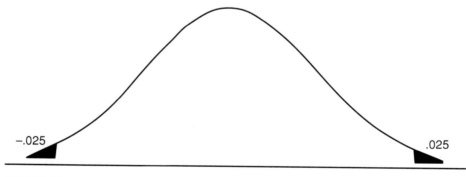

FIGURE J.2
Normal Curve Showing Two-Tailed Test with .05 Level of Significance

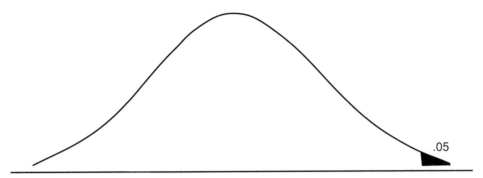

FIGURE J.3
Normal Curve Showing One-Tailed Test with Positive .05 Level of Significance

To determine if the difference between the mean of the control group (X_1) and the mean of the experimental group (X_2) is significant, we will apply the formula:

X_1	Frequency	Fx_1	X_1^2	Fx_1^2
5	1	5	25	25
6	1	6	36	36
3	2	6	9	18
2	2	4	4	16
Sum	6	21	74	113

X_2	Frequency	Fx_2	X_2^2	Fx_2^2
7	1	7	49	49
4	2	8	16	64
3	3	9	9	81
Sum	6	24	74	194

$$\overline{X}_1 = 3.5$$

$$\overline{X}_2 = 4$$

To find the value of t, we must substitute the symbols:

$$t = \frac{(3.5 - 4)}{\sqrt{\dfrac{\left(113 - \dfrac{(21)^2}{4} + 194 - \dfrac{(24)^2}{3}\right)\left(\dfrac{1}{4} + \dfrac{1}{3}\right)}{(4 + 3) - 2}}}$$

$$t = \frac{-0.5}{\sqrt{\dfrac{(113 - 110.25 + 194 - 192)(0.25 + 0.33)}{5}}}$$

$$t = \frac{-0.5}{\sqrt{\dfrac{(2.75)(.58)}{5}}}$$

$$t = \frac{-0.5}{\sqrt{\dfrac{1.595}{5}}}$$

$$t = \frac{-0.5}{\dfrac{1.26}{5}}$$

$$t = -1.984$$

Using a t table, we find that a t of -1.984 with 5 degrees of freedom is not statistically significant at the .05 level of significance. We can then conclude that there are no significant differences between the treatments in the experimental and the control groups.

Sometimes investigators use the same set of individuals as both the experimental and the control group by measuring changes of scores before and after treatment. In other cases, investigators may match two groups of individuals using one or more characteristics. In this case the formula for determining if there is a significant difference between the scores of two independent groups is not valid. The following formula may be used if the t-test is used to determine if there is a significant difference between the means of two matched or correlated groups.

$$t = \frac{\Sigma D}{\sqrt{\dfrac{[N\Sigma D - (\Sigma D)^2]}{N - 1}}}$$

where N = number of subjects
         D = difference betweeen scores

Suppose we want to determine if instruction in self-care procedures has made a significant difference in patients' knowledge concerning their condition. First we would give a pretest to determine the patients' knowledge about their condition. Then we would provide instruction in self-care procedures.

Finally, we would retest the patients to determine if their knowledge had changed significantly. Let's assume that the following scores are obtained:

Subject	Score before Instruction	Score after Instruction	Difference	Difference Squared
A	6	7	1	1
B	8	8	0	0
C	5	8	3	9
D	4	6	2	4
E	7	5	−2	4
F	7	8	1	1
G	3	7	4	16
H	6	6	0	0
I	6	9	3	9
J	4	5	1	1
Sum			13	45

Substituting numbers for symbols, we find:

$$t = \frac{13}{\sqrt{\dfrac{10 \times 45 - (13)^2}{9}}}$$

$$t = \frac{13}{\sqrt{\dfrac{450 - 169}{9}}}$$

$$t = \frac{13}{\sqrt{\dfrac{281}{9}}}$$

$$t = \frac{13}{\sqrt{31.22}}$$

$$t = \frac{13}{5.59}$$

$$t = 2.32$$

Looking up a t value of 2.32 with 9 degrees of freedom (N − 1), we find that there is a statistically significant difference at the .05 level on a one-tailed test. We could then conclude that instruction in self-care procedures made a significant difference in patients' knowledge concerning their condition.

One-Way Analysis of Variance. The *variance* is defined as the square of the standard deviation. The larger the variance, the greater the variability of the scores; that is, the more the scores are scattered or distributed from the mean. Analysis of variance is used when there are two or more treatments used simultaneously by the experimenter. If all of the treatments are compared two at a time by using the *t*-test, the experimenter increases the chances of committing a type II error. That is, the experimenter rejects the null hypothesis when there really is no significant difference between the means of the groups. A type I error occurs when the experimenter accepts the null hypothesis when there really is a significant difference between the means of two or more groups. Analysis of variance is reported as the *F* ratio, and what it really means is

$$\frac{\text{Variance between groups}}{\text{Variance within groups}}$$

Computing this seemingly simple formula requires a bit of arithmetic. Let us assume that we have three groups receiving different treatments for the same condition. Their scores (X) as a result of the treatments might look like this.

			Scores		
Group A		*Group B*		*Group C*	
X	X^2	X	X^2	X	X^2
8	64	4	16	3	9
7	49	4	16	3	9
6	36	5	25	4	16
		6	36	5	25
		3	9		
$\Sigma X_A = 21$ $\Sigma X_A^2 = 149$		$\Sigma X_B = 22$ $\Sigma X_B^2 = 102$		$\Sigma X_C = 15$ $\Sigma X_C^2 = 59$	
$N_A = 3$		$N_B = 6$		$N_C = 5$	

We must find the sums of squares for the total group, between groups, and within groups. This means that there are three separate steps of computation.

First, for the sum of squares for the total group. The formula looks like this:

$$t_{ss} = X_t^2 - \frac{(\Sigma X_t)^2}{N_t}$$

$$t = \text{total}$$

Substituting numbers for symbols we find:

$$\text{Total SS} = 310 - \frac{(58)^2}{14} = 310 - \frac{3364}{14}$$

$$= 310 - 240.29$$

$$\text{Total SS} = 69.71$$

To find the sum of squares within groups, we use the following formula:

$$\text{WSS} = \Sigma \left(\Sigma X_g^2 - \frac{(\Sigma X_g)^2}{N_g} \right)$$

$$g = \text{group}$$

Substituting numbers for symbols, we find:

$$\text{Within SS} = \left(149 - \frac{(21)^2}{3} \right) + \left(102 - \frac{(22)^2}{6} \right) + \left(59 - \frac{(15)^2}{5} \right)$$

$$= (149 - 147) + (102 - 80.67) + (59 - 45)$$

$$= 2 + 21.33 + 14$$

$$\text{Within SS} = 37.33$$

Finally, we find the between-groups sum of squares. This is the formula

$$\text{BSS} = \Sigma \frac{(\Sigma X_g)^2}{N_g} - \frac{(\Sigma X_t)^2}{N_t}$$

Substituting numbers for symbols, we find:

$$\text{Between SS} = \frac{21}{3} + \frac{22}{6} + \frac{15}{5} - \frac{(58)^2}{14}$$

$$= (147 + 80.67 + 45) - \frac{3364}{14}$$

$$= (147 + 80.67 + 45) - 240.19$$

$$= 272.67 - 240.29$$

$$\text{Between SS} = 32.38$$

We computed the total sum of squares to provide a check for the sum of squares between and within groups. The between groups sum of squares added to the within groups sum of square should yield the same total as the total sum of squares.

To compute mean squares, we must divide the within sum of squares by the degrees of freedom (DF_W) and between sum of squares by the degrees of freedom (DF_B).

The formulas look like this:

$$\bar{X}_W = \frac{\Sigma \left(\Sigma X_g^2 - \frac{(\Sigma X_g)^2}{N_g} \right)}{DF_W} \qquad \bar{X}B = \frac{\Sigma \left(\frac{(\Sigma X_g^2)}{N_g} - \frac{(\Sigma X_t)^2}{N_t} \right)}{DF_B}$$

To compute the degrees of freedom for between-groups, we subtract 1 from the number of groups or, in this case, $3 - 1 = 2$. To compute the degrees of freedom for within-groups, we subtract the number of groups from the total number of subjects, or $14 - 3 = 11$.

$$\text{Mean square between groups} = \frac{32.38}{11} = 2.94$$

$$\text{Mean square within groups} = \frac{37.33}{3} = 12.44$$

$$F = \frac{2.94}{12.44}$$

$$F = 0.24$$

Looking at a table of F ratios, we see that with 3 and 11 degrees of freedom, when $F = 0.24$, there is no significant difference at the .05 level. We can then conclude that there is no significant difference among the scores as a result of the treatments between the three groups.

If we had found a significant difference, we could apply one of several tests to determine between which sets of means the significance was really located. Among the tests are the Newman-Keuls test, the Tukey HSD test, the Scheffé test, and Dunnett's test. Each has advantages and limitations that should be noted before applying a specific test to your data. For further information, consult an advanced statistics text or a statistician.

Nonparametric Statistical Tests

Nonparametric statistical tests are used when the assumptions underlying parametric statistics cannot be ascribed to the data being analyzed. Nonparametric statistics do not require that the population be distributed in a normal fashion, and they allow the investigator to use nominal and ordinal levels of measurement. Generally, parametric methods are more powerful than nonparametric methods. This means that they will reject the null hypothesis more frequently than their nonparametric equivalents. For this reason, it is important to use parametric tests whenever the assumptions underlying their use can be met.

  The Chi-Square Test (x^2).   Sometimes we know only how many individuals occupy certain categories or groups. For example, male or female can be considered categories of gender, and each is exclusive of the other. The chi-square statistic can be used to determine whether observed frequencies of certain categories would be expected in a normal population or if the observed frequencies of the categories deviate from this expectation.
  Suppose that 90 people were asked to express their preference for one of three colors to be put on hospital walls, and their color preference came out as follows:

Yellow	Blue	Green
25	40	25

  The question to be answered is whether or not these observed differences are statistically significant from each other. To find this out, we must compute a chi-square:

$$x^2 = \frac{(O - E)^2}{E}$$

where O = observed frequencies
         E = expected frequencies

First we make a contingency table:

	Observed	Expected	Difference	Difference Squared
Yellow	25	30	5	25
Blue	40	30	10	100
Green	25	30	10	25

$$\frac{\text{Difference squared}}{\text{Expected frequencies}}$$

Yellow $\quad \dfrac{25}{30} = 0.803 \ldots$

Blue $\quad \dfrac{100}{30} = 3.333 \ldots$

Green $\quad \dfrac{25}{30} = 0.803 \ldots$

$$\chi^2 = 4.936 \ldots$$

Because there are two degrees of freedom (the number of categories minus one or $3 - 1 = 2$), a glance at a χ^2 table shows that there is no significant difference at the .05 level. We can therefore conclude that there is no statistically significant difference between the observed differences of the subjects' color preference and the expected differences of the subjects' color preference.

When there are several samples and several categories, the statistical computations remain the same. However, determining the expected frequencies in each cell requires an additional computation. If we use the same color categories as before but compare male and female preference, we might get something like this:

	Yellow		Blue		Green		Total
	O	E	O	E	O	E	
Male	10		20		15		35
Female	12		24		13		49
Total	22		44		28		83

To find the expected frequency, we multiply the total of the observed frequency of the column times the total of the observed frequencies of the row and divide by the total number in the sample:

$$EF = \frac{(C)(R)}{\text{Total}}$$

Male Expected Frequencies	Female Expected Frequencies

For yellow $\dfrac{(22)(35)}{83} = 9.28$ For yellow $\dfrac{(22)(49)}{83} = 12.99$

For green $\dfrac{(44)(35)}{83} = 18.55$ For green $\dfrac{(44)(49)}{83} = 25.98$

For blue $\dfrac{(28)(35)}{83} = 11.81$ For blue $\dfrac{(28)(49)}{83} = 16.53$

$O - E$	$(O - E)^2$	$\dfrac{(O - E)^2}{E}$	$O - E$	$(O - E)^2$	$\dfrac{(O - E)^2}{E}$
$10 - 9.28 = 0.72$	0.52	0.06	$12 - 12.99 = -0.99$	0.98	0.08
$20 - 18.55 = 1.45$	2.10	0.11	$24 - 25.98 = -1.98$	3.92	0.15
$15 - 11.81 = 3.19$	10.18	0.86	$13 - 16.53 = -3.53$	12.46	0.75

Summing all of the $\dfrac{(O - E)^2}{E}$ we find that $\chi^2 = 2.00$.

When we look at a χ^2 table, we find that 2.00 with four degrees of freedom = $p > .05$, so we can conclude that there is no significant difference between males and females in their choice of colors.

Investigators are cautioned that if more than 20 percent of the cells in the contingency table contain expected scores of less than 5, the chi-square result will not be accurate.

The Test Statistic. There is, however, another statistic that is more forgiving than the chi-square statistic. This is the test statistic (T). The test statistic is found in the same fashion as the chi-square and the result is read from the chi-square table. The test statistic allows the expected score in the cells to be as low as 1.[1]

The Mann-Whitney U Statistic. The Mann-Whitney U statistic provides a method for comparing the rankings of two different groups to determine if they differ from each other significantly. The formula looks like this:

$$U = (A)(B) + \frac{A(A + 1)}{2} - \Sigma RA$$

where $R = $ rank.

Suppose we had two groups with scores like this:

A	B
22	36
16	18
22	19
15	15
	19

First we rank all of the scores from lowest to highest. Note that tied scores assume the value of their combined ranks.

Scores	15	15	16	18	19	19	22	22	36
Rank	1.5	1.5	3	4	5.5	5.5	7.5	7.5	9

Scores by Rank

A Score	Rank	B Score	Rank
15	1.5	15	1.5
16	3	18	4
19	5.5	19	5.5
22	7.5	22	7.5
		36	9
Sum of ranks	17.5		27.5

Total A scores = 4 (N_1).   Total B scores = 5 (N_2).

$$U = (4)(5) + \frac{(4)(5)}{2} - 17.5 = 12.5$$

When we look at a Mann-Whitney U table where N = 4, we find that there is no U of 12.5. This means that we must recompute U by making A scores into B scores and B scores into A scores.

$$U = (5)(4) + \frac{(5)(4)}{2} - 27.5 = 7.5$$

We find that a U of 7.5 falls between 7 and 8 on the table and that a U of 7 yields a probability of .155 and a U of 8 yields a probability of .210. Since 7.5 falls between 7 and 8 and neither of these U's has a significance of p < .05, we can conclude that there is no statistically significant difference between the scores of the two groups.

Note that if N_2 is larger than 20, there is another formula used to compute U, and the value is read from a Z-score table.

The Kruskal-Wallis One-Way Analysis of Variance by Ranks. The Kruskal-Wallis statistic allows the analysis of variance using ranks rather than true scores. The statistic can also be used when very small groups are being compared. The Kruskal-Wallis statistic is read as H. The formula looks like this:

$$H = \left(\frac{12}{N(N+1)}\right) \left(\frac{\Sigma R_j^2}{N_j}\right) - 3(N-1)$$

where N = Total number of scores
        N_J = Number of scores in the Jth sample

Suppose that we have three groups of student nurses who were taught by three different instructors but were all given the same test. Were there any statistically significant differences between the scores of the three groups in terms of their knowledge? We rank the lowest score as 1 and continue to rank all scores on an ascending scale.

Group A		Group B		Group C	
Score	*Rank*	*Score*	*Rank*	*Score*	*Rank*
65	6	73	10	67	8
60	5	71	9	50	3
57	4	66	7	49	2
48	1				
Sum	16		26		13

$$H = \left(\frac{12}{(10)(11)}\right) \left(\frac{(16)^2}{4} + \frac{(26)^2}{3} + \frac{(13)^2}{3}\right) - 3(11)$$

$$= 0.10(64 + 225.33 + 56.33) - 33$$

$$= 34.57 - 33$$

$$H = 1.57$$

Consulting the table for the Kruskal-Wallis one-way analysis of variance, we find that 1.57 is not statistically significant at the .05 level or below. We can therefore conclude that there is no significant difference between the groups in terms of their knowledge on the test.

The Friedman Two-Way Analysis of Variance by Ranks. The Friedman two-way analysis of variance is designed to examine whether or not matched samples of subjects given different treatments differ significantly as the result of the different treatments. We use a chi-square table to determine the level of significance. The symbol for the Friedman two-way analysis of variance statistic is χ_r^2. The formula looks like this:

$$\chi_r^2 = \left[\frac{12}{NK(K + 1)} \Sigma (R_j)^2 \right] - 3N(K + 1)$$

where N = number of rows
       K = number of columns
       $(R_j)^2$ tells us to square and then sum all of the column rank totals.

Suppose we have one group of subjects receiving three different treatments and we want to determine if there is a statistically significant difference between the treatments. Their ranked scores as results of the treatments might look like this:

Treatment Subject	1 Rank	2 Rank	3 Rank
A	3	1	2
B	2	3	1
C	1	2	3
D	2	1	3
Sum of ranks	8	7	9

Applying the formula:

$$\chi_r^2 = \left(\frac{12}{(4)(3)(4)} \right) \left((8)^2 + (7)^2 + (9)^2 \right) - (3)(4)(4)$$

$$= \frac{12}{48} (64 + 49 + 81) - 48$$

$$= (0.25)(194) - 48$$

$$\chi_r^2 = 48.50 - 48 = 0.50$$

Consulting the table for the Friedman two-way analysis of variance for N = 4 and K = 3, we find that 0.50 yields a p of .931, which is far from statistically significant at the .05 level. We can therefore conclude that there is no significant difference between the treatments.

CORRELATIONS

Correlations measure the degree of relationship between two variables. The relationship between variables is expressed as the correlation coefficient. If the correlation coefficient is $+1$, the two variables are perfectly correlated in a positive way. If the correlation coefficient is -1, the two variables are perfectly correlated in a negative way. The closer a correlation coefficient is to 0, the less the variables are related.

Parametric Correlation

The Pearson Product-Moment Correlation. The principal parametric correlation coefficient is the Pearson product-moment, which is expressed as r and is frequently called the Pearson r or simply r. The formula for the Pearson product-moment looks like this:

$$r = \frac{\Sigma XY - \frac{(\Sigma X)(\Sigma Y)}{N}}{\sqrt{\left(\Sigma X^2 - \frac{(\Sigma X)^2}{N}\right)\left(\Sigma Y^2 - \frac{(\Sigma Y)^2}{N}\right)}}$$

Let's look at the scores of two variables (X and Y) and determine their relationship.

	X	Y	XY	X^2	Y^2
	6	3	18	36	9
	8	11	88	64	121
	12	9	108	144	81
	14	7	98	196	49
Sum	40	30	312	440	260

Substituting numbers for symbols:

$$r = \frac{312 - \frac{(40)(30)}{4}}{\sqrt{\left(440 - \frac{1,600}{4}\right)\left(260 - \frac{900}{4}\right)}}$$

$$= \frac{312 - 300}{\sqrt{(440 - 400)\ (260 - 225)}}$$

$$= \frac{12}{\sqrt{(40)(35)}}$$

$$= \frac{12}{\sqrt{1400}}$$

$$= \frac{12}{37.39}$$

$$r = 0.32$$

Nonparametric Correlation

The Spearman Rank Order Correlation.   The Spearman rank order correlation is often called the Spearman rho or simply rho. The symbol for the Spearman rho is r_s. This correlation is one of many nonparametric correlations. When the parametric assumptions of the Pearson product-moment cannot be met, many investigators choose to use the Spearman rho statistic. It is the only nonparametric correlation that we will show how to compute. The formula looks like this:

$$r_s = 1 - \frac{6\Sigma d^2}{N(N^2 - 1)}$$

where   N = Number of subjects
         d = Sum of the squared differences between the subjects' ranks

Suppose we had the following sets of scores for one group on two different tests and wish to determine how they are correlated: We rank from the highest to the lowest, with the highest score being 1.

	Test A			Test B			
Subject	Score	Rank		Score	Rank	d	d^2
A	15	1		14	2	−1	1
B	13	2		11	4	−2	4
C	12	3		15	1	2	4
D	11	4		12	3	1	1
E	8	5		10	5	0	0
							$\overline{10}$

$$r_s = 1 - \frac{6(10)}{5(24)}$$

$$= 1 - \frac{60}{120}$$

$$= 1 - .5$$

$$r_s = .5$$

Thus, we can say the correlation between the two tests is .5.

This concludes our statistical primer, in which we have presented a few of the commonly used statistical tests. Since there are many more tests reported in the literature, we strongly urge you to study more advanced texts or to consult a statistician if you wish to explore tests not discussed in this primer.

REFERENCE

1. Conover, W. J. 1980. *Practical Nonparamentric Statistics*. New York: Wiley, pp. 166–168.

BIBLIOGRAPHY AND SUGGESTED READINGS

Burns, N., and S. K. Grove. 1987. *The Practice of Nursing Research: Conduct, Critique and Utilization*. Philadelphia: W. B. Saunders.

Cochran, S., and J. Holliman. 1974. *Cheat Sheet for Stat*. Commerce, TX: Authors.

Conover, W. J. 1980. *Practical Nonparametric Statistics*. New York: Wiley.

Knapp, R. 1985. *Basic Statistics for Nurses*. New York: Wiley.

Munro, B. H., M. A. Visintainer, and E. B. Page. 1986. *Statistical Methods for Health Care Research*. Philadelphia: J. B. Lippincott.

Popham, W. J. 1967. *Educational Statistics*. New York: Harper & Row.

Siegel, S. 1956. *Nonparametric Statistics for the Behavioral Sciences*. New York: McGraw-Hill.

STATISTICAL TABLES

TABLE J.1
Areas of the Normal Curve in Terms of Z

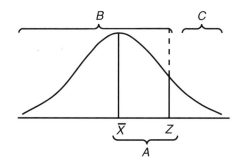

(1)	(2)	(3)	(4)	(1)	(2)	(3)	(4)
	A Area from Mean to	B Area in Larger	C Area in Smaller		A Area from Mean to	B Area in Larger	C Area in Smaller
z	z	Portion	Portion	z	z	Portion	Portion
0.00	.0000	.5000	.5000	0.30	.1179	.6179	.3821
0.01	.0040	.5040	.4960	0.31	.1217	.6217	.3783
0.02	.0080	.5080	.4920	0.32	.1255	.6255	.3745
0.03	.0120	.5120	.4880	0.33	.1293	.6293	.3707
0.04	.0160	.5160	.4840	0.34	.1331	.6331	.3669
0.05	.0199	.5199	.4801	0.35	.1368	.6368	.3632
0.06	.0239	.5239	.4761	0.36	.1406	.6406	.3594
0.07	.0279	.5279	.4721	0.37	.1443	.6443	.3557
0.08	.0319	.5319	.4681	0.38	.1480	.6480	.3520
0.09	.0359	.5359	.4641	0.39	.1517	.6517	.3483
0.10	.0398	.5398	.4602	0.40	.1554	.6554	.3446
0.11	.0438	.5438	.4562	0.41	.1591	.6591	.3409
0.12	.0478	.5478	.4522	0.42	.1628	.6628	.3372
0.13	.0517	.5517	.4483	0.43	.1664	.6664	.3336
0.14	.0557	.5557	.4443	0.44	.1700	.6700	.3300
0.15	.0596	.5596	.4404	0.45	.1736	.6736	.3264
0.16	.0636	.5636	.4364	0.46	.1772	.6772	.3228
0.17	.0675	.5675	.4325	0.47	.1808	.6808	.3192
0.18	.0714	.5714	.4286	0.48	.1844	.6844	.3156
0.19	.0753	.5753	.4247	0.49	.1879	.6879	.3121
0.20	.0793	.5793	.4207	0.50	.1915	.6915	.3085

(1)	(2)	(3)	(4)	(1)	(2)	(3)	(4)
	A Area from Mean to	B Area in Larger	C Area in Smaller		A Area from Mean to	B Area in Larger	C Area in Smaller
z	z	Portion	Portion	z	z	Portion	Portion
0.21	.0832	.5832	.4168	0.51	.1950	.6950	.3050
0.22	.0871	.5871	.4129	0.52	.1985	.6985	.3015
0.23	.0910	.5910	.4090	0.53	.2019	.7019	.2981
0.24	.0948	.5948	.4052	0.54	.2054	.7054	.2946
0.25	.0987	.5987	.4013	0.55	.2088	.7088	.2912
0.26	.1026	.6026	.3974	0.56	.2123	.7123	.2877
0.27	.1064	.6064	.3936	0.57	.2157	.7157	.2843
0.28	.1103	.6103	.3897	0.58	.2190	.7190	.2810
0.29	.1141	.6141	.3859	0.59	.2224	.7224	.2776
0.60	.2257	.7257	.2743	0.95	.3289	.8289	.1711
0.61	.2291	.7291	.2709	0.96	.3315	.8315	.1685
0.62	.2324	.7324	.2676	0.97	.3340	.8340	.1660
0.63	.2357	.7357	.2643	0.98	.3365	.8365	.1635
0.64	.2389	.7389	.2611	0.99	.3389	.8389	.1611
0.65	.2422	.7422	.2578	1.00	.3413	.8413	.1587
0.66	.2454	.7454	.2546	1.01	.3438	.8438	.1562
0.67	.2486	.7486	.2514	1.02	.3461	.8461	.1539
0.68	.2517	.7517	.2483	1.03	.3485	.8485	.1515
0.69	.2549	.7549	.2451	1.04	.3508	.8508	.1492
0.70	.2580	.7580	.2420	1.05	.3531	.8531	.1469
0.71	.2611	.7611	.2389	1.06	.3554	.8554	.1446
0.72	.2642	.7642	.2358	1.07	.3577	.8577	.1423
0.73	.2673	.7673	.2327	1.08	.3599	.8599	.1401
0.74	.2704	.7704	.2296	1.09	.3621	.8621	.1379
0.75	.2734	.7734	.2266	1.10	.3643	.8643	.1357
0.76	.2764	.7764	.2236	1.11	.3665	.8665	.1335
0.77	.2794	.7794	.2206	1.12	.3686	.8686	.1314
0.78	.2823	.7823	.2177	1.13	.3708	.8708	.1292
0.79	.2852	.7852	.2148	1.14	.3729	.8729	.1271
0.80	.2881	.7881	.2119	1.15	.3749	.8749	.1251
0.81	.2910	.7910	.2090	1.16	.3770	.8770	.1230
0.82	.2939	.7939	.2061	1.17	.3790	.8790	.1210
0.83	.2967	.7967	.2033	1.18	.3810	.8810	.1190
0.84	.2995	.7995	.2005	1.19	.3830	.8830	.1170
0.85	.3023	.8023	.1977	1.20	.3849	.8849	.1151
0.86	.3051	.8051	.1949	1.21	.3869	.8869	.1131

(continued)

TABLE J.1 (Continued)

(1)	(2)	(3)	(4)	(1)	(2)	(3)	(4)
z	A Area from Mean to z	B Area in Larger Portion	C Area in Smaller Portion	z	A Area from Mean to z	B Area in Larger Portion	C Area in Smaller Portion
0.87	.3078	.8078	.1922	1.22	.3888	.8888	.1112
0.88	.3106	.8106	.1894	1.23	.3907	.8907	.1093
0.89	.3133	.8133	.1867	1.24	.3925	.8925	.1075
0.90	.3159	.8159	.1841	1.25	.3944	.8944	.1056
0.91	.3186	.8186	.1814	1.26	.3962	.8962	.1038
0.92	.3212	.8212	.1788	1.27	.3980	.8980	.1020
0.93	.3238	.8238	.1762	1.28	.3997	.8997	.1003
0.94	.3264	.8264	.1736	1.29	.4015	.9015	.0985
1.30	.4032	.9032	.0968	1.65	.4505	.9505	.0495
1.31	.4049	.9049	.0951	1.66	.4515	.9515	.0485
1.32	.4066	.9066	.0934	1.67	.4525	.9525	.0475
1.33	.4082	.9082	.0918	1.68	.4535	.9535	.0465
1.34	.4099	.9099	.0901	1.69	.4545	.9545	.0455
1.35	.4115	.9115	.0885	1.70	.4554	.9554	.0446
1.36	.4131	.9131	.0869	1.71	.4564	.9564	.0436
1.37	.4147	.9147	.0853	1.72	.4573	.9573	.0427
1.38	.4162	.9162	.0838	1.73	.4582	.9582	.0418
1.39	.4177	.9177	.0823	1.74	.4591	.9591	.0409
1.40	.4192	.9192	.0808	1.75	.4599	.9599	.0401
1.41	.4207	.9207	.0793	1.76	.4608	.9608	.0392
1.42	.4222	.9222	.0778	1.77	.4616	.9616	.0384
1.43	.4236	.9236	.0764	1.78	.4625	.9625	.0375
1.44	.4251	.9251	.0749	1.79	.4633	.9633	.0367
1.45	.4265	.9265	.0735	1.80	.4641	.9641	.0359
1.46	.4279	.9279	.0721	1.81	.4649	.9649	.0351
1.47	.4292	.9292	.0708	1.82	.4656	.9656	.0344
1.48	.4306	.9306	.0694	1.83	.4664	.9664	.0336
1.49	.4319	.9319	.0681	1.84	.4671	.9671	.0329
1.50	.4332	.9332	.0668	1.85	.4678	.9678	.0322
1.51	.4345	.9345	.0655	1.86	.4686	.9686	.0314
1.52	.4357	.9357	.0643	1.87	.4693	.9693	.0307
1.53	.4370	.9370	.0630	1.88	.4699	.9699	.0301
1.54	.4382	.9382	.0618	1.89	.4706	.9706	.0294
1.55	.4394	.9394	.0606	1.90	.4713	.9713	.0287
1.56	.4406	.9406	.0594	1.91	.4719	.9719	.0281
1.57	.4418	.9418	.0582	1.92	.4726	.9726	.0274
1.58	.4429	.9429	.0571	1.93	.4732	.9732	.0268

(1)	(2)	(3)	(4)	(1)	(2)	(3)	(4)
z	A Area from Mean to z	B Area in Larger Portion	C Area in Smaller Portion	z	A Area from Mean to z	B Area in Larger Portion	C Area in Smaller Portion
1.59	.4441	.9441	.0559	1.94	.4738	.9738	.0262
1.60	.4452	.9452	.0548	1.95	.4744	.9744	.0256
1.61	.4463	.9463	.0537	1.96	.4750	.9750	.0250
1.62	.4474	.9474	.0526	1.97	.4756	.9756	.0244
1.63	.4484	.9484	.0516	1.98	.4761	.9761	.0239
1.64	.4495	.9495	.0505	1.99	.4767	.9767	.0233
2.00	.4772	.9772	.0228	2.35	.4906	.9906	.0094
2.01	.4778	.9778	.0222	2.36	.4909	.9909	.0091
2.02	.4783	.9783	.0217	2.37	.4911	.9911	.0089
2.03	.4788	.9788	.0212	2.38	.4913	.9913	.0087
2.04	.4793	.9793	.0207	2.39	.4916	.9916	.0084
2.05	.4798	.9798	.0202	2.40	.4918	.9918	.0082
2.06	.4803	.9803	.0197	2.41	.4920	.9920	.0080
2.07	.4808	.9808	.0192	2.42	.4922	.9922	.0078
2.08	.4812	.9812	.0188	2.43	.4925	.9925	.0075
2.09	.4817	.9817	.0183	2.44	.4927	.9927	.0073
2.10	.4821	.9821	.0179	2.45	.4929	.9929	.0071
2.11	.4826	.9826	.0174	2.46	.4931	.9931	.0069
2.12	.4830	.9830	.0170	2.47	.4932	.9932	.0068
2.13	.4834	.9834	.0166	2.48	.4934	.9934	.0066
2.14	.4838	.9838	.0162	2.49	.4936	.9936	.0064
2.15	.4842	.9842	.0158	2.50	.4938	.9938	.0062
2.16	.4846	.9846	.0154	2.51	.4940	.9940	.0060
2.17	.4850	.9850	.0150	2.52	.4941	.9941	.0059
2.18	.4854	.9854	.0146	2.53	.4943	.9943	.0057
2.19	.4857	.9857	.0143	2.54	.4945	.9945	.0055
2.20	.4861	.9861	.0139	2.55	.4946	.9946	.0054
2.21	.4864	.9864	.0136	2.56	.4948	.9948	.0052
2.22	.4868	.9868	.0132	2.57	.4949	.9949	.0051
2.23	.4871	.9871	.0129	2.58	.4951	.9951	.0049
2.24	.4875	.9875	.0125	2.59	.4952	.9952	.0048
2.25	.4878	.9878	.0122	2.60	.4953	.9953	.0047
2.26	.4881	.9881	.0119	2.61	.4955	.9955	.0045
2.27	.4884	.9884	.0116	2.62	.4956	.9956	.0044
2.28	.4887	.9887	.0113	2.63	.4957	.9957	.0043
2.29	.4890	.9890	.0110	2.64	.4959	.9959	.0041

(continued)

TABLE J.1 (Continued)

(1)	(2)	(3)	(4)	(1)	(2)	(3)	(4)
z	A Area from Mean to z	B Area in Larger Portion	C Area in Smaller Portion	z	A Area from Mean to z	B Area in Larger Portion	C Area in Smaller Portion
2.30	.4893	.9893	.0107	2.65	.4960	.9960	.0040
2.31	.4896	.9896	.0104	2.66	.4961	.9961	.0039
2.32	.4898	.9898	.0102	2.67	.4962	.9962	.0038
2.33	.4901	.9901	.0099	2.68	.4963	.9963	.0037
2.34	.4904	.9904	.0096	2.69	.4964	.9964	.0036
2.70	.4965	.9965	.0035	3.00	.4987	.9987	.0013
2.71	.4966	.9966	.0034	3.01	.4987	.9987	.0013
2.72	.4967	.9967	.0033	3.02	.4987	.9987	.0013
2.73	.4968	.9968	.0032	3.03	.4988	.9988	.0012
2.74	.4969	.9969	.0031	3.04	.4988	.9988	.0012
2.75	.4970	.9970	.0030	3.05	.4989	.9989	.0011
2.76	.4971	.9971	.0029	3.06	.4989	.9989	.0011
2.77	.4972	.9972	.0028	3.07	.4989	.9989	.0011
2.78	.4973	.9973	.0027	3.08	.4990	.9990	.0010
2.79	.4974	.9974	.0026	3.09	.4990	.9990	.0010
2.80	.4974	.9974	.0026	3.10	.4990	.9990	.0010
2.81	.4975	.9975	.0025	3.11	.4991	.9991	.0009
2.82	.4976	.9976	.0024	3.12	.4991	.9991	.0009
2.83	.4977	.9977	.0023	3.13	.4991	.9991	.0009
2.84	.4977	.9977	.0023	3.14	.4992	.9992	.0008
2.85	.4978	.9978	.0022	3.15	.4992	.9992	.0008
2.86	.4979	.9979	.0021	3.16	.4992	.9992	.0008
2.87	.4979	.9979	.0021	3.17	.4992	.9992	.0008
2.88	.4980	.9980	.0020	3.18	.4993	.9993	.0007
2.89	.4981	.9981	.0019	3.19	.4993	.9993	.0007
2.90	.4981	.9981	.0019	3.20	.4993	.9993	.0007
2.91	.4982	.9982	.0018	3.21	.4993	.9993	.0007
2.92	.4982	.9982	.0018	3.22	.4994	.9994	.0006
2.93	.4983	.9983	.0017	3.23	.4994	.9994	.0006
2.94	.4984	.9984	.0016	3.24	.4994	.9994	.0006
2.95	.4984	.9984	.0016	3.30	.4995	.9995	.0005
2.96	.4985	.9985	.0015	3.40	.4997	.9997	.0003
2.97	.4985	.9985	.0015	3.50	.4998	.9998	.0002
2.98	.4986	.9986	.0014	3.60	.4998	.9998	.0002
2.99	.4986	.9986	.0014	3.70	.4999	.9999	.0001

Source: Joseph H. Porter and Robert J. Hamm, *Statistics: Applications for the Behavioral Sciences,* 1986, Table A, pp. 384–388. Reprinted by permission of Brooks/Cole Publishing Company, Pacific Grove, CA 93950.

ABLE J.2
he Student t Distribution

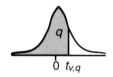

q v	0.600	0.700	0.750	0.800	0.850	0.900	0.925	0.950	0.975	0.990	0.995	0.999	.9995
1	0.325	0.727	1.000	1.376	1.963	3.078	4.165	6.314	12.71	31.82	63.66	318.3	636.6
2	0.289	0.617	0.816	1.061	1.386	1.886	2.282	2.920	4.303	6.965	9.925	22.33	31.60
3	0.277	0.584	0.765	0.978	1.250	1.638	1.924	2.353	3.182	4.541	5.841	20.21	12.92
4	0.271	0.569	0.741	0.941	1.190	1.533	1.778	2.132	2.776	3.747	4.604	7.173	8.610
5	0.267	0.559	0.727	0.920	1.156	1.476	1.699	2.015	2.571	3.365	4.032	5.893	6.869
6	0.265	0.553	0.718	0.906	1.134	1.440	1.650	1.943	2.447	3.143	3.707	5.208	5.959
7	0.263	0.549	0.711	0.896	1.119	1.415	1.617	1.895	2.365	2.998	3.499	4.785	5.408
8	0.262	0.546	0.706	0.889	1.108	1.397	1.592	1.860	2.306	2.896	3.355	4.501	5.041
9	0.261	0.543	0.703	0.883	1.100	1.383	1.574	1.833	2.262	2.821	3.250	4.297	4.781
10	0.260	0.542	0.700	0.879	1.093	1.372	1.559	1.812	2.228	2.764	3.169	4.144	4.587
11	0.260	0.540	0.697	0.876	1.088	1.363	1.548	1.796	2.201	2.718	3.106	4.025	4.437
12	0.259	0.539	0.695	0.873	1.083	1.356	1.538	1.782	2.179	2.681	3.055	3.930	4.318
13	0.259	0.538	0.694	0.870	1.079	1.350	1.530	1.771	2.160	2.650	3.012	3.852	4.221
14	0.258	0.537	0.692	0.868	1.076	1.345	1.523	1.761	2.145	2.624	2.977	3.787	4.140
15	0.258	0.536	0.691	0.866	1.074	1.341	1.517	1.753	2.131	2.602	2.947	3.733	4.073
16	0.258	0.535	0.690	0.865	1.071	1.337	1.512	1.746	2.120	2.583	2.921	3.686	4.015
17	0.257	0.534	0.689	0.863	1.069	1.333	1.508	1.740	2.110	2.567	2.898	3.646	3.965
18	0.257	0.534	0.688	0.862	1.067	1.330	1.504	1.734	2.101	2.552	2.878	3.610	3.922
19	0.257	0.533	0.688	0.861	1.066	1.328	1.500	1.729	2.093	2.539	2.861	3.579	3.883
20	0.257	0.533	0.687	0.860	1.064	1.325	1.497	1.725	2.086	2.528	2.845	3.552	3.850
21	0.257	0.532	0.686	0.859	1.063	1.323	1.494	1.721	2.080	2.518	2.831	3.527	3.819
22	0.256	0.532	0.686	0.858	1.061	1.321	1.492	1.717	2.074	2.508	2.819	3.505	3.792
23	0.256	0.532	0.685	0.858	1.060	1.319	1.489	1.714	2.069	2.500	2.807	3.485	3.768
24	0.256	0.531	0.685	0.857	1.059	1.318	1.487	1.711	2.064	2.492	2.797	3.467	3.745
25	0.256	0.531	0.684	0.856	1.058	1.316	1.485	1.708	2.060	2.485	2.787	3.450	3.725
26	0.256	0.531	0.684	0.856	1.058	1.315	1.483	1.706	2.056	2.479	2.779	3.435	3.707
27	0.256	0.531	0.684	0.855	1.057	1.314	1.482	1.703	2.052	2.473	2.771	3.422	3.690
28	0.256	0.530	0.683	0.855	1.056	1.313	1.480	1.701	2.048	2.467	2.763	3.408	3.674
29	0.256	0.530	0.683	0.854	1.055	1.311	1.479	1.699	2.045	2.462	2.756	3.396	3.659
30	0.256	0.530	0.683	0.854	1.055	1.310	1.477	1.697	2.042	2.457	2.750	3.385	3.646
31	0.256	0.530	0.682	0.853	1.054	1.309	1.476	1.696	2.040	2.453	2.744	3.375	3.633
32	0.255	0.530	0.682	0.853	1.054	1.309	1.475	1.694	2.037	2.449	2.738	3.365	3.622
33	0.255	0.530	0.682	0.853	1.053	1.308	1.474	1.692	2.035	2.445	2.733	3.356	3.611
34	0.255	0.529	0.682	0.852	1.052	1.307	1.473	1.691	2.032	2.441	2.728	3.348	3.601
35	0.255	0.529	0.682	0.852	1.052	1.306	1.472	1.690	2.030	2.438	2.724	3.340	3.591
36	0.255	0.529	0.681	0.852	1.052	1.306	1.471	1.688	2.028	2.434	2.719	3.333	3.582

(continued)

TABLE J.2 (Continued)

v \ q	0.600	0.700	0.750	0.800	0.850	0.900	0.925	0.950	0.975	0.990	0.995	0.999	.9995
37	0.255	0.529	0.681	0.851	1.051	1.305	1.470	1.687	2.026	2.431	2.715	3.326	3.574
38	0.255	0.529	0.681	0.851	1.051	1.304	1.469	1.686	2.024	2.429	2.712	3.319	3.566
39	0.255	0.529	0.681	0.851	1.050	1.304	1.468	1.685	2.023	2.426	2.708	3.313	3.558
40	0.255	0.529	0.681	0.851	1.050	1.303	1.468	1.684	2.021	2.423	2.704	3.307	3.551
45	0.255	p.528	0.680	0.850	1.049	1.301	1.465	1.679	2.014	2.412	2.690	3.281	3.520
50	0.255	0.528	0.679	0.849	1.047	1.299	1.462	1.676	2.009	2.403	2.678	3.261	3.496
60	0.254	0.527	0.679	0.848	1.045	1.296	1.458	1.671	2.000	2.390	2.660	3.232	3.460
70	0.254	0.527	0.678	0.847	1.044	1.294	1.456	1.667	1.994	2.381	2.648	3.211	3.435
80	0.254	0.526	0.678	0.846	1.043	1.292	1.453	1.664	1.990	2.374	2.639	3.195	3.416
90	0.254	0.526	0.677	0.846	1.042	1.291	1.452	1.662	1.987	2.368	2.632	3.183	3.402
100	0.254	0.526	0.677	0.845	1.042	1.290	1.451	1.660	1.984	2.364	2.626	3.174	3.390
120	0.254	0.526	0.677	0.845	1.041	1.289	1.449	1.658	1.980	2.358	2.617	3.160	3.373
150	0.254	0.526	0.676	0.844	1.040	1.287	1.447	1.655	1.976	2.351	2.609	3.145	3.357
∞	0.253	0.524	0.674	0.842	1.036	1.282	1.440	1.645	1.960	2.326	2.576	3.090	3.291

Source: H. R. Neave, *Statistics Tables*, 1978, Table 3.1, "The Student t Distribution," p. 41. Copyright © 197 by Routledge. Reprinted by permissioon of the author and publisher.

TABLE J.3
The F Distribution

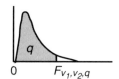

v_2	q	$v_1$1	2	3	4	5	6	7	8	9	10	12	15	20	30	50	∞
	.9	39.9	49.5	53.6	55.8	57.2	58.2	58.9	59.4	59.9	60.2	60.7	61.2	61/7	62.3	62.7	63.3
	.95	161	200	216	225	230	234	237	239	241	242	244	246	248	250	252	254
	.975	648	800	864	900	922	937	948	957	963	969	977	985	993	1001	1008	1018
	.990	4052	5000	5403	5625	5764	5859	5928	5981	6022	6056	6106	6157	7209	6261	6303	6366
	.995	1621	2000	2161	2250	2306	2344	2371	2393	2409	2422	2443	2463	2484	2504	2521	2546
	.999	4053	5000	5404	5625	5764	5859	5929	5981	6023	6056	6107	6158	6209	6261	6303	6366

For $v_2 = 1$: values for $q = 0.995$ should be multiplied by 10
values for $q = 0.999$ should be multiplied by 100

v_2	q	$v_1$1	2	3	4	5	6	7	8	9	10	12	15	20	30	50	∞
	.9	8.53	9.00	9.16	9.24	9.29	9.33	9.35	9.37	9.38	9.39	9.41	9.42	9.44	9.46	9.47	9.49
	.95	18.5	19.0	19.2	19.2	19.3	19.3	19.4	19.4	19.4	19.4	19.4	19.4	19.5	19.5	19.5	19.5
	.975	38.5	39.0	39.2	39.2	39.3	39.3	39.4	39.4	39.4	39.4	39.4	39.4	39.4	39.5	39.5	39.5
	.990	98.5	99.0	99.2	99.2	99.3	99.3	99.4	99.4	99.4	99.4	99.4	99.4	99.4	99.5	99.5	99.5
	.995	199	199	199	199	199	199	199	199	199	199	199	199	199	199	199	199
	.999	999	999	999	999	999	999	999	999	999	999	999	999	999	999	999	999
	.9	5.54	5.46	5.39	5.34	5.31	5.28	5.27	5.25	5.24	5.23	5.22	5.20	5.18	5.17	5.15	5.13
	.95	10.1	9.55	9.28	9.12	9.01	8.94	8.89	8.85	8.81	8.79	8.74	8.70	8.66	8.62	8.58	8.53
	.975	17.4	16.0	15.4	15.1	14.9	14.7	14.6	14.5	14.5	14.4	14.3	14.3	14.2	14.1	14.0	13.9
	.990	34.1	30.8	29.5	28.7	28.2	27.9	27.7	27.5	27.3	27.2	27.1	26.9	26.7	26.5	26.4	26.1
	.995	55.6	49.8	47.5	46.2	45.4	44.8	44.4	44.1	43.9	43.7	43.4	43.1	42.8	42.5	42.2	41.8
	.999	167	149	141	137	135	133	132	131	130	129	128	127	126	125	125	123
	.9	4.54	4.32	4.19	4.11	4.05	4.01	3.98	3.95	3.94	3.92	3.90	3.87	3.84	3.82	3.80	3.76
	.95	7.71	6.94	6.59	6.39	6.26	6.16	6.09	6.04	6.00	5.96	5.91	5.86	5.80	5.75	5.70	5.63
	.975	12.2	10.6	9.98	9.60	9.36	9.20	9.07	8.98	8.90	8.84	8.75	8.66	8.56	8.46	8.38	8.26
	.990	21.2	18.0	16.7	16.0	15.5	15.2	15.0	14.8	14.7	14.5	14.4	14.2	14.0	13.8	13.7	13.5
	.995	31.3	26.3	24.3	23.2	22.5	22.0	21.6	21.4	21.1	21.0	20.7	20.4	20.2	19.9	19.7	19.3
	.999	74.1	61.2	56.2	53.4	51.7	50.5	49.7	49.0	48.5	48.1	47.4	46.8	46.1	45.4	44.9	44.1
	.9	4.06	3.78	3.62	3.52	3.45	3.40	3.37	3.34	3.32	3.30	3.27	3.24	3.21	3.17	3.15	3.10
	.95	6.61	5.79	5.41	5.19	5.05	4.95	4.88	4.82	4.77	4.74	4.68	4.62	4.56	4.50	4.44	4.36
	.975	10.0	8.43	7.76	7.39	7.15	6.98	6.85	6.76	6.68	6.62	6.52	6.43	6.33	6.23	6.14	6.02
	.990	16.3	13.3	12.1	11.4	11.0	10.7	10.5	10.3	10.2	10.1	9.89	9.72	9.55	9.38	9.24	9.02
	.995	22.8	18.3	16.5	15.6	14.9	14.5	14.2	14.0	13.8	13.6	13.4	13.1	12.9	12.7	12.5	12.1
	.999	47.2	37.1	33.2	31.1	29.8	28.8	28.2	27.6	27.2	26.9	26.4	25.9	25.4	24.9	24.4	23.8

(continued)

TABLE J.3 (Continued)

v_2	q	$v_1$1	2	3	4	5	6	7	8	9	10	12	15	20	30	50	∞
6	.9	3.78	3.46	3.29	3.18	3.11	3.05	3.01	2.98	2.96	2.94	2.90	2.87	2.84	2.80	2.77	2.7
	.95	5.99	5.14	4.76	4.53	4.39	4.28	4.21	4.15	4.10	4.06	4.00	3.94	3.87	3.81	3.75	3.6
	.975	8.81	7.26	6.60	6.23	5.99	5.82	5.70	5.60	5.52	5.46	5.37	5.27	5.17	5.07	4.98	4.8
	.990	13.7	10.9	9.78	9.15	8.75	8.47	8.26	8.10	7.98	7.87	7.72	7.56	7.40	7.23	7.09	6.8
	.995	18.6	14.5	12.9	12.0	11.5	11.1	10.8	10.6	10.4	10.3	10.0	9.81	9.59	9.36	9.17	8.8
	.999	35.5	27.0	23.7	21.9	20.8	20.0	19.5	19.0	18.7	18.4	18.0	17.6	17.1	16.7	16.3	15.
7	.9	3.59	3.26	3.07	2.96	2.88	2.83	2.78	2.75	2.72	2.70	2.67	2.63	2.59	2.56	2.52	2.4
	.95	5.59	4.74	4.35	4.12	3.97	3.87	3.79	3.73	3.68	3.64	3.57	3.51	3.44	3.38	3.32	3.2
	.975	8.07	6.54	5.89	5.52	5.29	5.12	4.99	4.90	4.82	4.76	4.67	4.57	4.47	4.36	4.28	4.1
	.990	12.2	9.55	8.45	7.85	7.46	7.19	6.99	6.84	6.72	6.62	6.47	6.31	6.16	5.99	5.86	5.6
	.995	16.2	12.4	10.9	10.1	9.52	9.16	8.89	8.68	8.51	8.38	8.18	7.97	7.75	7.53	7.35	7.0
	.999	29.2	21.7	18.8	17.2	16.2	15.5	15.0	14.6	14.3	14.1	13.7	13.3	12.9	12.5	12.2	11.
8	.9	3.46	3.11	2.92	2.81	2.73	2.67	2.62	2.59	2.56	2.54	2.50	2.46	2.42	2.38	2.35	2.2
	.95	5.32	4.46	4.07	3.84	3.69	3.58	3.50	3.44	3.39	3.35	3.28	3.22	3.15	3.08	3.02	2.9
	.975	7.57	6.06	5.42	5.05	4.82	4.65	4.53	4.43	43.6	4.30	4.20	4.10	4.00	3.89	3.81	3.6
	.990	11.3	8.65	7.59	7.01	6.63	6.37	6.18	6.03	5.91	5.81	5.67	5.52	5.36	5.20	5.07	4.8
	.995	14.7	11.0	9.60	8.81	8.30	7.95	7.69	7.50	7.34	7.21	7.01	6.81	6.61	6.40	6.22	5.9
	.999	25.4	18.5	15.8	14.4	13.5	12.9	12.4	12.0	11.8	11.5	11.2	10.8	10.5	10.1	9.80	9.3
9	.9	3.36	3.01	2.81	2.69	2.61	2.55	2.51	2.47	2.44	2.42	2.38	2.34	2.30	2.25	2.22	2.1
	.95	5.12	4.26	3.86	3.63	3.48	3.37	3.29	3.23	3.18	3.14	3.07	3.01	2.94	2.86	2.80	2.7
	.975	7.21	5.71	5.08	4.72	4.48	4.32	4.20	4.10	4.03	3.96	3.87	3.77	3.67	3.56	3.47	3.3
	.990	10.6	8.02	6.99	6.42	6.06	5.80	5.61	5.47	5.35	5.26	5.11	4.96	4.81	4.65	4.52	4.3
	.995	13.6	10.1	8.72	7.96	7.47	7.13	6.88	6.69	6.54	6.42	6.23	6.03	5.83	5.62	5.45	5.1
	.999	22.9	16.4	13.9	12.6	11.7	11.1	10.7	10.4	10.1	9.89	9.57	9.24	8.90	8.55	8.26	7.8
10	.9	3.29	2.92	2.73	2.61	2.52	2.46	2.41	2.38	2.35	2.32	2.28	2.24	2.20	2.16	2.12	2.0
	.95	4.96	4.10	3.71	3.48	3.33	3.22	3.14	3.07	3.02	2.98	2.91	2.85	2.77	2.70	2.64	2.5
	.975	6.94	5.46	4.83	4.47	4.24	4.07	3.95	3.85	3.78	3.72	3.62	3.52	3.42	3.31	3.22	3.0
	.990	10.0	7.56	6.55	5.99	5.64	5.39	5.20	5.06	4.94	4.85	4.71	4.56	4.41	4.25	4.12	3.9
	.995	12.8	9.43	8.08	7.34	6.87	6.54	6.30	6.12	5.97	5.85	5.66	5.47	5.27	5.07	4.90	4.6
	.999	21.0	14.9	12.6	11.3	10.5	9.93	9.52	9.20	8.96	8.75	8.45	8.13	7.80	7.47	7.19	6.7
11	.9	3.23	2.86	2.66	2.54	2.45	2.39	2.34	2.30	2.27	2.25	2.21	2.17	2.12	2.08	2.04	1.9
	.95	4.84	3.98	3.59	3.36	3.20	3.09	3.01	2.95	2.90	2.85	2.79	2.72	2.65	2.57	2.51	2.4
	.975	6.72	5.26	4.63	4.28	4.04	3.88	3.76	3.66	3.59	3.53	3.43	3.33	3.23	3.12	3.03	2.8
	.990	9.65	7.21	6.22	5.67	5.32	5.07	4.89	4.74	4.63	4.54	4.40	4.25	4.10	3.94	3.81	3.6
	.995	12.2	8.91	7.60	6.88	6.42	6.10	5.86	5.68	5.54	5.42	5.24	5.05	4.86	4.65	4.49	4.2
	.999	19.7	13.8	11.6	10.3	9.58	9.05	8.66	8.35	8.12	7.92	7.63	7.32	7.01	6.68	6.42	6.0
12	.9	3.18	2.81	2.61	2.48	2.39	2.33	2.28	2.24	2.21	2.19	2.15	2.10	2.06	2.01	1.97	1.9
	.95	4.75	3.89	3.49	3.26	3.11	3.00	2.91	2.85	2.80	2.75	2.69	2.62	2.54	2.47	2.40	2.3
	.975	6.55	5.10	4.47	4.12	3.89	3.73	3.61	3.51	3.44	3.37	3.28	3.18	3.07	2.96	2.87	2.7
	.990	9.33	6.93	5.95	5.41	5.06	4.82	4.64	4.50	4.39	4.30	4.16	4.01	3.86	3.70	3.57	3.3
	.995	11.8	8.51	7.23	6.52	6.07	5.76	5.52	5.35	5.20	5.09	4.91	4.72	4.53	4.33	4.17	3.9
	.999	18.6	13.0	10.8	9.63	8.89	8.38	8.00	7.71	7.48	7.29	7.00	6.71	6.40	6.09	5.83	5.4

v_2	q	$v_1$1	2	3	4	5	6	7	8	9	10	12	15	20	30	50	∞
3	.9	3.14	2.76	2.56	2.43	2.35	2.28	2.23	2.20	2.16	2.14	2.10	2.05	2.01	1.96	1.92	1.85
	.95	4.67	3.81	3.41	3.18	3.03	2.92	2.83	2.77	2.71	2.67	2.60	2.53	2.46	2.38	2.31	2.21
	.975	6.41	4.97	4.35	4.00	3.77	3.60	3.48	3.39	3.31	3.25	3.15	3.05	2.95	2.84	2.74	2.60
	.990	9.07	6.70	5.74	5.21	4.86	4.62	4.44	4.30	4.19	4.10	3.96	3.82	3.66	3.51	3.38	3.17
	.995	11.4	8.19	6.93	6.23	5.79	5.48	5.25	5.08	4.94	4.82	4.64	4.46	4.27	4.07	3.91	3.65
	.999	17.8	12.3	10.2	9.07	8.35	7.86	7.49	7.21	6.98	6.80	6.52	5.23	5.93	5.63	5.37	4.97
4	.9	3.10	2.73	2.52	2.39	2.31	2.24	2.19	2.15	2.12	2.10	2.05	2.01	1.96	1.91	1.87	1.80
	.95	4.60	3.74	3.34	3.11	2.96	2.85	2.76	2.70	2.65	2.60	2.53	2.46	2.39	2.31	2.24	2.13
	.975	6.30	4.86	4.24	3.89	3.66	3.50	3.38	3.29	3.21	3.15	3.05	2.95	2.84	2.73	2.64	2.49
	.990	8.86	6.51	5.56	5.04	4.69	4.46	4.28	4.14	4.03	3.94	3.80	3.66	3.51	3.35	3.22	3.00
	.995	11.1	7.92	6.68	6.00	5.56	5.26	5.03	4.86	4.72	4.60	4.43	4.25	4.06	3.86	3.70	3.44
	.999	17.1	11.8	9.73	8.62	7.92	7.44	7.08	6.80	6.58	6.40	6.13	5.85	5.56	5.25	5.00	4.60
5	.9	3.07	2.70	2.49	2.36	2.27	2.21	2.16	2.12	2.09	2.06	2.02	1.97	1.92	1.87	1.83	1.76
	.95	4.54	3.68	3.29	3.06	2.90	2.79	2.71	2.64	2.59	2.54	2.48	2.40	2.33	2.25	2.18	2.07
	.975	6.20	4.77	4.15	3.80	3.58	3.41	3.29	3.20	3.12	3.06	2.96	2.86	2.76	2.64	2.55	2.40
	.990	8.68	6.36	5.42	4.89	4.56	4.32	4.14	4.00	3.89	3.80	3.67	3.52	3.37	3.21	3.08	2.87
	.995	10.8	7.70	6.48	5.80	5.37	5.07	4.85	4.67	4.54	4.42	4.25	4.07	3.88	3.69	3.52	3.26
	.999	16.6	11.3	9.34	8.25	7.57	7.09	6.74	6.47	6.26	6.08	5.81	5.54	5.25	4.95	4.70	4.31
6	.9	3.05	2.67	2.46	2.33	2.24	2.18	2.13	2.09	2.06	2.03	1.99	1.94	1.89	1.84	1.79	1.72
	.95	4.49	3.63	3.24	3.01	2.85	2.74	2.66	2.59	2.54	2.49	2.42	2.35	2.28	2.19	2.12	2.01
	.975	6.12	4.69	4.08	3.73	3.50	3.34	3.22	3.12	3.05	2.99	2.89	2.79	2.68	2.57	2.47	2.32
	.990	8.53	6.23	5.29	4.77	4.44	4.20	4.03	3.89	3.78	3.69	3.55	3.41	3.26	3.10	2.97	2.75
	.995	10.6	7.51	6.30	5.64	5.21	4.91	4.69	4.52	4.38	4.27	4.10	3.92	3.73	3.54	3.37	3.11
	.999	16.1	11.0	9.01	7.94	7.27	6.80	6.46	6.19	5.98	5.81	5.55	5.27	4.99	4.70	4.45	4.06
7	.9	3.03	2.64	2.44	2.31	2.22	2.15	2.10	2.06	2.03	2.00	1.96	1.91	1.86	1.81	1.76	1.69
	.95	4.45	3.59	3.20	2.96	2.81	2.70	2.61	2.55	2.49	2.45	2.38	2.31	2.23	2.15	2.08	1.96
	.975	6.04	4.62	4.01	3.66	3.44	3.28	3.16	3.06	2.98	2.92	2.82	2.72	2.62	2.50	2.41	2.25
	.990	8.40	6.11	5.18	4.67	4.34	4.10	3.93	3.79	3.68	3.59	3.46	3.31	3.16	3.00	2.87	2.65
	.995	10.4	7.35	6.16	5.50	5.07	4.78	4.56	4.39	4.25	4.14	3.97	3.79	3.61	3.41	3.25	2.98
	.999	15.7	10.7	8.73	7.68	7.02	6.56	6.22	5.96	5.75	5.58	5.32	5.05	4.78	4.48	4.24	3.85
8	.9	3.01	2.62	2.42	2.29	2.20	2.13	2.08	2.04	2.00	1.98	1.93	1.89	1.84	1.78	1.74	1.66
	.95	4.41	3.55	3.16	2.93	2.77	2.66	2.58	2.51	2.46	2.41	2.34	2.27	2.19	2.11	2.04	1.92
	.975	5.98	4.56	3.95	3.61	3.38	3.22	3.10	3.01	2.93	2.87	2.77	2.67	2.56	2.44	2.35	2.19
	.990	8.29	6.01	5.09	4.58	4.25	4.01	3.84	3.71	3.60	3.51	3.37	3.23	3.08	2.92	2.78	2.57
	.995	10.2	7.21	6.03	5.37	4.96	4.66	4.44	4.28	4.14	4.03	3.86	3.68	3.50	3.30	3.14	2.87
	.999	15.4	10.4	8.49	7.46	6.81	6.35	6.02	5.76	5.56	5.39	5.13	4.87	4.59	4.30	4.06	3.67
9	.9	2.99	2.61	2.40	2.27	2.18	2.11	2.06	2.02	1.98	1.96	1.91	1.86	1.81	1.76	1.71	1.63
	.95	4.38	3.52	3.13	2.90	2.74	2.63	2.54	2.48	2.42	2.38	2.31	2.23	2.16	2.07	2.00	1.88
	.975	5.92	4.51	3.90	3.56	3.33	3.17	3.05	2.96	2.88	2.82	2.72	2.62	2.51	2.39	2.30	2.13
	.990	8.18	5.93	5.01	4.50	4.17	3.94	3.77	3.63	3.52	3.43	3.30	3.15	3.00	2.84	2.71	2.49
	.995	10.1	7.09	5.92	5.27	4.85	4.56	4.34	4.18	4.04	3.93	3.76	3.59	3.40	3.21	3.04	2.78
	.999	15.1	10.2	8.28	7.27	6.62	6.18	5.85	5.59	5.39	5.22	4.97	4.70	4.43	4.14	3.90	3.51

(continued)

TABLE J.3 (Continued)

v_2	q	$v_1$1	2	3	4	5	6	7	8	9	10	12	15	20	30	50	∞
20	.9	2.97	2.59	2.38	2.25	2.16	2.09	2.04	2.00	1.96	1.94	1.89	1.84	1.79	1.74	1.69	1.6
	.95	4.35	3.49	3.10	2.87	2.71	2.60	2.51	2.45	2.39	2.35	2.28	2.20	2.12	2.04	1.97	1.8
	.975	5.87	4.46	3.86	3.51	3.29	3.13	3.01	2.91	2.84	2.77	2.68	2.57	2.46	2.35	2.25	2.0
	.990	8.10	5.85	4.94	4.43	4.10	3.87	3.70	3.56	3.46	3.37	3.23	3.09	2.94	2.78	2.64	2.4
	.995	9.94	6.99	5.82	5.17	4.76	4.47	4.26	4.09	3.96	3.85	3.68	3.50	3.32	3.12	2.96	2.6
	.999	14.8	9.95	8.10	7.10	6.46	6.02	5.69	5.44	5.24	5.08	4.82	4.56	4.29	4.00	3.77	3.3
21	.9	2.96	2.57	2.36	2.23	2.14	2.08	2.02	1.98	1.95	1.92	1.87	1.83	1.78	1.72	1.67	1.5
	.95	4.32	3.47	3.07	2.84	2.68	2.57	2.49	2.42	2.37	2.32	2.25	2.18	2.10	2.01	1.94	1.8
	.975	5.83	4.42	3.82	3.48	3.25	3.09	2.97	2.87	2.80	2.73	2.64	2.53	2.42	2.31	2.21	2.0
	.990	8.02	5.78	4.87	4.37	4.04	3.81	3.64	3.51	3.40	3.31	3.17	3.03	2.88	2.72	2.58	2.3
	.995	9.83	6.89	5.73	5.09	4.68	4.39	4.18	4.01	3.88	3.77	3.60	3.43	3.24	3.05	2.88	2.6
	.999	14.6	9.77	7.94	6.95	6.32	5.88	5.56	5.31	5.11	4.95	4.70	4.44	4.17	3.88	3.64	3.2
22	.9	2.95	2.56	2.35	2.22	2.13	2.06	2.01	1.97	1.93	1.90	1.86	1.81	1.76	1.70	1.65	1.5
	.95	4.30	3.44	3.05	2.82	2.66	2.55	2.46	2.40	2.34	2.30	2.23	2.15	2.07	1.98	1.91	1.7
	.975	5.79	4.38	3.78	3.44	3.22	3.05	2.93	2.84	2.76	2.70	2.60	2.50	2.39	2.27	2.17	2.0
	.990	7.95	5.72	4.82	4.31	3.99	3.76	3.59	3.45	3.35	3.26	3.12	2.98	2.83	2.67	2.53	2.3
	.995	9.73	6.81	5.65	5.02	4.61	4.32	4.11	3.94	3.81	3.70	3.54	3.36	3.18	2.98	2.82	2.5
	.999	14.4	9.61	7.80	6.81	6.19	5.76	5.44	5.19	4.99	4.83	4.58	4.33	4.06	3.78	3.54	3.1
23	.9	2.94	2.55	2.34	2.21	2.11	2.05	1.99	1.95	1.92	1.89	1.84	1.80	1.74	1.69	1.64	1.5
	.95	4.28	3.42	3.03	2.80	2.64	2.53	2.44	2.37	2.32	2.27	2.20	2.13	2.05	1.96	1.88	1.7
	.975	5.75	4.35	3.75	3.41	3.18	3.02	2.90	2.81	2.73	2.67	2.57	2.47	2.36	2.24	2.14	1.9
	.990	7.88	5.66	4.76	4.26	3.94	3.71	3.54	3.41	3.30	3.21	3.07	2.93	2.78	2.62	2.48	2.2
	.995	9.63	6.73	5.58	4.95	4.54	4.26	4.05	3.88	3.75	3.64	3.47	3.30	3.12	2.92	2.76	2.4
	.999	14.2	9.47	7.67	6.70	6.08	5.65	5.33	5.09	4.89	4.73	4.48	4.23	3.96	3.68	3.44	3.0
24	.9	2.93	2.54	2.33	2.19	2.10	2.04	1.98	1.94	1.91	1.88	1.83	1.78	1.73	1.67	1.62	1.5
	.95	4.26	3.40	3.01	2.78	2.62	2.51	2.42	2.36	2.30	2.25	2.18	2.11	2.03	1.94	1.86	1.7
	.975	5.72	4.32	3.72	3.38	3.15	2.99	2.87	2.78	2.70	2.64	2.54	2.44	2.33	2.21	2.11	1.9
	.990	7.82	5.61	4.72	4.22	3.90	3.67	3.50	3.36	3.26	3.17	3.03	2.89	2.74	2.58	2.44	2.2
	.995	9.55	6.66	5.52	4.89	4.49	4.20	3.99	3.83	3.69	3.59	3.42	3.25	3.06	2.87	2.70	2.4
	.999	14.0	9.34	7.55	6.59	5.98	5.55	5.23	4.99	4.80	4.64	4.39	4.14	3.87	3.59	3.36	2.9
25	.9	2.92	2.53	2.32	2.18	2.09	2.02	1.97	1.93	1.89	1.87	1.82	1.77	1.72	1.66	1.61	1.5
	.95	4.24	3.39	2.99	2.76	2.60	2.49	2.40	2.34	2.28	2.24	2.16	2.09	2.01	1.92	1.84	1.7
	.975	5.69	4.29	3.69	3.35	3.13	2.97	2.85	2.75	2.68	2.61	2.51	2.41	2.30	2.18	2.08	1.9
	.990	7.77	5.57	4.68	4.18	3.85	3.63	3.46	3.32	3.22	3.13	2.99	2.85	2.70	2.54	2.40	2.1
	.995	9.48	6.60	5.46	4.84	4.43	4.15	3.94	3.78	3.64	3.54	3.37	3.20	3.01	2.82	2.65	2.3
	.999	13.9	9.22	7.45	6.49	5.89	5.46	5.15	4.91	4.71	4.56	4.31	4.06	3.79	3.52	3.28	2.8
30	.9	2.88	2.49	2.28	2.14	2.05	1.98	1.93	1.88	1.85	1.82	1.77	1.72	1.67	1.61	1.55	1.4
	.95	4.17	3.32	2.92	2.69	2.53	2.42	2.33	2.27	2.21	2.16	2.09	2.01	1.93	1.84	1.76	1.6
	.975	5.57	4.18	3.59	3.25	3.03	2.87	2.75	2.65	2.57	2.51	2.41	2.31	2.20	2.07	1.97	1.7
	.990	7.56	5.39	4.51	4.02	3.70	3.47	3.30	3.17	3.07	2.98	2.84	2.70	2.55	2.39	2.25	2.0
	.995	9.18	6.35	5.24	4.62	4.23	3.95	3.74	3.58	3.45	3.34	3.18	3.01	2.82	2.63	2.46	2.1
	.999	13.3	8.77	7.05	6.12	5.53	5.12	4.82	4.58	4.39	4.24	4.00	3.75	3.49	3.22	2.98	2.5

v_2	q	$v_1$1	2	3	4	5	6	7	8	9	10	12	15	20	30	50	∞
35	.9	2.85	2.46	2.25	2.11	2.02	1.95	1.90	1.85	1.82	1.79	1.74	1.69	1.63	1.57	1.51	1.41
	.95	4.12	3.27	2.87	2.64	2.49	2.37	2.29	2.22	2.16	2.11	2.04	1.96	1.88	1.79	1.70	1.56
	.975	5.48	4.11	3.52	3.18	2.96	2.80	2.68	2.58	2.50	2.44	2.34	2.23	2.12	2.00	1.89	1.70
	.990	7.42	5.27	4.40	3.91	3.59	3.37	3.20	3.07	2.96	2.88	2.74	2.60	2.44	2.28	2.14	1.89
	.995	8.98	6.19	5.09	4.48	4.09	3.81	3.61	3.45	3.32	3.21	3.05	2.88	2.69	2.50	2.33	2.04
	.999	12.9	8.47	6.79	5.88	5.30	4.89	4.59	4.36	4.18	4.03	3.79	3.55	3.29	3.02	2.78	2.38
40	.9	2.84	2.44	2.23	2.09	2.00	1.93	1.87	1.83	1.79	1.76	1.71	1.66	1.61	1.54	1.48	1.38
	.95	4.08	3.23	2.84	2.61	2.45	2.34	2.25	2.18	2.12	2.08	2.00	1.92	1.84	1.74	1.66	1.51
	.975	5.42	4.05	3.46	3.13	2.90	2.74	2.62	2.53	2.45	2.39	2.29	2.18	2.07	1.94	1.83	1.64
	.990	7.31	5.18	4.31	3.83	3.51	3.29	3.12	2.99	2.89	2.80	2.66	2.52	2.37	2.20	2.06	1.80
	.995	8.83	6.07	4.98	4.37	3.99	3.71	3.51	3.35	3.22	3.12	2.95	2.78	2.60	2.40	2.23	1.93
	.999	12.6	8.25	6.59	5.70	5.13	4.73	4.44	4.21	4.02	3.87	3.64	3.40	3.14	2.87	2.64	2.23
45	.9	2.82	2.42	2.21	2.07	1.98	1.91	1.85	1.81	1.77	1.74	1.70	1.64	1.58	1.52	1.46	1.35
	.95	4.06	3.20	2.81	2.58	2.42	2.31	2.22	2.15	2.10	2.05	1.97	1.89	1.81	1.71	1.63	1.47
	.975	5.38	4.01	3.42	3.09	2.86	2.70	2.58	2.49	2.41	2.35	2.25	2.14	2.03	1.90	1.79	1.59
	.990	7.23	5.11	4.25	3.77	3.45	3.23	3.07	2.94	2.83	2.74	2.61	2.46	2.31	2.14	2.00	1.74
	.995	8.71	5.97	4.89	4.29	3.91	3.64	3.43	3.28	3.15	3.04	2.88	2.71	2.53	2.33	2.16	1.85
	.999	12.4	8.09	6.45	5.56	5.00	4.61	4.32	4.09	3.91	3.76	3.53	3.29	3.04	2.76	2.53	2.12
50	.9	2.81	2.41	2.20	2.06	1.97	1.90	1.84	1.80	1.76	1.73	1.68	1.63	1.57	1.50	1.44	1.33
	.95	4.03	3.18	2.79	2.56	2.40	2.29	2.20	2.13	2.07	2.03	1.95	1.87	1.78	1.69	1.60	1.44
	.975	5.34	3.97	3.39	3.05	2.83	2.67	2.55	2.46	2.38	2.32	2.22	2.11	1.99	1.87	1.75	1.55
	.990	7.17	5.06	4.20	3.72	3.41	3.19	3.02	2.89	2.78	2.70	2.56	2.42	2.27	2.10	1.95	1.68
	.995	8.63	5.90	4.83	4.23	3.85	3.58	3.38	3.22	3.09	2.99	2.82	2.65	2.47	2.27	2.10	1.79
	.999	12.2	7.96	6.34	5.46	4.90	4.51	4.22	4.00	3.82	3.67	3.44	3.20	2.95	2.68	2.44	2.03
60	.9	2.79	2.39	2.18	2.04	1.95	1.87	1.82	1.77	1.74	1.71	1.66	1.60	1.54	1.48	1.41	1.29
	.95	4.00	3.15	2.76	2.53	2.37	2.25	2.17	2.10	2.04	1.99	1.92	1.84	1.75	1.65	1.56	1.39
	.975	5.29	3.93	3.34	3.01	2.79	2.63	2.51	2.41	2.33	2.27	2.17	2.06	1.94	1.82	1.70	1.48
	.990	7.08	4.98	4.13	3.65	3.34	3.12	2.95	2.82	2.72	2.63	2.50	2.35	2.20	2.03	1.88	1.60
	.995	8.49	5.79	4.73	4.14	3.76	3.49	3.29	3.13	3.01	2.90	2.74	2.57	2.39	2.19	2.01	1.69
	.999	12.0	7.77	6.17	5.31	4.76	4.37	4.09	3.86	3.69	3.54	3.32	3.08	2.83	2.55	2.32	1.89
80	.9	2.77	2.37	2.15	2.02	1.92	1.85	1.79	1.75	1.71	1.68	1.63	1.57	1.51	1.44	1.38	1.24
	.95	3.96	3.11	2.72	2.49	2.33	2.21	2.13	2.06	2.00	1.95	1.88	1.79	1.70	1.60	1.51	1.32
	.975	5.22	3.86	3.28	2.95	2.73	2.57	2.45	2.35	2.28	2.21	2.11	2.00	1.88	1.75	1.63	1.40
	.990	6.96	4.88	4.04	3.56	3.26	3.04	2.87	2.74	2.64	2.55	2.42	2.27	2.12	1.94	1.79	1.49
	.995	8.33	5.67	4.61	4.03	3.65	3.39	3.19	3.03	2.91	2.80	2.64	2.47	2.29	2.08	1.90	1.56
	.999	11.7	7.54	5.97	5.12	4.58	4.20	3.92	3.70	3.53	3.39	3.16	2.93	2.68	2.41	2.16	1.72
100	.9	2.76	2.36	2.14	2.00	1.91	1.83	1.78	1.73	1.69	1.66	1.61	1.56	1.49	1.42	1.35	1.21
	.95	3.94	3.09	2.70	2.46	2.31	2.19	2.10	2.03	1.97	1.93	1.85	1.77	1.68	1.57	1.48	1.28
	.975	5.18	3.83	3.25	2.92	2.70	2.54	2.42	2.32	2.24	2.18	2.08	1.97	1.85	1.71	1.59	1.35
	.990	6.90	4.82	3.98	3.51	3.21	2.99	2.82	2.69	2.59	2.50	2.37	2.22	2.07	1.89	1.74	1.43
	.995	8.24	5.59	4.54	3.96	3.59	3.33	3.13	2.97	2.85	2.74	2.58	2.41	2.23	2.02	1.84	1.49
	.999	11.5	7.41	5.86	5.02	4.48	4.11	3.83	3.61	3.44	3.30	3.07	2.84	2.59	2.32	2.08	1.62

(continued)

TABLE J.3 (Continued)

v_2	q	$v_1$1	2	3	4	5	6	7	8	9	10	12	15	20	30	50	∞
120	.9	2.75	2.35	2.13	1.99	1.90	1.82	1.77	1.72	1.68	1.65	1.60	1.55	1.48	1.41	1.34	1.19
	.95	3.92	3.07	2.68	2.45	2.29	2.18	2.09	2.02	1.96	1.91	1.83	1.75	1.66	1.55	1.46	1.25
	.975	5.15	3.80	3.23	2.89	2.67	2.52	2.39	2.30	2.22	2.16	2.05	1.94	1.82	1.69	1.56	1.31
	.990	6.85	4.79	3.95	3.48	3.17	2.96	2.79	2.66	2.56	2.47	2.34	2.19	2.03	1.86	1.70	1.38
	.995	8.18	5.54	4.50	3.92	3.55	3.28	3.09	2.93	2.81	2.71	2.54	2.37	2.19	1.98	1.80	1.43
	.999	11.4	7.32	5.78	4.95	4.42	4.04	3.77	3.55	3.38	3.24	3.02	2.78	2.53	2.26	2.02	1.54
∞	.9	2.71	2.30	2.08	1.94	1.85	1.77	1.72	1.67	1.63	1.60	1.55	1.49	1.42	1.34	1.26	1.00
	.95	3.84	3.00	2.60	2.37	2.21	2.10	2.01	1.94	1.88	1.83	1.75	1.67	1.57	1.46	1.35	1.00
	.975	5.02	3.69	3.12	2.79	2.57	2.41	2.29	2.19	2.11	2.05	1.94	1.83	1.71	1.57	1.43	1.00
	.990	6.63	4.61	3.78	3.32	3.02	2.80	2.64	2.51	2.41	2.32	2.18	2.04	1.88	1.70	1.52	1.00
	.995	7.88	5.30	4.28	3.72	3.35	3.09	2.90	2.74	2.62	2.52	2.36	2.19	2.00	1.79	1.59	1.00
	.999	10.8	6.91	5.42	4.62	4.10	3.74	3.47	3.27	3.10	2.96	2.74	2.51	2.27	1.99	1.73	1.00

Source: H. R. Neave, *Statistics Tables*, 1978, Table 3.3, "The F Distribution," pp. 44–47. Copyright © 1978 by Routledge. Reprinted by permission of the author and publisher.

TABLE J.4
The χ^2 (Chi-Squared) Distribution

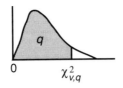

$$0 \qquad \chi^2_{v,q}$$

q \ v	.0005	0.001	0.005	0.010	0.025	0.050	0.075	0.100	0.150	0.200	0.300	0.400
1	$.0^6393$	$.0^5157$	$.0^4393$	$.0^3157$	$.0^3982$	.00393	.00886	.0158	.0358	.0642	0.148	0.275
2	.00100	.00200	0.0100	0.0201	0.0506	0.103	0.156	0.211	0.325	0.446	0.713	1.022
3	0.0153	0.0243	0.0717	0.115	0.216	0.352	0.472	0.584	0.798	1.005	1.424	1.869
4	0.0639	0.0908	0.207	0.297	0.484	0.711	0.897	1.064	1.366	1.649	2.195	2.753
5	0.158	0.210	0.412	0.554	0.831	1.145	1.394	1.610	1.994	2.343	3.000	3.655
6	0.299	0.381	0.676	0.872	1.237	1.635	1.941	2.204	2.661	3.070	3.828	4.570
7	0.485	0.598	0.989	1.239	1.690	2.167	2.528	2.833	3.358	3.822	4.671	5.493
8	0.710	0.857	1.344	1.646	2.180	2.733	3.144	3.490	4.078	4.594	5.527	6.423
9	0.972	1.152	1.735	2.088	2.700	3.325	3.785	4.168	4.817	5.380	6.393	7.357
10	1.265	1.479	2.156	2.558	3.247	3.940	4.446	4.865	5.570	6.179	7.267	8.295
11	1.587	1.834	2.603	3.053	3.816	4.575	5.124	5.578	6.336	6.989	8.148	9.237
12	1.934	2.214	3.074	3.571	4.404	5.226	5.818	6.304	7.114	7.807	9.034	10.18
13	2.305	2.617	3.565	4.107	5.009	5.892	6.524	7.042	7.901	8.634	9.926	11.13
14	2.697	3.041	4.075	4.660	5.629	6.571	7.242	7.790	8.696	9.467	10.82	12.08
15	3.108	3.483	4.601	5.229	6.262	7.261	7.969	8.547	9.499	10.31	11.72	13.03
16	3.536	3.942	5.142	5.812	6.908	7.962	8.707	9.312	10.31	11.15	12.62	13.98
17	3.980	4.416	5.697	6.408	7.564	8.672	9.452	10.09	11.12	12.00	13.53	14.94
18	4.439	4.905	6.265	7.015	8.231	9.390	10.21	10.86	11.95	12.86	14.44	15.89
19	4.912	5.407	6.844	7.633	8.907	10.12	10.97	11.65	12.77	13.72	15.35	16.85
20	5.398	5.921	7.434	8.260	9.591	10.85	11.73	12.44	13.60	14.58	16.27	17.81
21	5.896	6.447	8.034	8.897	10.28	11.59	12.50	13.24	14.44	15.44	17.18	18.77
22	6.404	6.983	8.643	9.542	10.98	12.34	13.28	14.04	15.28	16.31	18.10	19.73
23	6.924	7.529	9.260	10.20	11.69	13.09	14.06	14.85	16.12	17.19	19.02	20.69
24	7.453	8.085	9.886	10.86	12.40	13.85	14.85	15.66	16.97	18.06	19.94	21.65
25	7.991	8.649	10.52	11.52	13.12	14.61	15.64	16.47	17.82	18.94	20.87	22.62
26	8.538	9.222	11.16	12.20	13.84	15.38	16.44	17.29	18.67	19.82	21.79	23.58
27	9.093	9.803	11.81	12.88	14.57	16.15	17.24	18.11	19.53	20.70	22.72	24.54
28	9.656	10.39	12.46	13.56	15.31	16.93	18.05	18.94	20.39	21.59	23.65	25.51
29	10.23	10.99	13.12	14.26	16.05	17.71	18.85	19.77	21.25	22.48	24.58	26.48
30	10.80	11.59	13.79	14.95	16.79	18.49	19.66	20.60	22.11	23.36	25.51	27.44
31	11.39	12.20	14.46	15.66	17.54	19.28	20.48	21.43	22.98	24.26	26.44	28.41
32	11.98	12.81	15.13	16.36	18.29	20.07	21.30	22.27	23.84	25.15	27.37	29.38
33	12.58	13.43	15.82	17.07	19.05	20.87	22.12	23.11	24.71	26.04	28.31	30.34
34	13.18	14.06	16.50	17.79	19.81	21.66	22.94	23.95	25.59	26.94	29.24	31.31
35	13.79	14.69	17.19	18.51	20.57	22.47	23.76	24.80	26.46	27.84	30.18	32.28
36	14.40	15.32	17.89	19.23	21.34	23.27	24.59	25.64	27.34	28.73	31.12	33.25
37	15.02	15.97	18.59	19.96	22.11	24.07	25.42	26.49	28.21	29.64	32.05	34.22
38	15.64	16.61	19.29	20.69	22.88	24.88	26.25	27.34	29.09	30.54	32.99	35.19
39	16.27	17.26	20.00	21.43	23.65	25.70	27.09	28.20	29.97	31.44	33.93	36.16
40	16.91	17.92	20.71	22.16	24.43	26.51	27.93	29.05	30.86	32.34	34.87	37.13
45	20.14	21.25	24.31	25.90	28.37	30.61	32.14	33.35	35.29	36.88	39.58	42.00
50	23.46	24.67	27.99	29.71	32.36	34.76	36.40	37.69	39.75	41.45	44.31	46.86
60	30.34	31.74	35.53	37.48	40.48	43.19	45.02	46.46	48.76	50.64	53.81	56.62
70	37.47	39.04	43.28	45.44	48.76	51.74	53.75	55.33	57.84	59.90	53.35	66.40
80	44.79	46.52	51.17	53.54	57.15	60.39	62.57	64.28	66.99	69.21	72.92	76.19
90	52.28	54.16	59.20	61.75	65.65	69.13	71.46	73.29	76.20	78.56	82.51	85.99
100	59.90	61.92	67.33	70.06	74.22	77.93	80.41	82.36	85.44	87.95	92.13	95.81
120	75.47	77.76	83.85	86.92	91.57	95.70	98.46	100.6	104.0	106.8	111.4	115.5
150	99.46	102.1	109.1	112.7	118.0	122.7	215.8	128.3	132.1	135.3	140.5	145.0
200	140.7	143.8	152.2	156.4	162.7	168.3	172.0	174.8	179.4	183.0	189.0	194.3

(continued)

TABLE J.4 (Continued)

v \ q	0.500	0.600	0.700	0.800	0.850	0.900	0.925	0.950	0.975	0.990	0.995	0.999	.999
1	0.455	0.708	1.074	1.642	2.072	2.706	3.170	3.841	5.024	6.635	7.879	10.83	12.12
2	1.386	1.833	2.408	3.219	3.794	4.605	5.181	5.991	7.378	9.210	10.60	13.82	15.20
3	2.366	2.946	3.665	4.642	5.317	6.251	6.905	7.815	9.348	11.34	12.84	16.27	17.73
4	3.357	4.045	4.878	5.989	6.745	7.779	8.496	9.488	11.14	13.28	14.86	18.47	20.00
5	4.351	5.132	6.064	7.289	8.115	9.236	10.01	11.07	12.83	15.09	16.75	20.52	22.11
6	5.348	6.211	7.231	8.558	9.446	10.64	11.47	12.59	14.45	16.81	18.55	22.46	24.10
7	6.346	7.283	8.383	9.803	10.75	12.02	12.88	14.07	16.01	18.48	20.28	24.32	26.02
8	7.344	8.351	9.524	11.03	12.03	13.36	14.27	15.51	17.53	20.09	21.95	26.12	27.87
9	8.343	9.414	10.66	12.24	13.29	14.68	15.63	16.92	19.02	21.67	23.59	27.88	29.67
10	9.342	10.47	11.78	13.44	14.53	15.99	16.97	18.31	20.48	23.21	25.19	29.59	31.42
11	10.34	11.53	12.90	14.63	15.77	17.28	18.29	19.68	21.92	24.72	26.76	31.26	33.14
12	11.34	12.58	14.01	15.81	16.99	18.55	19.60	21.03	23.34	26.22	28.30	32.91	34.82
13	12.34	13.64	15.12	16.98	18.20	19.81	20.90	22.36	24.74	27.69	29.82	34.53	36.48
14	13.34	14.69	16.22	18.15	19.41	21.06	22.18	23.68	26.12	29.14	31.32	36.12	38.11
15	14.34	15.73	17.32	19.31	20.60	22.31	23.45	25.00	27.49	30.58	32.80	37.70	39.72
16	15.34	16.78	18.42	20.47	21.79	23.54	24.72	26.30	28.85	32.00	34.27	39.25	41.31
17	16.34	17.82	19.51	21.61	22.98	24.77	25.97	27.59	30.19	33.41	35.72	40.79	42.88
18	17.34	18.87	20.60	22.76	24.16	25.99	27.22	28.87	31.53	34.81	37.16	42.31	44.43
19	18.34	19.91	21.69	23.90	25.33	27.20	28.46	30.14	32.85	36.19	38.58	43.82	45.97
20	19.34	20.95	22.77	25.04	26.50	28.41	29.69	31.41	34.17	37.57	40.00	45.31	47.50
21	20.34	21.99	23.86	26.17	27.66	29.62	30.92	32.67	35.48	38.93	41.40	46.80	49.01
22	21.34	23.03	24.94	27.30	28.82	30.81	32.14	33.92	36.78	40.29	42.80	48.27	50.51
23	22.34	24.07	26.02	28.43	29.98	32.01	33.36	35.17	38.08	41.64	44.18	49.73	52.00
24	23.34	25.11	27.10	29.55	31.13	33.20	34.57	36.42	39.36	42.98	45.56	51.18	53.48
25	24.34	26.14	28.17	30.68	32.28	34.38	35.78	37.65	40.65	44.31	46.93	52.62	54.95
26	25.34	27.18	29.25	31.79	33.43	35.56	36.98	38.89	41.92	45.64	48.29	54.05	56.41
27	26.34	28.21	30.32	32.91	34.57	36.74	38.18	40.11	43.19	46.96	49.64	55.48	57.86
28	27.34	29.25	31.39	34.03	35.71	37.92	39.38	41.34	44.46	48.28	50.99	56.89	59.30
29	28.34	30.28	32.46	35.14	36.85	39.09	40.57	42.56	45.72	49.59	52.34	58.30	60.73
30	29.34	31.32	33.53	36.25	37.99	40.26	41.76	43.77	46.98	50.89	53.67	59.70	62.16
31	30.34	32.35	34.60	37.36	39.12	41.42	42.95	44.99	48.23	52.19	55.00	61.10	63.58
32	31.34	33.38	35.66	38.47	40.26	42.58	44.13	46.19	49.48	53.49	56.33	62.49	65.00
33	32.34	34.41	36.73	39.57	41.39	43.75	45.31	47.40	50.73	54.78	57.65	63.87	66.40
34	33.34	35.44	37.80	40.68	42.51	44.90	46.48	48.60	51.97	56.06	58.96	65.25	67.80
35	34.34	36.47	38.86	41.78	43.64	46.06	47.66	49.80	53.20	57.34	60.27	66.62	69.20
36	35.34	37.50	39.92	42.88	44.76	47.21	48.84	51.00	54.44	58.62	61.58	67.99	70.59
37	36.34	38.53	40.98	43.98	45.89	48.36	50.01	52.19	55.67	59.89	62.88	59.35	71.97
38	37.34	39.56	42.05	45.08	47.01	49.51	51.17	53.38	56.90	61.16	64.18	70.70	73.35
39	38.34	40.59	43.11	46.17	48.13	50.66	52.34	54.57	58.12	62.43	65.48	72.05	74.73
40	39.34	41.62	44.16	47.27	49.24	51.81	53.50	55.76	59.34	63.69	66.77	73.40	76.09
45	44.34	46.76	49.45	52.73	54.81	57.51	59.29	61.66	65.41	69.96	73.17	80.08	82.88
50	49.33	51.89	54.72	58.16	60.35	63.17	65.03	67.50	71.42	76.15	79.49	86.66	89.56
60	59.33	62.13	65.23	68.97	71.34	74.40	76.41	79.08	83.30	88.38	91.95	99.61	102.7
70	69.33	72.36	75.69	79.71	82.26	85.53	87.68	90.53	95.02	100.4	104.2	112.3	115.6
80	79.33	82.57	86.12	90.41	93.11	96.58	98.86	101.9	106.6	112.3	116.3	124.8	128.3
90	89.33	92.76	96.52	101.1	103.9	107.6	110.0	113.1	118.1	124.1	128.3	137.2	140.8
100	99.33	102.9	106.9	111.7	114.7	118.5	121.0	124.3	129.6	135.8	140.2	149.4	153.2
120	119.3	123.3	127.6	132.8	136.1	140.2	143.0	146.6	152.2	159.0	163.6	173.6	177.6
150	149.3	153.8	158.6	164.3	168.0	172.6	175.6	179.6	185.8	193.2	198.4	209.3	213.6
200	199.3	204.4	210.0	216.6	220.7	226.0	229.5	234.0	241.1	249.4	255.3	267.5	272.4

Source: H. R. Neave, *Statistics Tables*, 1978, Table 3.2, ''The χ^2 (Chi-Squared) Distribution,'' pp. 42–43. Copyright © 1978 by Routledge. Reprinted by permission of the author and publisher.

TABLE J.5

Mann-Whitney U Values: Critical values of the Mann-Whitney U statistic for a one-tailed test at $\alpha = .01$ (roman type) and $\alpha = .005$ (boldface type) and for a two-tailed test at $\alpha = .02$ (roman type) and $\alpha = .01$ (boldface type)*

n_2 \ n_1	1	2	3	4	5	6	7	8	9	10	11	12	13	14	15	16	17	18	19	20
1	—	—	—	—	—	—	—	—	—	—	—	—	—	—	—	—	—	—	—	—
2	—	—	—	—	—	—	—	—	—	—	—	—	0	0	0	0	0	0	1	1
																			0	**0**
3	—	—	—	—	—	—	0	0	1	1	1	2	2	2	3	3	4	4	4	5
							—	—	**0**	**0**	**0**	**1**	**1**	**1**	**2**	**2**	**2**	**2**	**3**	**3**
4	—	—	—	—	0	1	1	2	3	3	4	5	5	6	7	7	8	9	9	10
					—	**0**	**0**	**1**	**1**	**2**	**2**	**3**	**3**	**4**	**5**	**5**	**6**	**6**	**7**	**8**
5	—	—	—	0	1	2	3	4	5	6	7	8	9	10	11	12	13	14	15	16
				—	**0**	**1**	**1**	**2**	**3**	**4**	**5**	**6**	**7**	**7**	**8**	**9**	**10**	**11**	**12**	**13**
6	—	—	—	1	2	3	4	6	—	8	9	11	12	13	15	16	18	19	20	22
				0	**1**	**2**	**3**	**4**	**5**	**6**	**7**	**9**	**10**	**11**	**12**	**13**	**15**	**16**	**17**	**18**
7	—	—	0	1	3	4	6	7	9	11	12	14	16	17	19	21	23	24	26	28
			—	**0**	**1**	**3**	**4**	**6**	**7**	**9**	**10**	**12**	**13**	**15**	**16**	**18**	**19**	**21**	**22**	**24**
8	—	—	0	2	4	6	7	9	11	13	15	17	20	22	24	26	28	30	32	34
			—	**1**	**2**	**4**	**6**	**7**	**9**	**11**	**13**	**15**	**17**	**18**	**20**	**22**	**24**	**26**	**28**	**30**
9	—	—	1	3	5	7	9	11	14	16	18	21	23	26	28	31	33	36	38	40
			0	**1**	**3**	**5**	**7**	**9**	**11**	**13**	**16**	**18**	**20**	**22**	**24**	**27**	**29**	**31**	**33**	**36**
10	—	—	1	3	6	8	11	13	16	19	22	24	27	30	33	36	38	41	44	47
			0	**2**	**4**	**6**	**9**	**11**	**13**	**16**	**18**	**21**	**24**	**26**	**29**	**31**	**34**	**37**	**39**	**42**
11	—	—	1	4	7	9	12	15	18	22	25	28	31	34	37	41	44	47	50	53
			0	**2**	**5**	**7**	**10**	**13**	**16**	**18**	**21**	**24**	**27**	**30**	**33**	**36**	**39**	**42**	**45**	**48**
12	—	—	2	5	8	11	14	17	21	24	28	31	35	38	42	46	49	53	56	60
			1	**3**	**6**	**9**	**12**	**15**	**18**	**21**	**24**	**27**	**31**	**34**	**37**	**41**	**44**	**47**	**51**	**54**
13	—	0	2	5	9	12	16	20	23	27	31	35	39	43	47	51	55	59	63	67
	—	**1**	**3**	**7**	**10**	**13**	**17**	**20**	**24**	**27**	**31**	**34**	**38**	**42**	**45**	**49**	**53**	**56**	**60**
14	—	0	2	6	10	13	17	22	26	30	34	38	43	47	51	56	60	65	69	73
	—	**1**	**4**	**7**	**11**	**15**	**18**	**22**	**26**	**30**	**34**	**38**	**42**	**46**	**50**	**54**	**58**	**63**	**67**
15	—	0	3	7	11	15	19	24	28	33	37	42	47	51	56	61	66	70	75	80
	—	**2**	**5**	**8**	**12**	**16**	**20**	**24**	**29**	**33**	**37**	**42**	**46**	**51**	**55**	**60**	**64**	**69**	**73**
16	—	0	3	7	12	16	21	26	31	36	41	46	51	56	61	66	71	76	82	87
	—	**2**	**5**	**9**	**13**	**18**	**22**	**27**	**31**	**36**	**41**	**45**	**50**	**55**	**60**	**65**	**70**	**74**	**79**
17	—	0	4	8	13	18	23	28	33	38	44	49	55	60	66	71	77	82	88	93
	—	**2**	**6**	**10**	**15**	**19**	**24**	**29**	**34**	**39**	**44**	**49**	**54**	**60**	**65**	**70**	**75**	**81**	**86**
18	—	0	4	9	14	19	24	30	36	41	47	53	59	65	70	76	82	88	94	100
	—	**2**	**6**	**11**	**16**	**21**	**26**	**31**	**37**	**42**	**47**	**53**	**58**	**64**	**70**	**75**	**81**	**87**	**92**
19	—	1	4	9	15	20	26	32	38	44	50	56	63	69	75	82	88	94	101	107
	0	**3**	**7**	**12**	**17**	**22**	**28**	**33**	**39**	**45**	**51**	**56**	**63**	**69**	**74**	**81**	**87**	**93**	**99**
20	—	1	5	10	16	22	28	34	40	47	53	60	67	73	80	87	93	100	107	114
	0	**3**	**8**	**13**	**18**	**24**	**30**	**36**	**42**	**48**	**54**	**60**	**67**	**73**	**79**	**86**	**92**	**99**	**105**

(continued)

TABLE J.5 (Continued)

n_2 \ n_1	1	2	3	4	5	6	7	8	9	10	11	12	13	14	15	16	17	18	19	20
1	—	—	—	—	—	—	—	—	—	—	—	—	—	—	—	—	—	—	0	0
																			—	—
2	—	—	—	—	0	0	0	1	1	1	1	2	2	2	3	3	3	4	4	4
					—	—	—	0	0	0	0	1	1	1	1	1	2	2	2	2
3	—	—	0	0	1	2	2	3	3	4	5	5	6	7	7	8	8	9	10	11
	—	—	—	—	0	1	1	2	2	3	3	4	4	5	5	6	6	7	7	8
4	—	—	0	1	2	3	4	5	6	7	8	9	10	11	12	14	15	16	17	18
	—	—	—	0	1	2	3	4	4	5	6	7	8	9	10	11	11	12	13	13
5	—	0	1	2	4	5	6	8	9	11	12	13	15	16	18	19	20	22	23	25
	—	—	0	1	2	3	5	6	7	8	9	11	12	13	14	15	17	18	19	20
6	—	0	2	3	5	7	8	10	12	14	16	17	19	21	23	25	26	28	30	32
	—	—	1	2	3	5	6	8	10	11	13	14	16	17	19	21	22	24	25	27
7	—	0	2	4	6	8	11	13	15	17	19	21	24	26	28	30	33	35	37	39
	—	—	1	3	5	6	8	10	12	14	16	18	20	22	24	26	28	30	32	34
8	—	1	3	5	8	10	13	15	18	20	23	26	28	31	33	36	39	41	44	47
	—	0	2	4	6	8	10	13	15	17	19	22	24	26	29	31	34	36	38	41
9	—	1	3	6	9	12	15	18	21	24	27	30	33	36	39	42	45	48	51	54
	—	0	2	4	7	10	12	15	17	20	23	26	28	31	34	37	39	42	45	48
10	—	1	4	7	11	14	17	20	24	27	31	34	37	41	44	48	51	55	58	62
	—	0	3	5	8	11	14	17	20	23	26	29	33	36	39	42	45	48	52	55
11	—	1	5	8	12	16	19	23	27	31	34	38	42	46	50	54	57	61	65	69
	—	0	3	6	9	13	16	19	23	26	30	33	37	40	44	47	51	55	58	62
12	—	2	5	9	13	17	21	26	30	34	38	42	47	51	55	60	64	68	72	77
	—	1	4	7	11	14	18	22	26	29	33	37	41	45	49	53	57	61	65	69
13	—	2	6	10	15	19	24	28	33	37	42	47	51	56	61	65	70	75	80	84
	—	1	4	8	12	16	20	24	28	33	37	41	45	50	54	59	63	67	72	76
14	—	2	7	11	16	21	26	31	36	41	46	51	56	61	66	71	77	82	87	92
	—	1	5	9	13	17	22	26	31	36	40	45	50	55	59	64	67	74	78	83
15	—	3	7	12	18	23	28	33	39	44	50	55	61	66	72	77	83	88	94	100
	—	1	5	10	14	19	24	29	34	39	44	49	54	59	64	70	75	80	85	90
16	—	3	8	14	19	25	30	36	42	48	54	60	65	71	77	83	89	95	101	107
	—	1	6	11	15	21	26	31	37	42	47	53	59	64	70	75	81	86	92	98
17	—	3	9	15	20	26	33	39	45	51	57	64	70	77	83	89	96	102	109	115
	—	2	6	11	17	22	28	34	39	45	51	57	63	67	75	81	87	93	99	105
18	—	4	9	16	22	28	35	41	48	55	61	68	75	82	88	95	102	109	116	123
	—	2	7	12	18	24	30	36	42	48	55	61	67	74	80	86	93	99	106	112
19	0	4	10	17	23	30	37	44	51	58	65	72	80	87	94	101	109	116	123	130
	—	2	7	13	19	25	32	38	45	52	58	65	72	78	85	92	99	106	113	119
20	0	4	11	18	25	32	39	47	54	62	69	77	84	92	100	107	115	123	130	138
	—	2	8	13	20	27	34	41	48	55	62	69	76	83	90	98	105	112	119	127

*Dashes in the body of the table indicate that no decision is possible at the stated level of significance.
Source: Joseph H. Porter and Robert J. Hamm, *Statistics: Applications for the Behavioral Sciences,* 1986, Table D, pp. 392–393. Reprinted by permission of Brooks/Cole Publishing Company, Pacific Grove, CA 93950.

TABLE J.6
Critical Values for the Kruskal-Wallis Test (small sample sizes)

Unequal sample sizes

$$H = \frac{12}{N(N+1)} \sum_{i=1}^{k} \frac{R_i^2}{n_i} - 3(N+1)$$

	k = 3			k = 4		
Sample sizes	α = 5%	1%		Sample sizes	α = 5%	1%
2 2 2	—	—		2 1 1 1	—	—
				2 2 1 1	—	—
3 2 1	—	—		2 2 2 1	5.679	—
3 2 2	4.714	—		2 2 2 2	6.167	6.667
3 3 1	5.143	—				
3 3 2	5.361	—		3 1 1 1	—	—
3 3 3	5.600	7.200		3 2 1 1	—	—
				3 2 2 1	5.833	—
4 1 1	—	—		3 2 2 2	6.333	7.133
4 2 1	—	—		3 3 2 1	6.244	7.200
4 2 2	5.333	—		3 3 2 2	6.527	7.636
4 3 1	5.208	—		3 3 3 1	6.600	7.400
4 3 2	5.444	6.444		3 3 3 2	6.727	8.015
4 3 3	5.791	6.745		3 3 3 3	7.000	8.538
4 4 1	5.455	7.036				
4 4 3	5.598	7.144		4 1 1 1	—	—
4 4 4	5.692	7.564		4 2 1 1	5.833	—
				4 2 2 1	6.133	7.000
5 1 1	—	—		4 2 2 2	6.545	7.391
5 2 1	5.000	—		4 3 1 1	6.178	7.067
5 2 2	5.160	6.533		4 3 2 1	6.309	7.455
5 3 1	4.960	—		4 3 2 2	6.621	7.871
5 3 2	5.251	6.909		4 3 3 1	6.545	7.758
5 3 3	5.648	7.079		4 3 3 2	6.795	8.333
5 4 1	4.985	6.955		4 3 3 3	6.984	8.659
5 4 2	5.273	7.205		4 4 1 1	5.945	7.909
5 4 3	5.656	7.445		4 4 2 1	6.386	7.909
5 4 4	5.657	7.760		4 4 2 2	6.731	8.346
5 5 1	5.127	7.309		4 4 3 1	6.635	8.231
5 5 2	5.338	7.338		4 4 3 2	6.874	8.621
5 5 3	5.705	7.578		4 4 3 3	7.038	8.876
5 5 4	5.666	7.823		4 4 4 1	6.725	8.588
5 5 5	5.780	8.000		4 4 4 2	6.957	8.871
6 1 1	—	—				
6 2 1	4.822	—				
6 2 2	5.345	6.655				
6 3 1	4.855	6.873				
6 3 2	5.348	6.970				
6 3 3	5.615	7.410				
6 4 1	4.947	7.106				

(continued)

Unequal sample sizes	k = 3			k = 4		
	Sample sizes	α = 5%	1%	Sample sizes	α = 5%	1%
	6 4 3	5.610	7.500			
	6 4 4	5.681	7.795			
	6 5 1	4.990	7.182			
	6 5 2	5.338	7.376			
	6 5 3	5.602	7.590			
	6 5 4	5.661	7.936			
	6 5 5	5.729	8.028			
	6 6 1	4.945	7.121			
	6 6 2	5.410	7.467			
	6 6 3	5.625	7.725			
	6 6 4	5.724	8.000			
	6 6 5	5.765	8.124			
	6 6 6	5.801	8.222			
	1 1 1 1 1	—	—	1 1 1 1 1 1	—	—
	2 1 1 1 1	—	—	2 1 1 1 1 1	—	—
	2 2 1 1 1	—	—	2 2 1 1 1 1	—	—
	2 2 2 1 1	6.750	—	2 2 2 1 1 1	7.600	—
	2 2 2 2 1	7.133	7.533	2 2 2 2 1 1	8.018	8.618
	2 2 2 2 2	7.418	8.291	2 2 2 2 2 1	8.455	9.227
				2 2 2 2 2 2	8.846	9.846
	3 1 1 1 1	—	—			
	3 2 1 1 1	6.583	—	3 1 1 1 1 1	—	—
	3 2 2 1 1	6.800	7.600	3 2 1 1 1 1	7.467	—
	3 2 2 2 1	7.309	8.127	3 2 2 1 1 1	7.945	8.509
	3 2 2 2 2	7.682	8.682	3 2 2 2 1 1	8.348	9.136
	3 3 1 1 1	7.111	—	3 2 2 2 2 1	8.731	9.692
	3 3 2 1 1	7.200	8.073	3 2 2 2 2 2	9.033	10.22
	3 3 2 2 1	7.591	8.576	3 3 1 1 1 1	7.909	8.564
	3 3 2 2 2	7.910	9.115	3 3 2 1 1 1	8.303	9.045
	3 3 3 1 1	7.576	8.424	3 3 2 2 1 1	8.615	9.628
	3 3 3 2 1	7.769	9.051	3 3 2 2 2 1	8.923	10.15
	3 3 3 2 2	8.044	9.505	3 3 3 1 1 1	8.461	9.564
	3 3 3 3 1	8.000	9.451	3 3 3 2 1 1	8.835	10.08
	4 1 1 1 1	—	—	4 1 1 1 1 1	7.333	—
	4 2 1 1 1	6.733	—	4 2 1 1 1 1	7.827	8.400
				4 2 2 1 1 1	8.205	9.000
				4 2 2 2 1 1	8.558	9.538
				4 2 2 2 2 1	8.868	10.07
				4 3 1 1 1 1	8.053	9.023
				4 3 2 1 1 1	8.429	9.506
				4 3 2 2 1 1	8.742	10.01
				4 3 3 1 1 1	8.654	9.934
				4 4 1 1 1 1	8.231	9.538
				4 4 2 1 1 1	8.571	9.940
				5 1 1 1 1 1	7.909	—
				5 2 1 1 1 1	7.891	8.682

Equal sample sizes

$$H = \frac{12}{n^2 k(nk+1)} \sum_{i=1}^{k} R_i^2 - 3(nk+1)$$

	k = 3		k = 4		k = 5		k = 6	
n	α = 5%	1%	α = 5%	1%	α = 5%	1%	α = 5%	1%
2	—	—	6.167	6.667	7.418	8.291	8.846	9.846
3	5.600	7.200	7.000	8.538	8.333	10.20	9.789	11.82
4	5.692	7.654	7.235	9.287	8.685	11.07	10.14	12.72
5	5.780	8.000	7.377	9.789	8.876	11.57	10.36	13.26
6	5.801	8.222	7.453	10.09	9.002	11.91	10.50	13.60
7	5.819	8.378	7.501	10.25	9.080	12.14	10.59	13.84
8	5.805	8.465	7.534	10.42	9.126	12.29	10.66	13.99
9	5.831	8.529	7.557	10.53	9.166	12.41	10.71	14.13
10	5.853	8.607	7.586	1062	9.200	12.50	10.75	14.24
11	5.885	8.648	7.623	10.69	9.242	12.58	10.76	14.32
12	5.872	8.712	7.629	10.75	9.274	12.63	10.79	14.38
13	5.901	8.735	7.645	10.80	9.303	12.69	10.83	14.44
14	5.896	8.754	7.658	10.84	9.307	12.74	10.84	14.49
15	5.902	8.821	7.676	10.87	9.302	12.77	10.86	14.53
16	5.909	8.822	7.678	10.90	9.313	12.79	10.88	14.56
17	5.915	8.856	7.682	10.92	9.325	12.83	10.88	14.60
18	5.932	8.865	7.698	10.95	9.334	12.85	10.89	14.63
19	5.923	8.887	7.701	10.98	9.342	12.87	10.90	14.64
20	5.926	8.905	7.703	10.98	9.353	12.91	10.92	14.67
∞	5.991	9.210	7.815	11.34	9.488	13.28	11.07	15.09

Source: H. R. Neave and P. L. Worthington, *Distribution-Free Tests*, 1988, Table N, ''Critical Values for the Kruskal-Wallis Test,'' pp. 392–394. Copyright © 1988 by Routledge. Reprinted by permission of the authors and publisher.

TABLE J.7
Critical Values for Friedman's Test

$$M = \frac{12}{nk(k+1)} \sum_{i=1}^{k} R_i^2 - 3n(k+1)$$

n	k = 3 $\alpha = 5\%$	1%	k = 4 $\alpha = 5\%$	1%	k = 5 $\alpha = 5\%$	1%	k = 6 $\alpha = 5\%$	1%
2	—	—	6.000	—	7.600	8.000	9.143	9.714
3	6.000	—	7.400	9.000	8.533	10.13	9.857	11.76
4	6.500	8.000	7.800	9.600	8.800	11.20	10.29	12.71
5	6.400	8.400	7.800	9.960	8.960	11.68	10.49	13.23
6	7.000	9.000	7.600	10.20	9.067	11.87	10.57	13.62
7	7.143	8.857	7.800	10.54	9.143	12.11	10.67	13.86
8	6.250	9.000	7.650	10.50	9.200	13.20	10.71	14.00
9	6.222	9.556	7.667	10.73	9.244	12.44	10.78	14.14
10	6.200	9.600	7.680	10.68	9.280	12.48	10.80	14.23
11	6.545	9.455	7.691	10.75	9.309	12.58	10.84	14.32
12	6.500	9.500	7.700	10.80	9.333	12.60	10.86	14.38
13	6.615	9.385	7.800	10.85	9.354	12.68	10.89	14.45
14	6.143	9.143	7.714	10.89	9.371	12.74	10.90	14.49
15	6.400	8.933	7.720	10.92	9.387	12.80	10.92	14.54
16	6.500	9.375	7.800	10.95	9.400	12.80	10.96	14.57
17	6.118	9.294	7.800	10.05	9.412	12.85	10.95	14.61
18	6.333	9.000	7.733	10.93	9.422	12.89	10.95	14.63
19	6.421	9.579	7.863	11.02	9.432	12.88	11.00	14.67
20	6.300	9.300	7.800	11.10	9.400	12.92	11.00	14.66
∞	5.991	9.210	7.815	11.34	9.488	13.28	11.07	15.09

Source: H. R. Neave and P. L. Worthington, *Distribution-Free Tests,* 1988, Table O, "Critical Values for Friedman's Tests," p. 395. Copyright © 1988 by Routledge. Reprinted by permission of the authors and publisher.

Glossary

Abstract: A concise summary of a study.

Accidental sampling: Nonprobability sampling method in which the sampling units are selected because they are available to the investigator at the time of data collection. Also called *convenience sampling.*

Alternate forms reliability: Method of determining reliability in which two different forms of an instrument are administered to the same individuals and the two sets of scores are then correlated. Also called *equivalent forms reliability.*

Analysis of covariance (ANCOVA): Parametric statistical test to determine the differences between the means of two or more groups by removing the effects of one or more confounding variables.

Analysis of variance (ANOVA): Parametric statistical test to determine the differences between the means of two or more groups.

Anonymity: Protection of the rights of the study subjects so that the respondents are not directly linked to their responses.

Applied research: Research conducted to generate new knowledge that can be applied in practical settings without undue delay.

Assumption: A statement whose correctness or validity is taken for granted.

Attrition: Loss of subjects during a research study.

Basic research: Research designed to formulate theory rather than be utilized for immediate application.

Case studies: In-depth studies of individuals or small groups.

Chi-square (χ^2): A statistical technique used to determine if observed frequencies differ from expected frequencies.

Cliometrics: Use of statistical analysis in historical research.

Cluster sampling: A probability sample in which the cluster is the primary sampling unit. Clusters consist of groups that have the same characteristic(s).

Concept: A single idea (often one word) that represents several related ideas (e.g., *grief*).

Conceptual framework: Discussion of the relationship of concepts that underlie the study problem and support the rationale (reason) for conducting the study.

Confidentiality: Responses of study subjects are not linked with the individuals who provided them when the study results are communicated.

Confounding variables: Variables that may interfere with the direct causal relationship of independent variables to dependent variables.

Construct: Hypothetical grouping of abstract concepts (prejudice, intelligence).

Construct validity: The degree to which a measuring instrument measures a specific hypothetical trait, such as intelligence.

Content analysis: ''. . . the technique that provides a systematic means of measuring the frequency, order, or intensity of words, phrases or sentences.''[1]

Content validity: A method for determining the validity of a measuring instrument that utilizes the consensus of a judge panel of experts. The panel agrees that the measuring instrument measures what it is said to measure.

Control: Elimination or reduction of extraneous variables that could influence the dependent variable under investigation.

Convenience sampling: See *Accidental sampling*.

Control group: The group in which the experimental treatment is not introduced.

Correlation: The strength of the quantifiable relationship between two or more variables.

Correlation coefficient: The number that represents the strength of the quantifiable relationship between two or more variables.

Criterion-related validity: The general term that includes concurrent and predictive validity. Refers to the relationship of the measuring instrument to some already known external criterion or other valid instrument.

Criterion variable: A preestablished measure of success. Sometimes called the *dependent variable*.

Cross-sectional study: A research technique in which data are collected at a certain point in time.

Datum: A unit of information (plural: *data*).

Debriefing: Providing subjects of the study with information about the study after the study has been concluded.

Deductive: Method of reasoning that moves from the general to the specific.

Delphi technique: A research methodology for predicting or emphasizing the main concerns of a group.

Dependent variable: The variable that changes as the independent variable is manipulated by the researcher; sometimes called the *criterion variable*.

Descriptive research approach: Research approach that is present-oriented and designed to answer questions based on the ongoing events of the present.

Descriptive statistics: Statistics used to describe and summarize data.

Direct definition: Definition of a term taken from the dictionary.

Double blind study: Experimental strategy in which neither the subjects nor those who collect the data know which subjects are in the experimental group and which subjects are in the control group.

Empirical evidence: Data gathered to generate new knowledge. It must be rooted in objective reality and gathered directly or indirectly through human senses.

Empirical generalization: A principle derived from empirical evidence.

Ethnography: Inductive research approach for in-depth investigation of a culture or cultures in which data related to the members of the culture are collected, analyzed, and described.

Experimental research approach: Research approach in which the independent variable(s) is manipulated under controlled conditions to determine the effect on the dependent variable(s); also characterized by random assignment of study subjects to treatment conditions.

Exploratory study (pilot study): A preliminary study used to determine strengths and weaknesses of a planned project; may also be used as the basis of future studies.

Ex post facto research: Type of research design in which the independent variable is not manipulated because changes in the independent variable have already occurred prior to the study.

External criticism: The evaluation of the validity of historical data.

Extraneous variable: Uncontrolled variables outside the purpose of the study that influence the study's results.

Face validity: A subjective method for determining validity of a measuring instrument. It is determined by inspection of the items to see that the instrument contains important items that measure the variables being studied.

Frequency distribution: The arrangement of the scores or values of characteristics from the highest to the lowest or in a systematic way.

Friedman two-way analysis of variance by ranks: Nonparametric statistical test using ordinal-level data to determine whether related samples have come from the same population by determining mean ranks.

Generalizability: See *Inference.*

Grounded theory: Inductive research approach that generates the theoretical underpinnings of the research by "grounding" or basing the theory in the data being collected.

H₀: See *Null hypothesis.*

Hawthorne effect: Term used to describe the psychological reactions to the presence of the investigator, or to special treatment during a research study, which tend to alter the responses of the subject.

Historical research approach: Research approach that deals with what has happened in the past and how those happenings affect the present.

Hypothesis: A statement of predicted relationships between the variables under study; an educated or calculated guess by the researcher. It is the testable component of the research (plural: *hypotheses*).

Independent variable: The variable that is purposely manipulated or changed by the researcher; also called the *manipulated variable.*

Inductive: Method of reasoning that moves from the specific to the general.

Inference: Information gathered from a sample is generalized to a population.

Inferential statistics: Statistical tests used to make inferences (generalizations) to the larger population from which the sample was drawn.

Informed consent: Voluntary agreement by a study subject to participate in a research study after being informed about the study and the rights of the subjects who participate.

Institutional Review Board (IRB): A committee appointed by an agency to review research being conducted within the agency to ensure protection of the rights of subjects participating in a research study.

Internal criticism: The evaluation of the reliability or accuracy of what is stated in a historical document.

Interrater reliability: Method for determining reliability in which the strength of agreement between the observations made by two or more observers is determined. Also called *interobserver reliability.*

Interval data scale: Data based on a scale that has equal intervals.

Interview: Verbal questioning of respondents by the investigator in order to collect data. Requires interaction between people.

Judgment sampling: See *Purposive sampling.*

Kruskal-Wallis one-way analysis of variance by ranks: A nonparametric statistical test that ranks ordinal-level data to determine whether independent samples were drawn from the same continuous population.

Level of significance: The probability level used to reject the null hypothesis.

Likert scale: A scale for rating attitudes in which each statement usually has five possible responses: strongly agree, agree, uncertain, disagree, strongly disagree.

Longitudinal study: A research design in which data are collected from the same subjects over a period of time.

Manipulated variable: See *Independent variable.*

Mann-Whitney U: Nonparametric statistical test that uses ordinal data (ranks) to determine if two independent samples have been drawn from the same population.

Mean: The arithmetic average.

Measures of central tendency: See *Mean, Median, Mode, Standard deviation.*

Median: The number above which 50 percent of the observations fall.

MEDLARS (Medical Literature Analysis and Retrieval System): The computerized literature retrieval service of the National Library of Medicine.

MEDLINE: A computerized data base that references biomedical journal articles.

Meta-analysis: ''The statistical analysis of a large collection of results from individual studies for the purpose of integrating the findings into a single, generalizable finding.''[2]

Mode: The most frequently occurring score or number value.

Multiple analysis of variance (MANOVA): Parametric statistical test to determine interaction effects between two or more independent variables and two or more dependent variables.

Nominal data scale: Data that can be separated only into mutually exclusive categories.

Nonparametric statistics: ''A general class of inferential statistics that does not involve rigorous assumptions about the distribution of the critical variables: most often used when the data are measured on the nominal or ordinal scales.''[3]

Nonprobability sampling: Sampling approach in which the investigator has no ability to estimate the probability that each element of the population will be included in the sample, or even that it has some chance of being included.

Normal curve: A theoretical bell-shaped curve with most measurement clustered about the center and a few measurements at the extreme ends.

Null hypothesis (H$_0$): The most commonly used method of stating the way the relationship between the variables being studied will be tested. The null hypothesis is stated as follows: ''There is no statistically significant difference between the experimental and the control group.'' Also termed *statistical hypothesis.*

Nursing research: Research conducted to answer questions or find solutions to problems specifically related to nursing. It has the purpose of developing an organized body of scientific knowledge unique to nursing.

Observation: Watching and noting actions and reactions.

Operational definition: The researcher's definition of a term that provides a description of the method for studying the concept by citing the necessary operations (manipulations and observations) to be used.

Opinionnaire: A questionnaire designed to elicit opinions.

Ordinal data scale: Data that are ordered, but for which there is no zero starting point, and the intervals between individual data are not equal. *Big, bigger,* and *biggest* are ordinal data.

Parametric statistics: ''. . . a class of inferential statistics that involves (a) assumptions about the distribution of the variables, (b) the estimation of a parameter, and (c) the use of interval measures.''[4]

Participant observation: Observation techniques in which the observer becomes a participant in the situation being observed.

Pearson r (Pearson product-moment correlation coefficient): A frequently used correlation statistic. Correlation coefficients expressed as r's range from -1 to $+1$.

Percentile rank: Descriptive statistic indicating the point below which a percentage of scores occurs.

Phenomenology: Inductive research approach based on the philosophy of phenomenology, which proposes to understand the whole human being through "the lived experience."

Pilot study: See *Exploratory study.*

Population: See *Target population.*

Population element: A single unit or member of the target population.

Pretest: (1) The process of testing out the effectiveness of a measuring instrument in gathering appropriate data. (2) In an experimental study, the data collection procedure prior to the experimental phase of the study.

Primary source: First-hand information obtained from original material; not interpretive or hearsay information.

Probability sampling: Sampling approach in which the investigator is able to specify, for each population element, the probability that it will be included in the sample. That is, there is a *known* probability of each element being included in the sample.

Projective tests: Psychological tests that require the subjects to respond to ambiguous situations.

Protocol: See *Research-based clinical protocol.*

Purposive sampling: Nonprobability sampling method in which subjects are selected according to specific criteria established by the investigator. Also called *judgmental sampling.*

Qualitative data: Data characterized by words (*pale, cyanotic,* etc.)

Quantitative data: Data characterized by numbers.

Quasi-experimental research: Research approach in which the independent variable is manipulated to determine the effect on the dependent variable, but subjects are not randomly assigned to treatment conditions.

Questionnaire: A paper-and-pencil data collection instrument that is completed by the study subjects themselves to elicit their attitudes or feelings.

Quota sampling: Nonprobability sampling method in which the investigator specifies a percentage for subjects' characteristics to be included in the sample to ensure adequate representation of those characteristics.

r: See *Pearson r.*

Randomization: Assignment of subjects to treatment conditions in such a manner that each population element is assigned by chance alone rather than by some purposive method.

Random sample: See *Simple random sample* or *Stratified random sample.*

Range: The distribution of scores from the lowest to highest; the high score minus the low score.

Rating scale: A scale that allows respondents to make a qualitative judgment. Rating scales yield ordinal data.

Ratio data scale: Data based on a scale that has equal intervals and an absolute zero starting point.

Reliability: The degree to which a measuring instrument obtains consistent results when it is reused.

Replication: Repeating a study using the same study design but different study subjects.

Research: A scientific process of inquiry and/or experimentation that involves purposeful, systematic, and rigorous collection, analysis, and interpretation of data in order to gain new knowledge or add to the existing body of scientific knowledge.

Research-based clinical protocol: A written document that organizes and transforms research-based knowledge so that it can be used to direct clinical practice activities.

Research hypothesis: Method of stating the hypothesis so that the relationship between the variables that the researcher expects as the study's outcome is specified.

Research utilization: Transferring research-based knowledge into actual practice.

Sample: A smaller part of the target population selected in such a way that the individuals in the sample represent (as nearly as possible) the characteristics of the target population.

Sampling: Process of selecting a sample from the target population.

Sampling unit: See *Population element.*

Scientific method: An orderly process that utilizes the principles of science and requires the use of certain sequential steps to acquire dependable information in the solving of problems.

Secondary source: An interpretive or hearsay source of data.

Serendipitous findings: Unplanned and unexpected discovery of significant results in a research study not related to the purpose of the study.

Simple random sampling: A probability sample in which the required number of sampling units is selected at random from the population in such a manner that each population element has an equal chance (probability) of being selected.

Single blind study: Experimental strategy carried out in either of two ways: (1) The study subjects know whether they are in the experimental or control group, but the data collectors do not know; (2) the data collectors know whether subjects are in the experimental or control group, but the subjects do not know.

Spearman's rho (r_s): A nonparametric measure of correlation.

Split-half reliability: Method for determining reliability in which responses to a measuring instrument are divided in half, scored separately, and then correlated. Also called odd–even reliability.

Spurious correlations: Correlations that yield high relationship values, but where no relationship actually exists.

Standard deviation: The general indicator of dispersion from the mean.

Statistical hypothesis: See *Null hypothesis.*

Statistical inference: Statistical analysis that permits conclusions to be drawn about a population based on examination of only a portion (sample) of the population.

Statistics: The techniques used to assemble, describe, and make inferences from numerical data.

Stratified random sampling: A variation of the simple random sample in which the target population is divided into two or more strata (categories of the characteristic), and a simple random sample is taken from each stratum (category).

Structured interview: An interview that has a set series of questions.

Student's t-test: See *t-Test.*

Survey research: Collection of data about present conditions directly from the study subjects, usually by questionnaire or interview.

Symbols: Those signs used to substitute for whole words or concepts, such as χ^2 for chi-square or r for Pearson product-moment correlation coefficient.

Target population: The total group of individual people or things meeting the designated set of criteria of interest to the researcher.

t-Test: A parametric statistical measure to determine the differences between the means of two groups.

Test of significance: Statistical test utilized to determine differences between groups.

Test–retest reliability: Method for determining reliability in which the same instrument is administered to the same individuals at different times and the two sets of scores are then correlated.

Test statistic (T):   A test similar to the chi-square test but which allows expected cell values to be as low as 1 in more than 20 percent of the cells.

Theoretical definition: Definition of a term using the specific language of the theory being used.

Theoretical framework: Discussion of one theory or interrelated theories being tested in order to support the rationale (reason) for conducting the study.

Theory: A set of statements, called *propositions*, that are stated in such a way as to form a logically interrelated deductive system. Used to summarize existing knowledge and to explain and/or predict phenomena and their relationships.

Type I error: Rejection of the null hypothesis when it should be accepted. Also called the *alpha error.*

Type II error: Acceptance of the null hypothesis when it should be rejected. Also called the *beta error.*

Unstructured interview: An interview that has a general framework for eliciting data but does not have a fixed pattern of questions.

Utilization: See *Research utilization.*

Validity: The extent to which a data-gathering instrument measures what it is supposed to measure by obtaining data relevant to what is being measured.

Variable: A multivalued entity. The attribute or characteristic under study that varies in some dimension.

Variance: The square of the standard deviation. It reflects the distance of individual scores from the mean.

χ^2:   See *Chi-square.*

Z-score: A number reflecting the distance that an individual score is from the mean in standard deviation units. Also termed standard score.

REFERENCES

1.   Burns, N., and S. K. Grove. 1987. *The Practice of Nursing Research: Conduct, Critique and Utilization.* Philadelphia: W. B. Saunders, p. 743.
2.   Lynn, M. R. 1989. ''Meta-Analysis: Appropriate Tool for Integration of Nursing Research?'' *Nursing Research,* 38(September–October): 302.
3.   Polit, D., and B. Hungler. 1987. *Nursing Research: Principles and Methods.* Philadelphia: J. B. Lippincott, p. 533.
4.   Ibid., p. 534.

Index

[321]